METHODS IN MOLECULAR BIOLOGY™

Series Editor
John M. Walker
School of Life Sciences
University of Hertfordshire
Hatfield, Hertfordshire, AL10 9AB, UK

For further volumes:
http://www.springer.com/series/7651

Quantitative Trait Loci (QTL)

Methods and Protocols

Edited by

Scott A. Rifkin

University of Californa, San Diego, CA, USA

Humana Press

Editor
Scott A. Rifkin, Ph.D.
University of Californa
San Diego, CA, USA

ISSN 1064-3745 ISSN 1940-6029 (electronic)
ISBN 978-1-4939-5832-0 ISBN 978-1-61779-785-9 (eBook)
DOI 10.1007/978-1-61779-785-9
Springer New York Heidelberg Dordrecht London

Printed on acid-free paper

Humana Press is a brand of Springer
Springer is part of Springer Science+Business Media (www.springer.com)

Preface

For over a century, biologists have searched for the genetic bases of phenotypic variation. While this program has been quite successful for simple Mendelian traits, most traits are complex, shaped by context-dependent interactions between multiple loci and the environment. Over the last 2 decades, leaps in genotyping technology, coupled with the development of sophisticated quantitative genetic analytical techniques, have made it possible to dissect complex traits and link quantitative variation in traits to allelic variation on chromosomes or *quantitative trait loci* (QTLs). Propelled by the genome projects and their spinoff technologies, QTL analyses have pervaded all fields of biology and form the backbone for the recent explosion of studies tying specific alleles to human disease. As sequencing becomes ever cheaper and easier, QTL studies will make it possible to relatively quickly identify key genes underlying traits even in non-model organisms, paving the way for discovering new biology.

As with any expanding field, the original QTL methodologies have been elaborated into a host of alternative and complementary techniques. A QTL experiment has many components—preparing the experimental mapping population, genotyping, measuring traits, analyzing the data and identifying QTLs, and feeding this information to downstream analyses—and its success depends upon each part fitting together and being appropriate for answering the motivating question. This volume contains chapters that focus on specific components of the entire process and also a set of case studies at the end where these individual components are linked together into an entire study.

This book is intended to serve as a practical resource for researchers interested in links between phenotypic and genotypic variation in fields from medicine to agriculture and from molecular biology to evolution to ecology. Many of the methods are similar between fields. QTL studies often involve multiple authors with complementary expertise, and the case studies in particular are intended to facilitate communication between scientists working on different parts of a project and to give a broader perspective on how each piece fits into the whole. QTL techniques will continue to be developed and further refined and extended. As phenotyping technology improves and as genotyping technology continues to accelerate, statistical approaches to dissecting the genotype–phenotype map will become increasingly important and powerful tools for biological research.

San Diego, CA, USA *Scott A. Rifkin*

Contents

Preface . . . . *v*
Contributors . . . . *ix*

PART I SETTING UP MAPPING POPULATIONS

1 Backcross Populations and Near Isogenic Lines 3
Rik Kooke, Erik Wijnker, and Joost J.B. Keurentjes
2 F_2 Designs for QTL Analysis 17
Yuan-Ming Zhang
3 Design and Construction of Recombinant Inbred Lines 31
Daniel A. Pollard
4 Two Flavors of Bulk Segregant Analysis in Yeast 41
Maitreya J. Dunham
5 Selecting Markers and Evaluating Coverage 55
Matthew A. Cleveland and Nader Deeb

PART II IDENTIFYING QUANTITATIVE TRAIT LOCI

6 Composite Interval Mapping and Multiple Interval Mapping: Procedures and Guidelines for Using Windows QTL Cartographer 75
Luciano Da Costa E. Silva, Shengchu Wang, and Zhao-Bang Zeng
7 Design Database for Quantitative Trait Loci (QTL) Data Warehouse, Data Mining, and Meta-Analysis 121
Zhi-Liang Hu, James M. Reecy, and Xiao-Lin Wu
8 Meta-analysis of QTL Mapping Experiments 145
Xiao-Lin Wu and Zhi-Liang Hu

PART III EXTENDING THE POWER OF QUANTITATIVE TRAIT LOCUS ANALYSIS

9 Using eQTLs to Reconstruct Gene Regulatory Networks 175
Lin S. Chen
10 Estimation and Interpretation of Genetic Effects with Epistasis Using the NOIA Model 191
José M. Álvarez-Castro, Örjan Carlborg, and Lars Rönnegård
11 Identifying QTL for Multiple Complex Traits in Experimental Crosses 205
Samprit Banerjee and Nengjun Yi
12 Functional Mapping of Developmental Processes: Theory, Applications, and Prospects 227
Kiranmoy Das, Zhongwen Huang, Jingyuan Liu, Guifang Fu, Jiahan Li, Yao Li, Chunfa Tong, Junyi Gai, and Rongling Wu

13 Statistical Models for Genetic Mapping in Polyploids: Challenges and Opportunities 245
Jiahan Li, Kiranmoy Das, Jingyuan Liu, Guifang Fu, Yao Li, Christian Tobias, and Rongling Wu

PART IV CASE STUDIES

14 eQTL 265
Lun Li, Xianghua Zhang, and Hongyu Zhao

15 Genetic Mapping of Quantitative Trait Loci for Disease-Related Phenotypes 281
Marcella Devoto and Mario Falchi

16 Quantitative Trait Locus Analysis in Haplodiploid Hymenoptera 313
Jürgen Gadau, Christof Pietsch, and Leo W. Beukeboom

Index *329*

Contributors

JOSÉ M. ÁLVAREZ-CASTRO • *Department of Genetics, University of Santiago de Compostela, Lugo, Galiza, Spain*
SAMPRIT BANERJEE • *Division of Biostatistics and Epidemiology, Department of Public Health, Weill Cornell Medical College, New York, NY, USA*
LEO W. BEUKEBOOM • *Evolutionary Genetics, Centre for Ecological and Evolutionary Studies, University of Groningen, NL-9750 AA Haren, The Netherlands*
ÖRJAN CARLBORG • *Department of Animal Breeding and Genetics, Swedish University of Agricultural Sciences, Uppsala, Sweden; Department of Cell and Molecular Biology, Uppsala University, Uppsala, Sweden*
LIN S. CHEN • *Department of Health Studies, The University of Chicago, Chicago, IL, USA*
MATTHEW A. CLEVELAND • *Genus plc, 100 Bluegrass Commons Boulevard, Suite 2200, Hendersonville, TN 37075, USA*
LUCIANO DA COSTA E. SILVA • *Department of Statistics and Bioinformatics Research Center, North Carolina State University, Raleigh, NC, USA*
KIRANMOY DAS • *Department of Statistics and Center for Statistical Genetics, Pennsylvania State University, Hershey, PA 17033, USA*
MARCELLA DEVOTO • *Division of Genetics, The Children's Hospital of Philadelphia, Philadelphia, PA, USA; Department of Pediatrics and CCEB, University of Pennsylvania, Philadelphia, PA, USA; Dipartimento di Medicina Molecolare, Universita' degli Studi La Sapienza, Roma, Italy*
NADER DEEB • *Genus plc., 100 Bluegrass Commons Boulevard, Suite 2200, Hendersonville, TN 37075, USA*
MAITREYA J. DUNHAM • *Department of Genome Sciences, University of Washington, Seattle, WA, USA*
MARIO FALCHI • *Department of Genomics of Common Disease, School of Public Health, Imperial College, London, UK*
GUIFANG FU • *Department of Statistics and Center for Statistical Genetics, Pennsylvania State University, Hershey, PA 17033, USA*
JUNYI GAI • *Soybean Research Institute of Nanjing Agricultural University, National Center for Soybean Improvement, National Key Laboratory for Crop Genetics and Germplasm Enhancement, Nanjing 210095, China*
JÜRGEN GADAU • *School of Life Sciences, Arizona State University, Tempe, AZ 58285, USA*
YUNQIAN GUO • *Center for Computational Biology, Beijing Forestry University, Beijing, China*
ZHI-LIANG HU • *Department of Animal Science, Center for Integrated Animal Genomics Iowa State University, 2255 Kildee Hall, Ames, IA 50011-3150, USA*

ZHONGWEN HUANG • *Department of Agronomy, Henan Institute of Science and Technology, Xinxiang 453003, China*
JOOST J.B. KEURENTJES • *Laboratory of Plant Physiology, Wageningen University, Wageningen, The Netherlands; Laboratory of Genetics, Wageningen University, Wageningen, The Netherlands*
RIK KOOKE • *Laboratory of Plant Physiology, Wageningen University, Wageningen, The Netherlands*
JIAHAN LI • *Department of Statistics and Center for Statistical Genetics, Pennsylvania State University, Hershey, PA 17033, USA*
LUN LI • *Hubei Bioinformatics and Molecular Imaging Key Laboratory, Huazhong University of Science and Technology, Wuhan, Hubei, China; Department of Epidemiology and Public Health, Yale University, New Haven, CT, USA*
YAO LI • *Department of Statistics, West Virginia University, Morgantown, WV 26506, USA*
JINGYUAN LIU • *Center for Statistical Genetics, The Pennsylvania State University, Hershey, PA, USA*
CHRISTOF PIETSCH • *Institute of Plant Genetics and Crop Plant Research (IPK), Correnstrasse 3 D-06466, Gatersleben, Germany*
DANIEL A. POLLARD • *Division of Biology, University of California, San Diego, La Jolla, CA 92093, USA*
JAMES M. REECY • *Department of Animal Science, Iowa State University, Ames, IA, USA*
LARS RÖNNEGÅRD • *Statistics Unit, Dalarna University, Borlänge, Sweden*
CHRISTIAN TOBIAS • *Genomics and Gene Discovery Research Unit, USDA-ARS Western Regional Research Center, Albany, CA 94710, USA*
CHUNFA TONG • *Center for Statistical Genetics, The Pennsylvania State University, Hershey, PA, USA*
SHENGCHU WANG • *Department of Statistics and Bioinformatics Research Center, North Carolina State University, Raleigh, NC, USA*
ERIK WIJNKER • *Laboratory of Genetics, Wageningen University, Wageningen, The Netherlands*
RONGLING WU • *Department of Statistics and Center for Statistical Genetics, Pennsylvania State University, Hershey, PA 17033, USA*
XIAO-LIN WU • *Departments of Animal Sciences & Dairy Science, UW-Madison, Madison, WI, USA*
NENGJUN YI • *Section of Statistical Genetics, Department of Biostatistics, University of Alabama at Birmingham, Birmingham, AL, USA*
ZHAO-BANG ZENG • *Department of Statistics and Bioinformatics Research Center, North Carolina State University, Raleigh, NC, USA; Department of Genetics, North Carolina State University, Raleigh, NC, USA*
XIANGHUA ZHANG • *Department of Electronic Science and Technology, University of Science and Technology of China, Hefei, Anhui, China; Department of Epidemiology and Public Health, Yale University, New Haven, CT, USA*

YUAN-MING ZHANG • *Section on Statistical Genomics, State Key Laboratory of Crop Genetics and Germplasm Enhancement, Nanjing Agricultural University, Nanjing 210095, China*
HONGYU ZHAO • *Department of Epidemiology and Public Health, Yale University, New Haven, CT, USA*

Part I

Setting Up Mapping Populations

Chapter 1

Backcross Populations and Near Isogenic Lines

Rik Kooke, Erik Wijnker, and Joost J.B. Keurentjes

Abstract

The development of near isogenic lines (NILs) through repeated backcrossing of genetically distinct parental lines is rather straightforward. Nonetheless, depending on the available resources and the purpose of the lines to be generated, several choices can be made to guide the design of such inbred populations. Here we outline the implications of these choices and provide recommendations for the efficient and proper development of NILs for a number of common scenarios.

Key words: Near isogenic lines, Chromosome substitution strains, Heterogeneous inbred families, Bulk segregant analysis, Marker-assisted selection, Genetic mapping

1. Introduction

For many purposes, it can be very useful to swap genomic regions of different species or species varieties. For instance, one may want to test different regions for allelic differences in a trait of interest and confirm the effect of predicted differences or breed in exotic properties in elite lines. The size and number of genomic regions depends on the objective, but generally a single small segment is transferred from a donor parent into the genetic background of a recipient parent. The resulting lines are called introgression lines (ILs) or, because of their prevailing mode of construction, backcross inbred lines (BILs). However, alternative ways are also in use, and we therefore prefer to use the term near isogenic lines (NILs) because of their genetic resemblance to the recipient parent. Although initially derived from heterogeneous progeny of selected crosses, NILs preferably are homozygous. The genetic make-up is then fixed in "immortal" lines which can be used endlessly and in many replications in various experiments.

As mentioned, NILs can be constructed through a variety of methods depending on the available resources. In their simplest

Scott A. Rifkin (ed.), *Quantitative Trait Loci (QTL): Methods and Protocols*, Methods in Molecular Biology, vol. 871,
DOI 10.1007/978-1-61779-785-9_1, © Springer Science+Business Media New York 2012

form, introgression lines carry a single target locus from a donor variety in an otherwise recurrent genetic background, i.e., isogenic to the recipient parent. In plant and animal breeding, the recipient parent is usually an enduring variety or inbred line/strain that has thrived for decades despite the introduction of new varieties in the field. Donor chromosomal regions can be taken from any resource, like congenic species (see Note 1), advanced backcrosses (BCs), recombinant inbred lines (RILs), doubled haploids (DHs) (see Note 2), heterogeneous inbred families (HIFs), or other mapping populations (F_2/F_3) (e.g., (1–3)). In all instances, however, the point of departure is a cross between two genotypes which segregate in subsequent generations and, in most cases, one to several rounds of backcrossing and/or selfing are necessary to eventually retrieve the desired genomic constitution.

NILs can serve many functions, ranging from breeding purposes to genetic analyses of complex quantitative traits. The ultimate objective of the lines determines for a large part the choice of starting material, crossing scheme, and eventually the genomic composition. For instance, for the confirmation of a QTL detected in an RIL population (see Chapter 3), a relatively large introgression is sufficient which can be derived from backcrossing a selected RIL to one of its parents. On the other hand, to avoid linkage drag, i.e., the simultaneous introgression of closely linked undesired genetic factors, the inclusion of an exotic trait in an elite breeding line requires a very small introgression and several generations of backcrossing after the initial F_1. Other objectives such as (fine) mapping or disentangling the genetic architecture of traits yet again require different approaches and accompanying selection criteria.

Despite their different functions, the efficient generation of small, targeted introgressions strongly depends on the employed selection method. NILs preferably have a genomic fragment on the targeted so-called carrier chromosome without additional donor genomic regions on noncarrier chromosomes (4). Therefore, applying the right approaches in generating NILs is one thing, employing efficient selection methods is another. Whereas in earlier days phenotypic selection strategies were used, with the advent of molecular markers genotypic selection criteria are nowadays common practice. The choice of one selection strategy over another depends on many factors including the subjected species, the crossing scheme applied, the desired genomic make-up, and intended purpose of the derived lines as well as time or cost constraints.

In this chapter, we will discuss the construction and design of NILs for a number of purposes. We will take into account the consequences of the choice of resources and crossing schemes and suggest strategies for efficient selection of lines. We will further illustrate the effect of differences in introgression size and population structure for several scenarios. Finally, we will provide mathematical guidelines for the design and development of NILs.

2. Mendelizing Genetic Effects

In many instances, NILs are constructed and used to confirm previously identified genetic loci that explain part of the variation observed in a specific trait of interest. Because many (quantitative) traits are controlled by multiple loci, each locus must be isolated from its genetic background to be independently tested in a Mendelian fashion. This allows for classic genetic analyses including dominance and interaction effects. Depending on the available resources, NILs can be constructed in various ways which will be outlined below.

2.1. Phenotypic Selection

Before the advent of molecular markers, phenotypic selection was a common practice to create introgression lines. In breeding programs, phenotypic selection is still used frequently as an initial criterion to reduce the number of individuals for molecular profiling. The starting material is always derived from a cross between the donor and recipient parent, but can either be a segregating (e.g., F_2) or fixed (e.g., RIL) population. From this population, a line with the desired phenotype is selected and backcrossed to the recipient parent for several generations (Fig. 1). In every generation, the progeny of the backcross is phenotyped and only those showing the desired properties are retained and further backcrossed. Depending on the starting material, an isogenic recurrent background containing small causal donor introgressions can be achieved within two to eight rounds of backcrossing. Note that no prior information about the number and genomic position of causal loci is required for this strategy. That said, as selection is not targeted to a single locus, multiple synergistically acting additive loci might be introgressed and selected for, especially if trait values depend on epistatic interactions. However, the number of loci can easily be deduced from the segregation ratios in subsequent generations of backcrossing. Furthermore, if the donor exhibits redundant loci, NILs with similar effects but different introgressions may be obtained. These can be confirmed in complementation crosses.

2.2. Confirmation of Mapped Loci

For many species, mapping populations exist or can be created (see Chapters 1–5). These populations serve to identify genomic loci (QTLs: see Note 3) that explain quantitative variation that can be observed for traits that segregate among progeny of crosses of distinct parental lines. Whether derived from BC, DH, RIL, or any other segregating population, all individual lines in a mapping population are more or less densely genotyped. This enables the selection of individuals carrying a genomic donor segment at the exact location of mapped QTLs and preferably a low proportion in the remaining genome. By selecting different lines, each QTL can be Mendelized independently. The selected lines are repeatedly

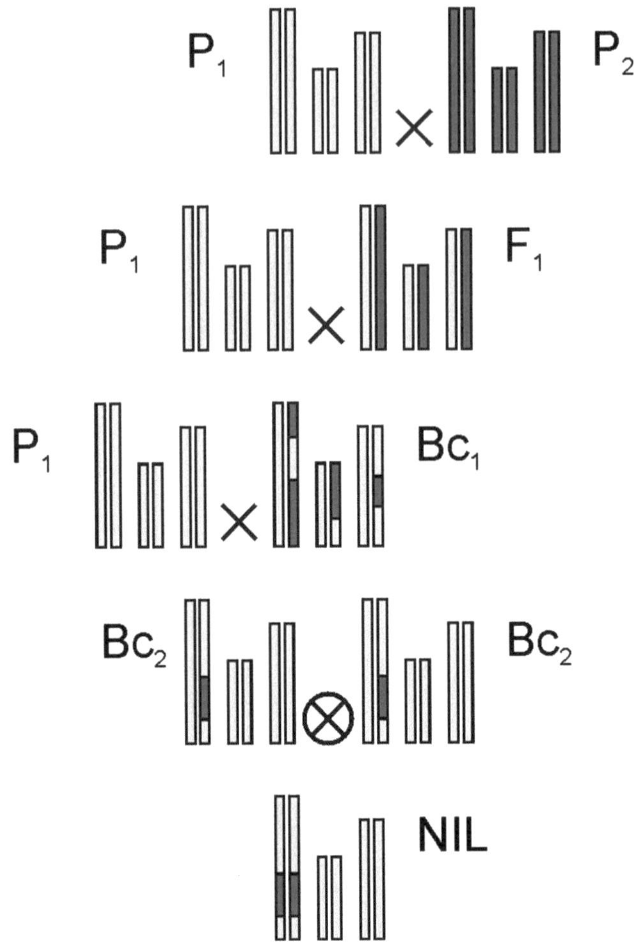

Fig. 1. The construction of NILs through repeated backcrossing. Crossing two genetically distinct parental lines results in a heterozygous offspring. By backcrossing the heterozygote to the recipient parent, the proportion of donor parental genome is reduced with 50%. In recurrent backcrosses, heterozygosity is further reduced to a small introgression followed by selfing or sibling mating to obtain a near isogenic line (NIL).

backcrossed to the recurrent parent until only the desired genomic donor segment remains and all other introgressions are lost. Since the genomic composition of the starting material is known, only a few markers targeted at the donor introgressions are sufficient to successfully monitor subsequent generations. Once a single introgression at the desired position remains, this line can be fixed by selfing or sibling mating after which the homozygous NIL can be phenotyped and compared to the recurrent parent to confirm the presence of a QTL in the introgressed region.

2.3. Fine Mapping and Cloning

Upon QTL detection and confirmation, NILs can be used to further fine map and ultimately clone the causal gene. For this, NILs spanning a QTL support interval are backcrossed to the recurrent parent to create lines heterozygous for the introgressed segment. Crossovers between the homologous chromosomes in these lines result in recombinants with smaller introgression sizes which can be phenotyped again to establish the presence or absence of the QTL in the reduced region. In an iterative process of backcrossing, recombinant selection, and phenotyping, the QTL is ultimately reduced to a single or a few genes which can then be tested using functional genomics approaches.

2.4. Heterogeneous Inbred Families

A special case of inbred lines are HIFs (3). After crossing two distinct parents, HIFs are inbred for five or six generations to create almost complete homozygous genotypes except for a few small regions (<5% of the genome size) (Fig. 2). A collection of HIFs can be used like any other mapping population to identify QTLs. Upon detection of a QTL, however, a single line containing a heterozygous region coinciding with the QTL but otherwise homozygous can be selected using the genotypic information of the population individuals. Progeny of this line will segregate only for the heterozygous region, creating homozygous lines with different genotypes at the QTL region in a single generation. These NILs can then be tested to compare the effect of the segregating region. A hallmark of HIFs is their genomic composition which, although homozygous, is a mosaic of the two parental lines. This offers the advantage that often more than one HIF can be selected which offers the possibility to evaluate the same locus in different genetic backgrounds. This allows testing QTLs for epistatic interactions with other genomic regions which otherwise can only be achieved by crossing pure introgression lines (5).

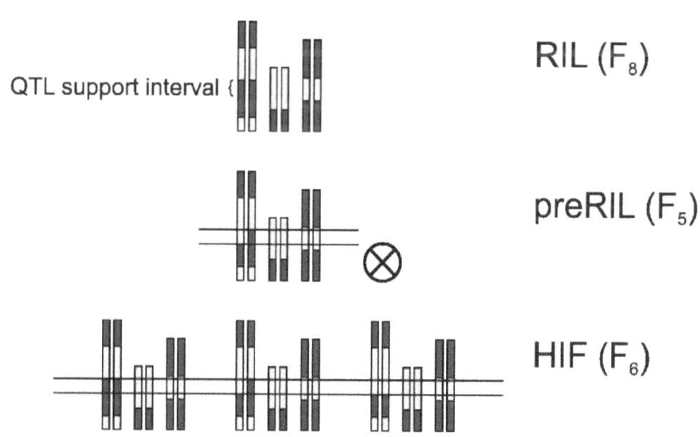

Fig. 2. The construction of heterogeneous inbred families (HIFs). A QTL detected in a RIL population can be confirmed by the use of HIFs. A predecessor of a RIL which is still heterozygous for the region of interest but otherwise homozygous is selfed after which the heterozygous region segregates in a Mendelian fashion. This enables the comparison of the trait of interest for that specific region for both parental genotypes in an isogenic background.

3. NIL Mapping Populations

In addition to confirming QTLs detected in mapping populations or introducing exotic traits in elite breeding lines, NILs can be used for mapping purposes themselves. A good indication of the presence of genetic factors explaining differences in quantitative traits is a comparison of distinct parental lines. In a sense, parental lines represent the largest possible NILs, i.e., the genome of one parent is completely replaced by that of another. To detect which part(s) is responsible for the observed phenotypic variation, the genome needs to be broken up into smaller introgressed segments divided over multiple lines which together provide genome-wide coverage. Depending on the species involved, the available resources, and the exact purpose of the developed lines, several strategies are in use which will be outlined below.

3.1. Bulk Segregant Analysis

Bulk segregant analysis (BSA) is often used in combination with phenotypic selection strategies (see above). This is probably the most basic form of genetic linkage mapping as it does not require a fully genotyped mapping population. Usually a few rounds of backcrossing and/or inbreeding are sufficient to create a segregating population. Trait values in such a genetic diverse population often show a wide distribution range. For qualitative traits, this will be a binominal distribution according to which the population can easily be divided into two discrete classes. For quantitative traits, however, the distribution will approximate normality due to the larger number of loci involved. Consequently, classifying population individuals on the basis of their phenotypes is much more difficult and arbitrary, but two methods for bulk segregation of quantitative distributions prevail. The first method simply splits the population on the basis of the mean, median, or mode (depending on the skewness) of the distribution. The second method is more strict and selects only the upper and lower quartile of the distribution. Both methods have their pros and cons. Splitting uses all lines of the population, and therefore includes all possible variation, but might misclassify individuals which reduces mapping power. Quartile classification, on the other hand, reduces the number of misclassified lines, but only uses half the population size and might only detect major effect loci. In all cases, however, two bulks are formed containing lines of either one of the two designated classes. In each bulk, all lines are pooled and the two resulting samples can then be genotyped genome-wide with molecular markers. Note that markers need to be codominant to quantify allelic frequencies; alternatively, each individual of the bulk can be genotyped separately. Genomic regions enriched for one of the two parental genotypes in either bulk then indicate QTLs for the trait of interest. In principle, all segregating populations can be subjected to BSA, but each will have their own specific properties (see Chapter 4).

3.2. Genome-Wide Coverage NIL Populations

For mapping purposes, NILs are most commonly used as sets of lines that together span the complete genome sequence (6). For many species, NILs are often the only alternative for immortal mapping populations, e.g., RIL populations often suffer from inbreeding distortion in outcrossing species (see Note 4). The advantage of NIL populations is that each line contains only a small section of the donor parent and can directly be compared to the recurrent parent without the need for sophisticated statistical tools. The construction of an NIL population covering the entire genome is a considerable investment and, depending on the use of the population, one can choose different designs. The largest and smallest possible introgressions are achieved when whole chromosomes (see below) and single-nucleotide polymorphisms (SNPs: see Chapter 5) are substituted, respectively. Between these two extremes, there are numerous more possibilities with different introgression sizes and with different amounts of overlap between introgression segments (Fig. 3). That said, there are a number of design issues that affect the mapping power and resolution of NIL populations. Although there is a large freedom of choice in population structures, practical and economic constraints, such as genome size, generation time, and maintenance or experimental costs, might direct the ultimate design. An obvious criterion is the size of the introgressed region in each of the individual NILs. Smaller introgressions provide a higher mapping resolution, but

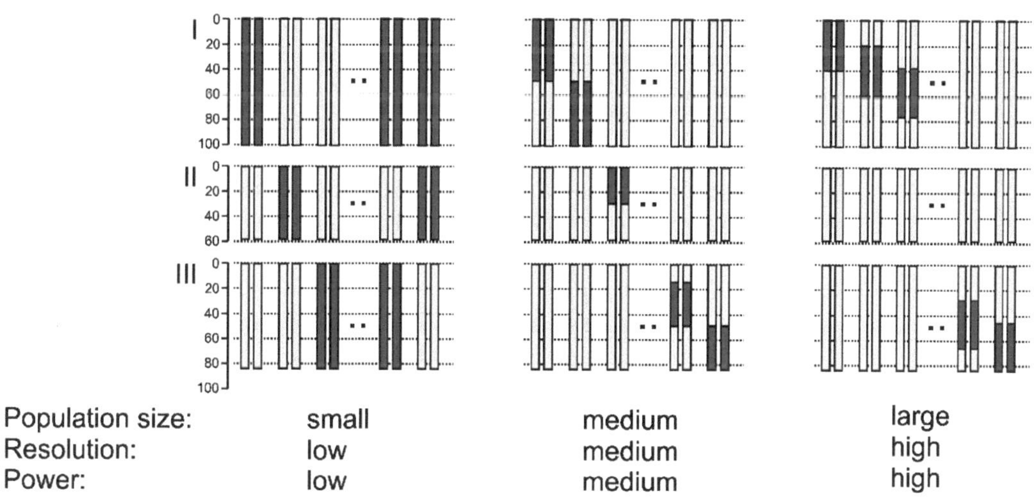

Fig. 3. Genome-wide coverage NIL populations. Different population designs can substantially affect population sizes, resolution, and power. Shown are three different designs, a reciprocal chromosome substitution library, a library with adjacent large introgressions, and a library with small overlapping introgressions.

larger population sizes, i.e., more lines, are needed to maintain genome-wide coverage. Especially for species with large genome sizes, this can considerably increase the number of lines to be maintained and hence experimentation costs. An alternative design consists of a population of NILs with overlapping introgressions in such a way that each genomic region is covered twice (or more). Such a population offers the experimenter the choice to exclude the overlapping lines at the cost of decreased power and resolution, but without losing genome-wide coverage (Fig. 3). Finally, one can choose to develop a one-way or a reciprocal population, i.e., each parental line serves both as recipient and donor parent in two separate collections of lines.

Once a certain design has been selected, NILs need to be developed in a concerted action. After generating an F_1, this will usually take several rounds of backcrossing (depending on the genome size, crossover frequencies (see Note 5 on heterochiasmy), and desired introgression sizes) followed by one or two generations of selfing or sibling mating. Eventually, NILs are selected by genotyping genomic regions using molecular markers. The efficiency of NIL construction can considerably be enhanced by using these markers in what is called marker-assisted selection (MAS). Different selection strategies have been defined based on marker selection applied to carrier and noncarrier chromosomes (7, 8). Two-stage selection is based on selection for the targeted segment on the carrier chromosome (foreground selection) and against donor genomic regions on noncarrier chromosomes (background selection). Three-stage selection involves one more step that selects for the amount of recombination between the target locus and its flanking markers and between the flanking markers and the telomeres on the carrier chromosome (8). Although in principle a desired genotype can be selected from a BC_1 population, this usually requires large population sizes, which exponentially increases with the genome size (see Subheading 4). Therefore, having more backcrosses is generally advantageous over genotyping more lines. Because the level of heterozygosity is highest in earlier generations, the number of backcrosses can substantially decrease genotyping costs. However, with each backcross, the average introgression size decreases, which needs to be considered when designing MAS strategies.

An example of using MAS in a crossing scheme could be to use two-stage selection in BC_1 and three-stage selection in advanced BC generations, minimizing both genotyping costs and the levels of donor parental DNA on noncarrier chromosomes (8). On noncarrier chromosomes, one can increase the number of markers in advanced generations and only use markers at the telomeres in early generations to reduce genotyping costs. Eventually all selected lines need to be genotyped at a resolution high enough to detect double crossovers (usually 10–20 cM). Finally, all desired lines which are still heterozygous for the introgressed region after backcrossing should be inbred to obtain a homozygous immortal mapping population.

3.3. Chromosome Substitution Strains

A special case of NILs are chromosome substitution strains (CSS): these carry the largest possible introgression of a single stretch of DNA into a recipient background. In such a strain, one of the chromosome pairs of the recipient parent has been substituted with that of another (donor) parent. Reasons for CSS construction may be multiple: First, a complete set of CSSs provides a crude mapping population for QTLs, assigning QTLs to whole chromosomes. Second, a CSS removes a lot of background noise from the population that greatly facilitates identification and fine mapping of QTLs ((9) and see above). Finally, a CSS provides an excellent starting point for the generation of smaller NILs. A CSS can be backcrossed to the recipient parent, introducing heterozygosity on only one chromosome pair. By subsequent backcrosses, the introgressed segment can be shortened until fixed by inbreeding.

The general approach in constructing CSSs is very similar to that described for NILs above. An alternative approach that works well for species with small genomes and large numbers of offspring is selecting lines carrying a nonrecombinant chromosome 1, screening the selected lines for a nonrecombinant chromosome 2, and so on for all chromosomes. This results in the elimination of approximately 50% of the individuals at every genotyping round, leaving a BC_1 population from which all CSS can be derived in the next generation (10).

4. Calculations

Although different criteria may apply for the diverse construction designs and purposes of NILs and backcross populations, a number of general rules are instrumental for the development of these resources. Because most designs follow basic Mendelian genetics, a standard set of statistical analyses can be applied to calculate segregation ratios, population sizes, genetic distances, etc.

4.1. Proportions of Parental Genomes in Backcrosses

The proportion of each parental genome depends on the number of backcrosses. The average proportion of the recurrent parental genome increases with every generation and is given by the formula: $(2^{(b+1)} - 1)/2^{(b+1)}$or $1 - \frac{1}{2}^{(b+1)}$ where b is the number of backcrosses assuming an infinite population size. The proportion of the donor genome then simply follows as $\frac{1}{2}^{(b+1)}$. Note that these proportions are independent of genome size and that the fraction of donor genome halves with every backcross: 50% in the F_1, 25% in BC_1, 12.5% in BC_2, etc.

4.2. Minimal Distance Between Markers

The genotype of individual lines at specific positions can be identified by molecular markers (see Chapter 5). The genotype at every other position, the marker intervals, needs to be estimated from its surrounding markers. To reliably estimate the genotype between two adjacent markers, their required maximal distance can be calculated. Incorrect estimates can result from double crossovers between adjacent markers which consequently will not be observed. The occurrence of double crossovers is therefore dependent on the recombination frequency between markers, which can be calculated using Haldane's mapping function: $r = \frac{1}{2}(1 - e^{(-2d/100)})$ where d is the distance between markers in cM. From this formula, it can easily be deduced that the probability of a single crossover event in a 20 cM region is 17% and a double crossover less than 3%. For a distance of 10 cM, the latter will be even less than 1%. For most purposes, a genetic distance of 10–20 cM between markers is therefore sufficient to reliably determine genome-wide genotypes. Note that the relationship between genetic and physical distances is not constant over the genome and can vary significantly between species.

4.3. Linkage Drag

The number of backcrosses needed to break undesired linkage between two loci with a given probability again depends on the genetic distance. The relationship is given by the formula: $N = \text{Log}_{(1-r)}(1 - P)$, where N is the number of backcrosses, r is the recombination frequency, and P is the probability of separation. To have 95% certainty that a crossover has occurred in a 20 cM interval would then take 17 generations of backcrossing. Equivalently, the probability of a crossover to occur between two loci at a given distance and number of backcrosses would read as $P = 1 - (1 - r)^N$. The chance of a single crossover after four backcrosses over a distance of 50 cM can then be calculated as 78%. Over a distance of 1 cM, this would be 4% (11). The examples given here of course represent random selections of single individuals. In practice, however, multiple individuals are often selected which increases the probability of crossover occurrence and therefore decreases the number of backcrosses needed. This is shown by the formula $P = 1 - (1 - p_1)^n$ where p_1 is the probability for a single individual and n the number of selected individuals. The chance that at least one out of ten individuals carries a crossover in a 1 cM interval after four generations of backcrossing would then be 34% (compare to 4% for a single individual).

4.4. Chromosome Substitution Strains

The generation of CSSs requires the transmission of whole chromosomes, and hence, depends upon the absence of crossovers. The chance of a certain chromosome not recombining is given by the function $e^{(-d/100)}$ where d is the length of the chromosome in cM, while assuming no crossover interference (9). The chance of finding a specific nonrecombinant donor chromosome in a BC_1 then equals $\frac{1}{2}e^{(-d/100)}$. When one wants to recover an individual carrying a nonrecombinant donor chromosome with a certainty of q, the required number of individuals can be calculated by solving $q = 1 - (1 - \frac{1}{2}e^{-d/100})^n$ for n.

For CSSs, all other chromosomes need to be of the recurrent parent genotype. The probability is described by $\frac{1}{2}(1 - r)^{(c-1)}$ where c is the number of chromosomes of the species and r is the recombination frequency according to Haldane's mapping function that assumes no interference between crossover events ($r = \frac{1}{2}(1 - e^{(-2d/100)})$ where d is the genetic distance in cM) (12). This probability can estimate the number of individuals that need to be genotyped in BC_1 to immediately obtain a pure CSS. The probability of obtaining a CSS is P(a non - recombinant target chromosome) $\times$ P (all other chromosomes recurrent) $= \frac{1}{2}e^{(-d/100)} \times \frac{1}{2}(1 - r)^{(c-1)}$. From this formula, it can be easily deduced that the number of individuals to be screened increases rapidly with the chromosome number of the species. For a species with only five chromosomes, fewer than 5000 BC_1 individuals need to be screened to obtain all possible CSSs. For a species with ten chromosomes, this would require millions of BC_1 individuals, and multiple generations of backcrossing and selection are therefore needed.

4.5. Fixing Heterozygous Segments

After backcrossing, all introgressed regions are heterozygous, and therefore selected lines require inbreeding to obtain immortal homozygous lines. The probability that a progeny carries a homozygous introgression after selfing is given by

$$P = (1 - r)^2/4 \quad \text{where } r = \frac{1}{2}(1 - e^{(-2d/100)})$$

when assuming no interference. The required population size to obtain the desired genotype with a probability of success q can then be calculated as: $n = \ln(1 - q)/\ln(1 - p)$ (13). For an introgressed segment of 20 cM, this means that more than 36 individuals (n) need to be screened to obtain 99.9% confidence (q) of selecting the desired homozygous line.

5. Notes

1. Congenic strains in animals.
   In animals, isogenic lines are often termed congenic strains. Especially in vertebrates, congenic strains are far more difficult to produce than, e.g., NILs in plants for a number of reasons. Vertebrates generally have a much longer generation time with lower numbers of offspring, suffer from inbreeding depression, and breeding is more costly. These drawbacks make it almost impossible to genotype a huge number of individuals and select

the most promising ones for further generations. Therefore, in animal research often more generations and intermediate selection are required to obtain a desired genotype.

2. Doubled haploids.
   A number of organisms, mostly plants but also certain animal species (e.g., *Drosophila* and certain fish species), allow for the production of doubled haploids (DHs). These are homozygous offspring derived from haploid individuals who underwent chromosome doubling. The unique properties of DHs lie in the fact that they allow for the direct fixation of the genetic content in (micro- or macro-) spores (gametes). DHs produce immortal lines and eliminate heterozygosity from offspring, thereby tremendously decreasing costs for genotyping. DH-production diminishes inbreeding steps and therefore the recovery of heterozygotes in inbreds. The use of DHs is widespread in agriculture where protocols have been developed for many crops (14).
3. Quantitative trait loci.
   Within plant and animal species, natural selection acting upon adaptations to different environmental conditions has led to a wide range of natural variation in quantitative traits. Most agronomical traits, such as yield, nutritional value, and biomass, are quantitatively inherited. These complex traits are affected by a large number of genes, by environmental variation and by genotype-by-environment interactions. For plant and animal breeding, it is of high importance to identify the genomic regions (QTLs) and genes that contribute to variation in these traits and use this knowledge to create new crop or strain varieties. QTL mapping is a powerful tool that can give a good indication of the different genomic regions contributing to the trait variation, the size of their effects, and epistatic interactions. Most often, QTL mapping is performed on crosses between two strains or accessions that vary strongly for a particular trait. In offspring populations, genomic regions of both genotypes segregate. With molecular markers, polymorphic for the two parents, each individual line can be genotyped. Statistical analyses then associate the genomic regions between the markers with the phenotypic trait under study (see also Chapter 3).
4. Interspecific crosses.
   In many breeding programs, attempts have been made to cross-reference lines with their wild relatives to map or introgress traits. Such crosses inherently cause a number of distinct problems which have been well documented (see (1) for an example in tomato breeding). Interspecific crosses can cause sterility and lethality problems in offspring caused by Dobzhansky-Muller incompatibilities. This may complicate

RIL construction or lead to RIL populations showing strong segregation distortions. NILs may then provide viable alternatives since in NILs the introduced donor genome fraction is much smaller.

Apart from zygote inviability, sequence divergence or chromosome rearrangements (such as inversions) can affect the meiotic behavior of chromosomes. Crossover recombination is less likely to occur between homeologous chromosome segments than between homologous chromosome segments. Again, work on tomato introgression lines is worth consulting (15). When small, homeologous chromosome segments are to be introgressed, selection should initially be aimed at obtaining the largest introgressions, and not (as one might intuitively think) for the smallest introgressions. The reason is that finding recombinants close to the locus of interest in later generations is much higher when the homeologous segment is large. Smaller introgressions may show strong suppression of crossover formation. For a review on crossover behavior, see (16).

5. Heterochiasmy.
   It may be worthwhile to pay attention to sexual differences in crossover frequencies since, depending on the species, these may vary (strongly) between sexes. In *Arabidopsis thaliana* for example, the number of crossovers during microsporogenesis is twofold higher as compared to megasporogenesis. This can have large consequences for the efficiency of breeding programs. When crossover incidence is to be maximized in the offspring of an *Arabidopsis* heterozygote, as is the case in the shortening of introgressed segments in backcross populations (NILs), the heterozygote should preferably be used as the male parent in crosses. When crossovers are not desired in a line, e.g., when constructing chromosome substitution lines, the heterozygote should be used as the female parent, which increases the chance of finding the required allele combinations twofold.

References

1. Eshed Y, Zamir D (1995) An introgression line population of *Lycopersicon pennellii* in the cultivated tomato enables the identification and fine mapping of yield-associated QTL. Genetics 141:1147–1162
2. Alonso-Blanco C, Bentsink L, Hanhart CJ, Vries HBE, Koornneef M (2003) Analysis of natural allelic variation at seed dormancy loci of *Arabidopsis thaliana*. Genetics 164:711–729
3. Tuinstra MR, Ejeta G, Goldsbrough PB (1997) Heterogeneous inbred family (HIF) analysis: a method for developing near-isogenic lines that differ at quantitative trait loci. Theor Appl Genet 95:1005–1011
4. Hospital F (2002) Marker-assisted backcross breeding: a case study in genotype building theory. In: Kang MS (ed) Quantitative genetics, genomics and plant breeding. CAB International, New York

5. Loudet O, Gaudon V, Trubuil A, Daniel-Vedele F (2005) Quantitative trait loci controlling root growth and architecture in *Arabidopsis thaliana* confirmed by heterogeneous inbred family. Theor Appl Genet 110:742–753
6. Keurentjes JJB, Bentsink L, Alonso-Blanco C, Hanhart CJ, Blankestijn-De Vries H, Effgen S et al (2007) Development of a near-isogenic line population of *Arabidopsis thaliana* and comparison of mapping power with a recombinant inbred line population. Genetics 175:891–905
7. Frisch M, Bohn M, Melchinger AE (1999) Comparison of selection strategies for marker-assisted backcrossing of a gene. Crop Sci 39:1295–1301
8. Falke KC, Miedaner T, Frisch M (2009) Selection strategies for the development of rye introgression libraries. Theor Appl Genet 119:595–603
9. Koumproglou R, Wilkes TM, Townson P, Wang XY, Beynon J, Pooni HS et al (2002) STAIRS: a new genetic resource for functional genomic studies of Arabidopsis. Plant J 31: 355–364
10. Allard RW (1960) Principles of plant breeding. Wiley, New York
11. Nadeau JH, Singer JB, Matin A, Lander ES (2000) Analysing complex genetic traits with chromosome substitution strains. Nat Genet 24:221–225
12. Visscher PM, Haley CS, Thompson R (1996) Marker-assisted introgression in backcross breeding programs. Genetics 144:1923–1932
13. Frisch M, Bohn M, Melchinger AE (1999) Minimum sample size and optimal positioning of flanking markers in marker-assisted backcrossing for transfer of a target gene. Crop Sci 39:967–975
14. Forster BP, Heberle-Bors E, Kasha KJ, Touraev A (2007) The resurgence of haploids in higher plants. Trends Plant Sci 12:368–375
15. Canady MA, Ji Y, Chetelat RT (2006) Homeologous recombination in *Solanum lycopersicoides* introgression lines of cultivated tomato. Genetics 174:1775–1788
16. Wijnker E, de Jong H (2008) Managing meiotic recombination in plant breeding. Trends Plant Sci 13:640–646

Chapter 2

F_2 Designs for QTL Analysis

Yuan-Ming Zhang

Abstract

This chapter covers the procedure of mapping quantitative trait loci (QTLs) in an F_2 breeding design. I describe genetic design, general methods and software, and several commonly used approaches. The genetic design section includes F_2 population construction. Widely used methods and software are introduced in the section of general methods and software. Finally, composite interval mapping, penalized maximum likelihood, and empirical Bayes are described in detail. Some issues related to the F_2 design are discussed.

Key words: F_2 design, Quantitative trait locus, Composite interval mapping, Penalized maximum likelihood, Empirical Bayes, Multiple quantitative trait loci model, Segregation analysis

1. Introduction

In modern quantitative genetics, phenotypic values, population structure, and marker information are used to infer the number of quantitative trait loci (QTLs) and to estimate their positions and effects. One key advance in QTL mapping was the introduction of interval mapping in a population from a cross between two inbred lines (1). Many variants of this approach have been developed, and they mainly focus on segregation populations such as F_2, backcross, double haploid (DH), and recombinant inbred line (RIL) populations ((2–7), Chapter 3).

F_2 populations play an important role in the genetic dissection of quantitative traits for several reasons. First, all kinds of genetic effects (additive, dominant, and all kinds of epistatic effects) can be estimated. Second, many genetic populations and designs are derived from the F_2, including the $F_{2:3}$ design, RIL, advanced intercross lines (AILs), and triple testcross (TTC) design. Third, a large F_2 population derived from two near-isogenic lines is frequently used in the fine mapping of QTL. In this chapter, we focus on the essential F_2 design for QTL analysis.

Scott A. Rifkin (ed.), *Quantitative Trait Loci (QTL): Methods and Protocols*, Methods in Molecular Biology, vol. 871, DOI 10.1007/978-1-61779-785-9_2,

2. Genetic Design

Several methods exist to construct an F_2 population. These approaches are described as below using plants as an example.

1. A female parent (inbred line, homozygous genotype) is crossed to a male parent (inbred line, homozygous genotype). The F_1 plants are selfed to develop F_2 seeds (Fig. 1). All F_2 seeds are planted to construct an F_2 plant population and these F_2 plants are genotyped for molecular markers and phenotyped for the trait. These phenotypic values along with molecular marker information are used to detect QTLs for quantitative traits. This is the most widely and commonly used method in coarse mapping of QTLs.
2. *Immortalized F_2 (IF_2) population*: This idea was first presented by Gardiner et al. (8). The heterozygosity of the F_2 population is "immortalized" by pooled random mating in the F_3 and subsequent generations, because the genotype of the F_2 is maintained in each pooled IF_2 family. The procedure is as follows. Forty F_3 seeds from each F_2 plant are planted in two rows. On successive pollinating days, pollen from five F_3 plants in one row is bulked and the bulked pollen is used to pollinate five F_3 plant in the same IF_2 family. A minimum of 20 ears are bulked to immortalize the F_2. Recently, another design for the IF_2 was proposed by Hua et al. (9) according to a double haploid (DH) or recombination inbred line (RIL) population (Fig. 2). In this design, all the DH lines or RILs are randomly divided into two groups with same sample size. The lines in each group are randomly numbered. The *i*th line in the first group is crossed to the *i*th line in the second group. Each of these lines is used only once in each round of pairing and

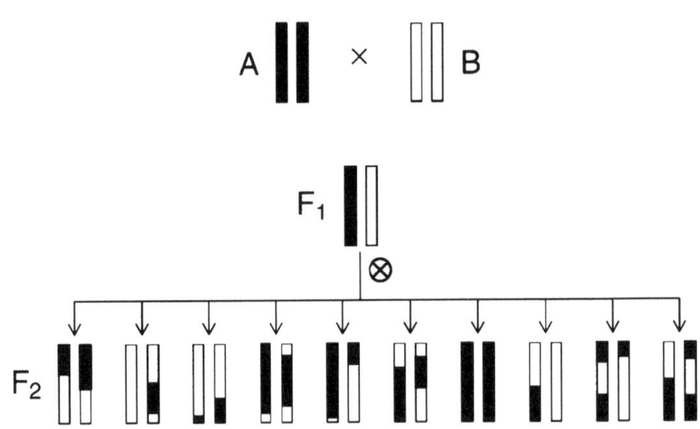

Fig. 1. Construction of an F2 population.

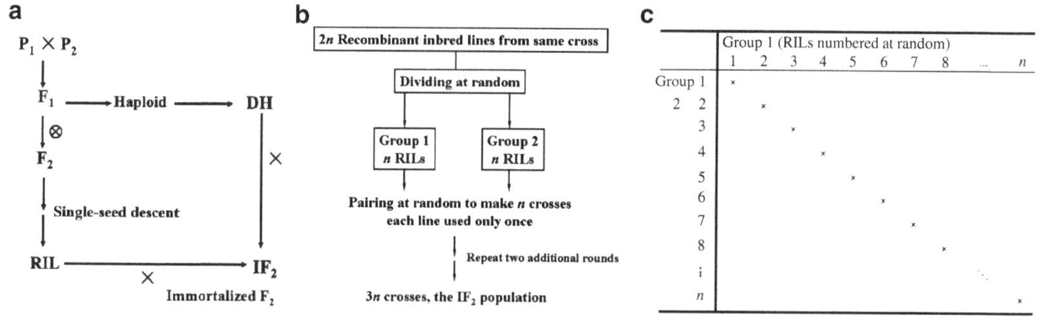

Fig. 2. Construction of an "immortalized F2" population. (**a**) The IF2 population is derived from a DH or RIL population; (**b**) the construction procedure; and (**c**) pairing between two RILs from different groups.

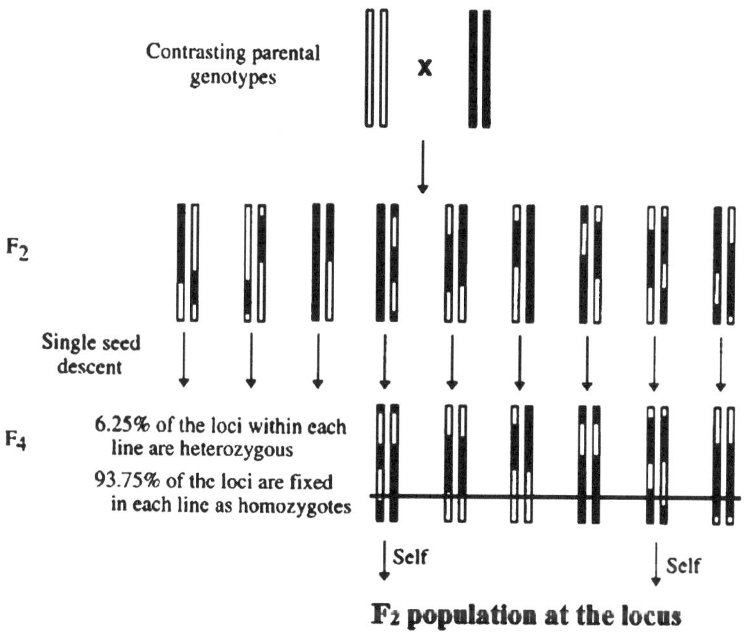

Fig. 3. Construction of an F2 population using residual heterozygous line.

crossing. In order to increase the sample size of the IF_2, the above procedure may be repeated multiple times. This population resembles an F_2 population in that the compositions and frequencies of single- and multilocus genotypes are similar to those of an F_2 population.

3. *Residual heterozygous line* (*RHL*): The RHL design was proposed by Yamanaka et al. (10) for fine mapping QTLs. It includes two steps (Fig. 3). First, a line is selected from an F_4 population such that its genome contains a heterozygous segment around a major QTL, but is homozygous in other regions, including other QTLs.

Second, the selected RHL is selfed to construct a large segregating F_2 population at the target region. This design is similar to the heterogeneous inbred family of Tuinstra et al. (11). However, the purpose of the latter is to develop near-isogenic lines that differ at the detected QTLs in order to confirm the QTLs.

4. The $F_{2:3}$ design: In the most widely used F_2 design above, all F_3 seeds from one F_2 plant are planted to construct an $F_{2:3}$ family and each $F_{2:3}$ family is phenotyped for quantitative trait. Thus, the strategy of using F_2 marker genotypes and $F_{2:3}$ average phenotypes for QTL mapping is named as the $F_{2:3}$ design (12).

3. General Methods and Software

There are a series of methods available for detecting QTLs in an F_2 population, such as interval mapping (1), composite interval mapping (13–15), multiple interval mapping (16), Bayesian analysis (5, 17), and penalized maximum likelihood (PML) method (18). Several packages (cataloged at: http://www.stat.wisc.edu/~yandell/statgen/software/biosci/qtl.html) have been developed to implement these methods, such as Windows QTL Cartographer V2.5_005 ((19), http://statgen.ncsu.edu/qtlcart/WQTLCart.htm), R/qtlbim v1.7.7 ((20), http://www.qtlbim.org), and QTL Network 2.0 ((21), http://ibi.zju.edu.cn/software/qtlnetwork/). Here we introduce three methods: composite interval mapping, the PML, and empirical Bayes ((22), http://www.statgen.ucr.edu/).

4. Composite Interval Mapping

4.1. Genetic Model

Consider one QTL on a marker interval (l, $l + 1$) in an F_2 population. Let us define the three possible genotypes by QQ, Qq, and qq. The phenotypic value of quantitative trait for the ith F_2 plant, y_i, may be described as below

$$y_i = \mu + x_i^* a^* + z_i^* d^* + \sum_{k \neq l, l+1} (x_{ik} a_k + z_{ik} d_k) + \varepsilon_i \qquad (1)$$

where μ is the model mean; a^* and d^* are additive and dominant effects of putative QTL, respectively; a_k and d_k are the partial regression coefficients of the phenotype y on the kth marker; x_i^* and z_i^* are indicator variables for the putative QTL in the ith individual, taking $x_i^* = 1$ and $z_i^* = 0$ for QQ, $x_i^* = 0$ and $z_i^* = 1$ for Qq, $x_i^* = -1$ and $z_i^* = 0$ for qq, and similar definition for x_{ik} and z_{ik}; and ε_i is a residual error with an assumed $N(0, \sigma^2)$ distribution.

4.2. Parameter Estimation

The distribution of y_i is a mixture of three normal distributions, so the likelihood function is given by

$$L(a^*, d^*, \mathbf{B}, \sigma^2) = \prod_{i=1}^{n} [p_{1i} f(y_i; \mathbf{X}_i\mathbf{B} + a^*, \sigma^2) + p_{2i} f(y_i; \mathbf{X}_i\mathbf{B} + d^*, \sigma^2) + p_{3i} f(y_i; \mathbf{X}_i\mathbf{B} - a^*, \sigma^2)] \quad (2)$$

where $f(t_1; t_2, t_3)$ represents the normal density of variable t_1 with mean t_2 and variance t_3; p_{1i}, p_{2i}, and p_{3i} are the probabilities of the three genotypes for the ith F_2 individual inferred from marker information. Therefore, the maximum likelihood estimates for the parameters are the solutions of

$$\begin{aligned}
a^* &= \sum_{i=1}^{n} (p_{1i}^* - p_{3i}^*)(y_i - \mathbf{X}_i\mathbf{B}) \Big/ \sum_{i=1}^{n} (p_{1i}^* + p_{3i}^*) \\
d^* &= \sum_{i=1}^{n} p_{2i}^*(y_i - \mathbf{X}_i\mathbf{B}) \Big/ \sum_{i=1}^{n} p_{2i}^* \\
\mathbf{B} &= (\mathbf{X}'\mathbf{X})^{-1}\mathbf{X}'[\mathbf{Y} - (\mathbf{P}_1^* - \mathbf{P}_2^*)a^* - \mathbf{P}_2^* d^*] \\
\sigma^2 &= \frac{1}{n} \sum_{i=1}^{n} [p_{1i}^*(y_i - \mathbf{X}_i\mathbf{B} - a^*)^2 + p_{2i}^*(y_i - \mathbf{X}_i\mathbf{B} - d^*)^2 \\
&\quad + p_{3i}^*(y_i - \mathbf{X}_i\mathbf{B} + a^*)^2]
\end{aligned} \quad (3)$$

where $\mathbf{X}_i$ is the ith row of matrix $\mathbf{X}$, $\mathbf{P}_s^* = (p_{si}^*)_{n\times 1}$ $(s = 1, 2, 3)$, $\mathbf{Y}^* = (y_i)_{n\times 1}$ and

$$p_{1i}^* = \frac{p_{1i} f(y_i; \mathbf{X}_i\mathbf{B} + a^*, \sigma^2)}{p_{1i} f(y_i; \mathbf{X}_i\mathbf{B} + a^*, \sigma^2) + p_{2i} f(y_i; \mathbf{X}_i\mathbf{B} + d^*, \sigma^2) + p_{3i} f(y_i; \mathbf{X}_i\mathbf{B} - a^*, \sigma^2)}$$

$$p_{2i}^* = \frac{p_{2i} f(y_i; \mathbf{X}_i\mathbf{B} + d^*, \sigma^2)}{p_{1i} f(y_i; \mathbf{X}_i\mathbf{B} + a^*, \sigma^2) + p_{2i} f(y_i; \mathbf{X}_i\mathbf{B} + d^*, \sigma^2) + p_{3i} f(y_i; \mathbf{X}_i\mathbf{B} - a^*, \sigma^2)}$$

$$p_{3i}^* = \frac{p_{3i} f(y_i; \mathbf{X}_i\mathbf{B} - a^*, \sigma^2)}{p_{1i} f(y_i; \mathbf{X}_i\mathbf{B} + a^*, \sigma^2) + p_{2i} f(y_i; \mathbf{X}_i\mathbf{B} + d^*, \sigma^2) + p_{3i} f(y_i; \mathbf{X}_i\mathbf{B} - a^*, \sigma^2)}$$

4.3. Likelihood Ratio Test

The hypotheses to be tested are $H_0 : a^* = d^* = 0$ and $H_1 : a^* \neq 0, d^* \neq 0$. The likelihood ratio statistic is

$$\mathrm{LOD} = \lg \frac{L(a^*, d^*, \mathbf{B}, \sigma^2)}{L(a^* = 0, d^* = 0, \tilde{\mathbf{B}}, \tilde{\sigma}^2)} \quad (4)$$

where

$$\tilde{\mathbf{B}} = (\mathbf{X}'\mathbf{X})^{-1}\mathbf{X}'\mathbf{Y}$$

and

$$\tilde{\sigma}^2 = \frac{1}{n}(\mathbf{Y} - \mathbf{X}\mathbf{B})'(\mathbf{Y} - \mathbf{X}\mathbf{B}).$$

The critical value for the LOD score obtained from 1,000 imputation experiments is often used to declare the presence of a putative QTL in a given genomic region. The QTL confidence interval (90–95%) is often defined as a map interval that corresponds to one LOD decline on either side of the peak.

This approach can be performed by Windows QTL Cartographer V2.5_005.

5. Penalized Maximum Likelihood Approach

5.1. Genetic Model

If several $F_{2:g}$ family populations derived from the direct and reciprocal crosses between two inbred lines are available, the average phenotypic value of a quantitative trait for the ith $F_{2:g}$ family of the $(g-2)$th family population of the kth cross $(i = 1, \cdots, n_{r-2};\ g = 3, \ldots, G;\ k = 1, 2)$, $y_{i(r-2)k}$, may be described by the following model:

$$y_{i(r-2)k} = \mu + x_c c + \mathrm{E} + \mathrm{G} + \mathrm{GE} + \mathrm{GC} + \varepsilon_i \tag{5}$$

where μ is the population mean, c is cytoplasmic effect, and the dummy variable x_c is defined as $x_c = 1$ for a direct cross and $x_c = -1$ for a reciprocal cross, E is environmental effect, G is genetic effect, GE is environment-by-QTL interaction effect, GC is cytoplasm-by-QTL interaction effect, ε_i is a residual error with an assumed $N(0, \sigma^2)$ distribution, and

$$\mathrm{E} = \sum_{j=1}^{R-1} x_{ij} r_j$$

$$\mathrm{G} = \sum_{l=1}^{m} \left(x_{i(R-1+2l-1)} a_l + x_{i(R-1+2l)} d_l\right)$$

$$\mathrm{GE} = \sum_{j=1}^{R-1} \sum_{l=1}^{m} \left[x_{ij} x_{i(R-1+2l-1)} (ae)_{jl} + x_{ij} x_{i(R-1+2l)} (de)_{jl}\right]$$

$$\mathrm{GC} = \sum_{l=1}^{m} \left[x_c x_{i(R-1+2l-1)} (ac)_l + x_c x_{i(R-1+2l)} (dc)_l\right]$$

where R and m are the numbers of environments and QTL, respectively, a is additive effect, d is dominant effect, ae is additive-by-environment interaction effect, de is dominant-by-environment interaction effect, ac is additive-by-cytoplasm interaction effect, dc is dominant-by-cytoplasm interaction effect, and x is a dummy variable for various effects. To reflect the genetic relationship among various generations, the value of x for a heterozygous F_g family is two times that for heterozygous F_{g-1} family. If the data are involved only in one of direct or reciprocal crosses, the cytoplasmic and cytoplasm-by-QTL interaction effects cannot be considered in the model (5). If the data are involved only in one environment, the environmental and environment-by-QTL interaction effects cannot be considered in the model (5).

Because all kinds of effects in model (5) are treated in the same way under the PML, model (5) can be rewritten for the sake of clarity as:

$$y_u = \sum_{l=1}^{p} z_{ul} b_l + \varepsilon_i \quad (u = 1, \cdots, n) \tag{6}$$

where $p = (R + 1)(2m + 1)$, and $n = 3 \times 504 = 1,512$. The pseudomarker approach uses the multimarker analysis with a slight modification by inserting virtual markers into all marker intervals >5 cM. Because of incomplete genotypic information in the real data analysis, multiple permutations for incomplete marker genotypes (23) can be adopted to simulate the incomplete genotypes. This requires multiple analyses of the data, one for each imputed dataset. Ten to fifty imputed datasets are usually sufficient. For each sample, the complete genotypes sampled are used to construct the design matrix for QTL effects in model (6).

If an IF_2 population is available, the molecular marker information of all the IF_2 plants is not needed, because the marker information for each IF_2 plant can be derived from its parents (Table 1). Therefore, the phenotypic values for IF_2 plants along with the deduced marker information are available in QTL mapping. The genetic model and corresponding methods are same as those in the F_2 design.

If RHL is available, the RHL is selfed to construct a new F_2 population. In the F_2 population, we scan only the target region of genome. Therefore, the information of markers on the target region along with the phenotypic value of a complex trait is used to perform fine mapping of QTL. The genetic model and corresponding methods are same as those in the F_2 design.

Table 1
Deduction of molecular marker genotypes of IF_2 plant from its parents

	Molecular marker				
Case	**1**	**2**	**3**	**4**	**5**
♀	AA	AA	aa	aa	aa
♂	aa	AA	AA	AA	aa
IF_2 individual	Aa	AA	Aa	Aa	aa

5.2. Parameter Estimation and Likelihood Ratio Test

All the effects in model (6) can be estimated by maximizing penalized log-likelihood

$$\psi = \sum_{i=1}^{n} \ln f(y_u; \sum_{l=1}^{p} z_{ul} b_l, \sigma^2) + \sum_{l=2}^{p} \{\ln f(b_l; \mu_l, \sigma_l^2) + \ln f(\mu_l; 0, \sigma_l^2/\eta)\} \quad (7)$$

with respect to parameters and hyperparameters simultaneously. Therefore, we get

$$b_t = \frac{1}{n}\sum_{u=1}^{n}(y_u - \sum_{l \neq t}^{p} z_{ul} b_l) \quad (t = 1, \cdots, R+1)$$

$$b_t = \left[\sum_{u=1}^{n} z_{ut}^2 + \sigma^2/\sigma_t^2\right]^{-1} \times \left[\sum_{u=1}^{n} z_{ut}(y_u - \sum_{l \neq t}^{p} z_{ul} b_l) + \mu_t \sigma^2/\sigma_t^2\right] \quad (t = R+2, \cdots, p) \quad (8)$$

$$\sigma^2 = \frac{1}{n}\sum_{u=1}^{n}(y_u - \sum_{l=1}^{p} z_{ul} b_l)^2$$

where $\mu_\tau = \beta_\tau/(\eta + 1)$, $\sigma_t^2 = \frac{1}{2}[(b_t - \mu_t)^2 + \eta\mu_t^2]$, and $\eta = 5$. In real data analysis, the procedure necessitates pretreatment to deal with dominant and missing markers and marker density. Marker imputation techniques may be used in the case of incomplete information marker data. They involve the calculation of the conditional probability of marker genotypes using a multipoint method and the sampling of a complete imputed data set for the marker genotypes. Usually, 30 imputed data sets are generated. Each data set is analyzed under the framework of model (6) with the PML method. Samples that have an LOD statistic of greater than 2.5 are counted. A QTL that had greater than 10% of the number of samples with an LOD > 2 compared to the total number of imputed samples (30) would be considered real. The QTL position is an average weighted by the total genetic variance of QTL detected. The reported result is the mean of estimates for each imputed data set. When marker density is too high, choosing one marker from the cluster of markers avoids a high degree of multicollinearity. When the markers are too sparse, virtual markers (treated as missing data) may be inserted. When the number of effects in the model (6) is much larger than sample size (e.g., 20 times), a two-stage method is proposed. In the first stage, a full model including all effects is divided into many reduced models, each with about 2,000 effects (or ten times sample size). In the second stage, the genetic model is modified so that only effects that have passed the first round of selection are included in the model, and PML can be used to reanalyze the data.

6. Empirical Bayes Approach

6.1. Genetic Model

The model (6) can be rewritten as

$$y = \mathbf{X}\beta + \sum_{l=1}^{p} Z_l \gamma_l + \varepsilon \tag{9}$$

where β is the non-QTL effect vector (e.g., the year effect), $\mathbf{X}$ is the corresponding design matrix, γ_l is a vector of genotypic effect for locus l, and Z_l is the corresponding incidence matrix determined by the genotypes of locus l. The residual error vector e is assumed to be distributed as $\varepsilon \sim N(0, \sigma^2 \mathbf{I}_n)$, where $\mathbf{I}_n$ is an $n \times n$ identity matrix and σ^2 is an unknown residual error variance.

6.2. Parameter Estimation

Using the standard procedure of mixed model methodology, the fixed effects and residual error variance are estimated by:

$$\begin{aligned} \beta &= (X'V^{-1}X)^{-1}X'V^{-1}y \\ \sigma^2 &= \frac{1}{n}(y - X\beta)'\left(y - X\beta - \sum_{l=1}^{p} Z_l E(\gamma_l)\right) \end{aligned} \tag{10}$$

where

$$\mathbf{V} = \sum_{l=1}^{p} Z_l Z_l' \sigma_l^2 + \mathbf{I}_n \sigma^2$$

and

$$p(\gamma_l | \sigma_l^2) = N(0, \sigma_l^2).$$

Xu's expectation and maximization (EM) algorithm treats regression coefficients as missing values (22). In the E-step, the expectation of the quadratic term required in the M-step is expressed as

$$E(\gamma_l' \gamma_l) = E(\gamma_l')E(\gamma_l) + \mathrm{tr}[\mathrm{var}(\gamma_l)] \tag{11}$$

where $E(\gamma_l) = \sigma_l^2 Z_l' \mathbf{V}^{-1}(y - \mathbf{X}\beta)$ and $\mathrm{var}(\gamma_l) = \mathbf{I}\sigma_l^2 - \sigma_l^2 Z_l' \mathbf{V}^{-1} Z_l \sigma_l^2$. In the M-step, update the fixed effects and residual error variance using Eq. (10) and σ_l^2 using equation

$$\sigma_l^2 = \frac{E(\gamma'_l \gamma_l) + \omega}{\tau + 3} \tag{12}$$

where

$$(\tau, \omega) = (0, 0).$$

7. Notes

7.1. F_2-Related Designs in QTL Mapping

Many genetic populations and designs are derived from the F_2. The first design is the $F_{2:3}$ design. Typical QTL statistics assume that each F_2 individual is genotyped for the marker and phenotyped for the trait. For plant traits with low heritability, it has been suggested that it is better to use the average phenotypic value of F_3 progeny derived from a same F_2 plant (or ear) in place of the F_2 phenotype itself. This strategy of using F_2 marker genotypes and $F_{2:3}$ average phenotypes for QTL mapping is named as the $F_{2:3}$ design and widely used in cotton, maize, and soybean (12). In real data analysis, there are two approaches. One is the classical $F_{2:3}$ design analysis, and the other is that fully takes advantage of the mixture distribution for $F_{2:3}$ families of heterozygous F_2 plants (12). Zhang and Xu show that incorporation of the mixture distribution information significantly increases the power of QTL detection relative to the classical $F_{2:3}$ design (12).

The second design is TTC design. It entails crossing the ith individual of an F_2 population to the same three testers, the two inbred lines (P_1 and P_2), and their F_1, to produce $3n$ families (L_{1i}, L_{2i}, and L_{3i}). The design provides separate tests for, and estimates of, the additive, dominance, and epistatic components of variability. Recently, we have developed a two-stage approach, which provides unbiased estimates for all the QTL effects.

There are some shortcomings for the F_2 design. First, the F_2 population is temporally limited and used only one time. To overcome this problem, the RIL population by single-seed descent and the IF_2 design are available. Second, there is rarely recombination in F_2 populations between closely linked loci because the gametes have undergone only a single cycle of recombination. AILs increase the number of recombination events. Recently, Kao and Zeng (24) have developed a statistical method for QTL mapping in advanced populations derived from two inbred lines, such as AILs. In molecular biology, SNP marker can be also used to overcome this issue. Third, most triploid endosperm trait loci mapping methods do not produce unbiased estimates of the two dominant effects of endosperm trait loci. A random hybridization design is an alternative method that may be used to overcome this problem (25). In addition, in any highly heterozygous outbred species, such as most trees and livestock, inbred lines cannot be developed and the cross between two heterozygous individuals is often named as pseudotestcross. This is because many markers are heterozygous in one parent, null in the other, and therefore segregate 1 : 1 in their F_1 progeny following a testcross configuration. If many markers are heterozygous in the two parents, their F_1 progeny will follow a F_2 configuration. In theory, it is more similar to four-way cross (26).

7.2. Mixed Major-Gene Plus Polygenes Inheritance Analysis

In the polygenic model of classical quantitative genetics, the genetic effect of a single locus is so small that it cannot be investigated separately, and loci must be studied collectively as a whole. However, QTL mapping and crop breeding have confirmed that the effects of genes responsible for quantitative traits are unequal and a gene may have a greater effect, making it a major gene. Thus, mixed major-gene plus polygenic inheritance is a useful alternative to classical quantitative genetics (27–29). In our studies, a series of genetic models are considered, such as one major gene (model A), two major genes (model B), pure polygenes (model C), one major gene plus polygenes (model D), and two major genes plus polygenes (model E). Taking gene action into account (additive-dominant and additive-dominant-epistasis), we construct model types within each class. In each genetic model, we assume that the frequency distribution of quantitative trait in a segregation population consists of several major-gene genotype component distributions; a likelihood function can be established and the maximum likelihood estimates of parameters are obtained through an expectation and iterated maximization (EIM) algorithm (28). Therefore, at least 24-model combinations are considered to select one model that best explain the quantitative trait variation by using both Akaike's information criterion and a set of tests of fitness. Finally, the estimates of genetic parameters are calculated from the estimates of component distributions in the optimal genetic model. All formulae and analytical procedures have been established for a single segregating population with or without its parents, including F_2 and $F_{2:3}$; for five generations of P_1, P_2, F_1, F_2, and $F_{2:3}$; and for six generations of P_1, P_2, F_1, BC_1, BC_2, and F_2 (29). This approach has been widely applied in China. However, this is a phenotypic analysis method, the major genes detected cannot be localized on chromosomes, and the estimates of genetic parameters have larger errors relative to QTL mapping.

7.3. Multi-QTL Joint Analysis

In interval mapping, the estimated position and effect of a putative QTL may be biased by the presence of other QTLs linked within the same chromosome, especially if the linkage is tight. In the extreme situation when the two linked QTLs have effects in opposite directions, the QTLs can cancel each other out and neither of them will be detected. On the other hand, if the two linked QTLs have effects in the same direction, a "ghost" QTL may be detected between the two real QTLs. To overcome the above issues, it is necessary to use a multi-QTL genetic model to estimate all QTL effects simultaneously in a single model. Jansen and Zeng independently proposed composite interval mapping (13–15). Thereafter, Kao et al. developed multiple interval mapping (16). Recently, various multi-QTL analyses have been successively developed, such as PML approach (18) and the empirical Bayes method (22).

The multi-QTL joint analysis approach differs from the classical methods. First, the joint analysis approach can jointly analyze a dataset with multiple environments or replicates. This increases sample size so that more QTLs can be detected using the new methods than for the classical methods (22, 30). Second, main and environmental effects and environmental and epistatic interactions are simultaneously considered in a single genetic model. A single-QTL model with the choice of markers to include as cofactors is tested once in composite interval mapping, while in multiple interval mapping a multi-QTL and interaction genetic model is studied. In other words, no interaction is included in the genetic model of composite interval mapping, and two common kinds of interactions—QTL-by-environment and interaction between the loci without main effects—are not evaluated in multiple interval mapping. Results show that the joint analysis seems to be more powerful. Therefore, we recommend the joint analysis approach.

Acknowledgments

The work was supported by the National Natural Science Foundation of China (30971848 and 30671333), the 111 Project (B08025), NCET (NCET-05-0489), and the Fundamental Research Funds for the Central Universities (KYT201002).

References

1. Lander ES, Botstein D (1989) Mapping Mendelian factors underlying quantitative traits using RFLP linkage maps. Genetics 121:185–199
2. Broman KW (2001) Review of statistical methods for QTL mapping in experimental crosses. Lab Anim 30:44–52
3. Knott SA (2005) Regression-based quantitative trait loci mapping: robust, efficient and effective. Phil Trans R Soc B 360:1435–1442
4. Zhang Y-M (2006) Advances on methods for mapping QTL in plants. Chin Sci Bull 51:2809–2818
5. Yi N, Shriner D (2008) Advances in Bayesian multiple quantitative trait loci mapping in experimental crosses. Heredity 100:240–252
6. Zou W, Zeng Z-B (2008) Statistical Methods for Mapping Multiple QTL. International Journal of Plant Genomics, Article ID 286561. doi:10.1155/2008/286561
7. Sorensen D (2009) Developments in statistical analysis in quantitative genetics. Genetica 136:319–322
8. Gardiner JM, Coe EH, Melia-Hancock S, Hoisington DA, Chao S (1993) Development of a core RFLP map in maize using an immortalized F_2 population. Genetics 134:917–930
9. Hua J, Xing Y, Wu W, Xu C, Sun X, Yu S, Zhang Q (2003) Single-locus heterotic effects and dominance by dominance interactions can adequately explain the genetic basis of heterosis in an elite rice hybrid. Proc Natl Acad Sci USA 100:2574–2579
10. Yamanaka N, Watanabe S, Toda K, Hayashi M, Huchigami H, Takahashi R, Harada K (2005) Fine mapping of the *FT1* locus for soybean flowering time using a residual heterozygous line derived from a recombinant inbred line. Theor Appl Genet 110:634–639
11. Tuinstra MR, Ejeta G, Goldsbrough PB (1997) Heterogeneous inbred family (HIF) analysis: a method for developing near-isogenic lines that differ at quantitative trait loci. Theor Appl Genet 95:1005–1011

12. Zhang Y-M, Xu S (2004) Mapping quantitative trait loci in F_2 incorporating phenotypes of F_3 progeny. Genetics 166:1981–1993
13. Jansen RC (1993) Interval mapping of multiple quantitative trait loci. Genetics 135:205–211
14. Zeng Z-B (1993) Theoretical basis for separation of multiple linked gene effects in mapping of quantitative trait loci. Proc Natl Acad Sci USA 90:10972–10976
15. Zeng Z-B (1994) Precision mapping of quantitative trait loci. Genetics 136:1457–1468
16. Kao C-H, Zeng Z-B, Teasdale RD (1999) Multiple interval mapping for quantitative trait loci. Genetics 152:1203–1216
17. Wang H, Zhang Y-M, Li X, Masinde GL, Mohan S, Baylink DJ, Xu S (2005) Bayesian shrinkage estimation of QTL parameters. Genetics 170:465–480
18. Zhang Y-M, Xu S (2005) A penalized maximum likelihood method for estimating epistatic effects of QTL. Heredity 95:96–104
19. Wang S, Basten CJ, Zeng Z-B (2010) Windows QTL Cartographer 2.5. Department of Statistics, North Carolina State University, Raleigh
20. Yandell BS, Mehta T, Banerjee S, Shriner D, Venkataraman R, Moon JY, Neely WW, Wu H, Smith R, Yi N (2007) R/qtlbim: QTL with Bayesian interval mapping in experimental crosses. Bioinformatics 23:641–643
21. Yang J, Zhu J, Williams RW (2007) Mapping the genetic architecture of complex traits in experimental populations. Bioinformatics 23:1527–1536
22. Xu S (2010) An expectation–maximization algorithm for the Lasso estimation of quantitative trait locus effects. Heredity 105: 483–494
23. Sen S, Churchill GA (2001) A statistical framework for quantitative trait mapping. Genetics 159:371–387
24. Kao C-K, Zeng M-H (2009) A study on the mapping of quantitative trait loci in advanced populations derived from two inbred lines. Genet Res 91:85–99
25. He X-H, Zhang Y-M (2008) Mapping epistatic QTL underlying endosperm traits using all markers on the entire genome in random hybridization design. Heredity 101:39–47
26. He X-H, Qin H, Hu Z, Zhang T, Zhang Y-M (2010) Mapping of epistatic quantitative trait loci in four-way crosses. Theor Appl Genet. doi:10.1007/s00122-010-1420-8
27. Elston RC, Steward J (1973) The analysis of quantitative traits for simple genetic models from parental, F_1 and backcross data. Genetics 73:695–711
28. Zhang Y-M, Gai J, Yang Y-H (2003) The EIM algorithm in the joint segregation analysis of quantitative traits. Genet Res 81:157–163
29. Gai J, Zhang Y-M, Wang JK (2003) The genetic system of quantitative traits in plants. Science Press, Beijing
30. Liu G, Li M, Wen J, Du Y, Zhang Y-M (2010) Functional mapping of quantitative trait loci associated with rice tillering. Mol Genet Genomics 284:263–271

Chapter 3

Design and Construction of Recombinant Inbred Lines

Daniel A. Pollard

Abstract

Recombinant inbred lines (RILs) are a collection of strains that can be used to map quantitative trait loci. Parent strains are crossed to create recombinants that are then inbred to isogenicity, resulting in a permanent resource for trait mapping and analysis. Here I describe the process of designing and constructing RILs. This consists of the following steps. Parent strains are selected based on phenotype, marker availability, and compatibility, and they may be genetically engineered to remove unwanted variation or to introduce reporters. A construction design scheme is determined, including the target population size, if and how advanced intercrossing will be done, and the number of generations of inbreeding. Parent crosses and F1 crosses are performed to create an F2 population. Depending on design, advanced intercrossing may be implemented to increase mapping resolution through the accumulation of additional meiotic crossover events. Finally, lines are inbred to create genetically stable recombinant lines. I discuss tips and techniques for maximizing mapping power and resolution and minimizing resource investment for each stage of the process.

Key words: Recombinant inbred line, Quantitative trait loci, Advanced intercross, Inbred line, Breeding design, Linkage map, Marker density, Mapping resolution, Mapping power, Drift

1. Introduction

The causative genetic loci underlying phenotypic traits can be mapped and studied using recombinant inbred lines (RILs) (1). RILs are a collection of strains derived from a cross of genetically divergent parent strains (see Fig. 1). Meiotic crossover events create a mosaic of parent genomes in each RIL. Phenotypes that quantitatively vary across the genetically distinct RILs can be mapped to their underlying causal loci, called quantitative trait loci (QTL). The mapping of QTL relies on markers, genotyped in each RIL, falling close enough to the causal loci (i.e., in linkage disequilibrium) to show a nonrandom association with the phenotype. Knowledge of the loci underlying phenotypic variation informs a large range of disciplines including medicine, agriculture, ecology, and evolution.

Scott A. Rifkin (ed.), *Quantitative Trait Loci (QTL): Methods and Protocols*, Methods in Molecular Biology, vol. 871,
DOI 10.1007/978-1-61779-785-9_3, © Springer Science+Business Media New York 2012

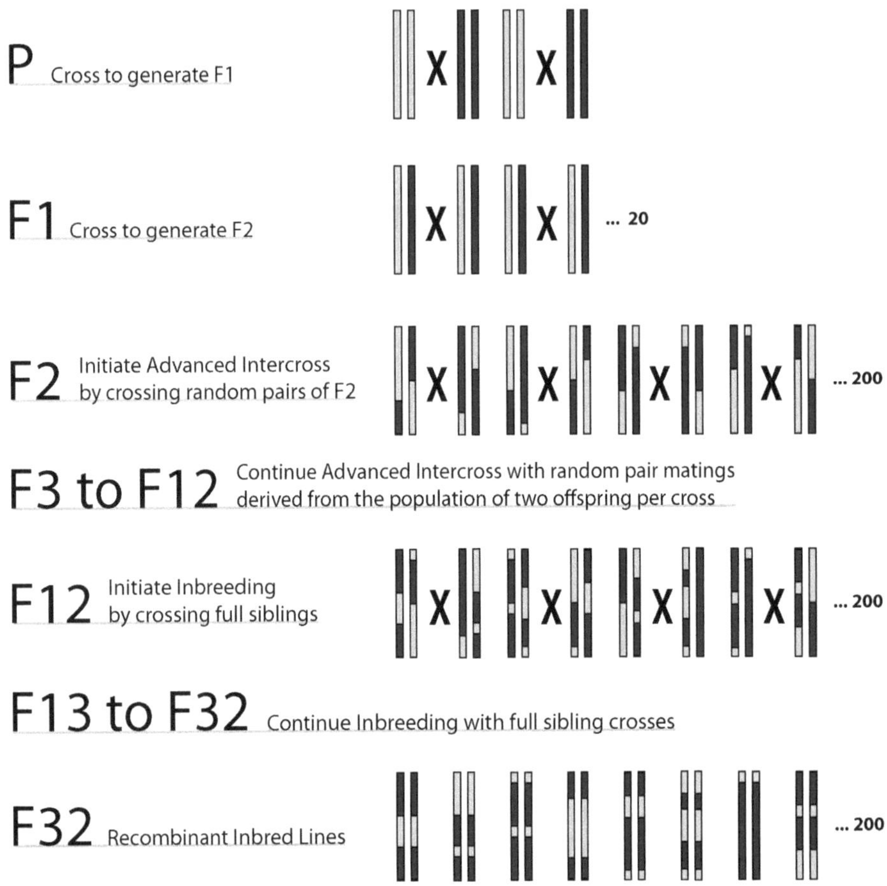

Fig. 1. Example of a RIL construction design. Two replicate parent crosses produce 40 F1. Twenty F1 crosses produce 400 F2. Two hundred random F2 crosses initiate the advanced intercross. Two hundred random pair matings of offspring (two from each cross) in each generation are performed for ten generations of intercrossing. Inbreeding of full siblings in all 200 lines begins at F12 and continues for 20 generations to F32. Individuals are represented by a set of diploid chromosomes. Each parent genotype is represented by either *light* or *dark grey*.

The step-by-step process of designing and constructing RILs for mapping phenotypes of interest is discussed in the following sections of this chapter:

2.1 Select Parent Strains

2.2 Select Construction Design

2.3 Parent Cross & F1 Cross

2.4 Advanced Intercross (Optional)

2.5 Inbreed

2.6 RIL Storage & Maintenance

Due to the enormous variation in species-specific techniques, we focus on the universal aspects of the process.

2. Methods

2.1. Select Parent Strains

The RIL design process begins with selecting parent strains that will be crossed to create the recombinants. While your parent strains may be predetermined, we outline several criteria to consider when options do exist.

1. Select strains with significant phenotypic divergence. Typically, significant divergence in the trait of interest is the initial criterion considered in selecting parent lines (see Note 1 for exceptions). Precisely defining your phenotype measurement assay and establishing the mean and variance of parent strains in your laboratory are prudent to accomplish prior to making a large resource investment in constructing a set of RILs.
2. Select strains with sufficient marker density. As described in detail in Chapter 5 on Map Making and Identifying QTL, mapping QTL depends on markers being in linkage disequilibrium with causal variants. Thus, it is important to select parent strains with a sufficient density of polymorphic markers for your QTL mapping purposes. What is sufficient? There is no universal answer to this question, though one can make some back of the envelope calculations to get a feeling for what to expect. First calculate the expected linkage map length resulting from your RIL construction design (linkage map length is the genetic distance spanned by all the chromosomes—a value that increases with increased recombination). Inbreeding to isogenicity through sibling matings (see Subheading 2.5) expands the F2 linkage map approximately fourfold, while inbreeding through selfing results in approximately twofold expansion (2). Advanced intercrossing for t generations (see Subheading 2.4) adds an additional map expansion of approximately $t/2 + 1$ (3). Given a linkage map of length L in your RILs, the number of randomly placed markers needed (n) to have fraction p loci within m map units of a random marker is:

$$n = \frac{\ln(1 - p)}{\ln\left(1 - \frac{2m}{L}\right)}$$

(See Note 2 for assumptions behind this derivation) (4). Plotting the number of markers (n) vs. m for different values of p and L can give an intuitive feeling for the relationship of these variables. Once a target number of markers is established, you can confirm that potential parent pairs have sufficient genotypic divergence for this marker density (see Note 3 for a discussion of the downside of extreme genotypic divergence between parents). Prior to RIL construction, the full set of markers should be selected and tested on the parents for accuracy and ease of genotyping.

3. Avoid incompatibility. Parent lines with known incompatibilities should be avoided as they will lead to the loss of some recombinants, resulting in allele frequency distortions, decreasing variation, and QTL detection power in the RILs. For example, RILs were constructed from two *Caenorhabditis elegans* strains with a previously unknown incompatibility that resulted in very strong allele frequency distortion across much of chromosome I (5).
4. Avoid segregation of other important traits. Some traits may be diverged in potential parent lines that would present an inconvenience for phenotyping and characterization of RILs. For example, divergence in a life history trait like developmental growth rate could make synchronizing strains challenging. Divergence in the efficiency of reverse genetic methods such as RNA inference could also present problems when validating causal variants (6). Careful testing of parent strains can produce a vastly more useful set of RILs.
5. Engineer parent strains. Given the resource investment in building RILs, it can be prudent to consider engineering transgenic parent strains. Such engineering could be for the purposes of removing existing variation in traits for which variation is not desirable (see Subheading 2.1, step 4) or for adding useful genes to both parents. For example, if a specific cell type will be the eventual focus of RIL phenotyping, one could engineer parent strains such that both contain transgenes expressing fluorescent markers for this cell type.
6. Inbreed parents. Ideally, parent lines should be inbred for a sufficient number of generations to be effectively isogenic (see Subheading 2.2, step 2). Inbreeding also provides the opportunity to remove recessive alleles that affect the trait of interest or life history traits.

2.2. Select Construction Design

Deciding on a design for the construction of a set of RILs requires some form of cost/benefit analysis. The major factors influencing this decision are the number of RILs produced, how many generations they are inbred, and if, how, and for how many generations they are intercrossed past the F2 generation. Different designs can require vastly different resources and can produce different mapping power and resolution, so each component of the design deserves careful consideration.

1. Determine the target RIL population size. Larger RIL populations have many advantages over smaller populations including reducing the influence of drift on allele frequencies (important for QTL detection power and mapping resolution) and increasing the number of crossing over events (important for mapping resolution). While increasing population size has different effects under different design schemes, it universally benefits

both power and resolution. Populations counted in the hundreds have negligible allele frequency drift and have high mapping resolution, while populations counted in the tens will have low mapping resolution and, as the population size approaches zero, will suffer from increasing allele frequency drift (7). Resource investment, however, scales nearly linearly with population size and must be made both during RIL construction as well as downstream for genotyping, phenotyping, and maintenance.

2. Determine the number of generations of inbreeding. Inbreeding both removes heterozygosity and generates additional independent crossing over events. After t generations of full sibling inbreeding, an initial level of heterozygosity, h_0, is approximately reduced to (8):

$$h_t = h_0 \times 1.17(0.809^t)$$

For selfing species, the expected homozygosity after t generations is $h_0/2^t$. In full sibling inbreeding, h_0 is reduced by 86% in 10 generations and 98.3% after 20 generations. In selfing inbreeding, h_0 is reduced by 99.9% in just 10 generations. With a few exceptions, 10 generations of selfing inbreeding and 20 generations of full sibling inbreeding should be sufficient. The inbreeding phase is highly valuable, straightforward to perform, and an unlikely target of resource economizing.

3. Determine if, how, and for how many generations to advance intercross. The F2 generation can be directly passaged through the inbreeding phase, or, if so desired, subject to a form of advanced intercrossing. Additional generations of intercrossing past the F2 generation has the potential to add many more crossing over events, which expands the linkage map and can improve the mapping resolution of the RILs by several fold (see Subheading 2.1, step 2). There are many schemes for deciding which line mates with which at each generation during the advanced intercross (e.g., circular (9), inbreeding avoidance (10), or random mating), but not all designs equally improve mapping resolution. Rockman and Kruglyak (7) showed through simulations that circular mating schemes and random mating schemes with variance in offspring number are relatively poor at improving mapping resolution compared to inbreeding avoidance and random mating with equal offspring number (11) (see Note 4 for an extreme example). Random mating with equal offspring number has an advantage over inbreeding avoidance in that it requires considerably less effort to implement and is unaffected by loss of lines during the intercross.

   Regardless of breeding scheme, one must determine how many generations to advanced intercross. Each generation of intercrossing expands the genetic map and improves QTL mapping resolution. However, intercrossing (including the parent cross) also provides opportunities for allele frequencies to drift. While some advanced intercross schemes reduce the effects of drift more than others, Rockman and Kruglyak (7) found that intercross scheme plays a minor role in determining the degree of drift compared to the dominant effect of population size. To avoid problems associated with drift, little to no advanced intercrossing should be used in small populations (counted in the tens), while many generations of advanced intercrossing can be used in large populations (counted in the hundreds). One additional concern for advanced intercrosses with many generations is mutation. Mutation plays a relatively small role in RILs without intercrossing because mutations accumulate independently in lines and will therefore be unlikely to affect QTL mapping. However, mutations that take place during the intercross phase can spread through the population, potentially confounding QTL mapping. So to decide whether and for how many generations to advanced intercross, the advantages of increased mapping resolution (assuming sufficient marker density) must be weighed against potential problems from drift (in small populations), shared mutations, and the resource expense of the additional generations of crossing.

2.3. Parent Cross and F1 Cross

The goal of the parent cross is to generate an F1 population with equal chromosomal contributions from each parent and that is sufficiently large to generate the desired F2 population.

1. Set up sufficient numbers of parent crosses. Replicate parent crosses are often needed to generate the desired RIL population (see Note 5 on reciprocal crosses). Given an average brood size of B, equal sex ratios, and monogamous outcrossing, the construction of a RIL population of size N will require at minimum $4N/B^2$ replicated parent crosses (see Fig. 1). For example, to construct a RIL population of 200 for a species with average brood sizes of 20, a minimum of 2 parent crosses are needed. For practical reasons, it is always recommended to set up more crosses than are needed to guarantee sufficient numbers of F1s.
2. F1 crosses. A minimum of $2N/B$ F1 crosses are required to generate the desired F2 population (see Fig. 1). From the example above ($N = 200$, $B = 20$), 20 F1 crosses are needed to generate an F2 population of 400 from which 200 inbreeding lines can be set up. As with the parent crosses, it is always recommended to set up more crosses than the minimum required to guarantee sufficient numbers of F2s.

2.4. Advanced Intercross (Optional)

The accurate and efficient implementation of an advanced intercrossing design depends on careful planning and organization. Even for a random mating design, you need to keep careful track of the provenance of every mated strain. See Note 6 for an important discussion of avoiding selection during intercrossing and inbreeding.

1. Initiate the intercross. Set up crosses from the F2 population (see Fig. 1). Use a simple naming scheme to give each mating a unique identifier. For example, use M1F2 for mating 1 in the F2 generation. Using a spreadsheet, record the names of the F2 crosses. As previously suggested, set up more crosses than your desired population size as some crosses might not produce offspring during the intercrossing and inbreeding. Note that many cross designs assume an even population size.
2. Plan the next intercross. Enumerate the next generation of crosses on your spreadsheet (based on your breeding design scheme). Indicate which plate will be crossed with which using the cross names. Assign new names to the new crosses. For example, you might indicate that mating 79 in the F3 generation is a cross of mating 1 and mating 164 from the F2 generation as M1F2 × M164F2 = M79F3. By planning ahead and printing out a spreadsheet that tells you what to do and what to name everything, you will have a clear record and you will minimize errors.
3. Implement the next cross. Follow your planned instructions and set up the next generation of crosses. See Note 7 on lost crosses and lines.
4. Repeat steps 2 and 3. Continue until the planned number of advanced intercross generations has been reached.

2.5. Inbreed

Inbreeding is a straightforward process of sibling pair mating (or singling for selfing species) for the desired number of generations (see Fig. 1). See Note 6 for an important discussion on avoiding selection during intercrossing and inbreeding.

1. Initiate inbreeding. Initiation of inbreeding from an F2 population involves the random pairing of F2 individuals (or singling F2 individuals for selfing species). Nothing needs to be done to initiate inbreeding from an advanced intercrossed population because they are already organized into lines and simply need to be switched to sibling pair mating or singling. Assign a unique name to each inbreeding line. Also, record which cross the inbreeding line was derived from if initiating from an advanced intercross.
2. Repeat. Continue inbreeding through sibling mating or singling until the desired number of generations has been reached.

2.6. RIL Storage and Maintenance

1. Store RILs if you can. Upon completion of the construction of the RILs, it is very important to protect your valuable resource. For organisms where storage is possible (e.g., seeds for plants or freezing microorganisms and worms), it is important to do this quickly to minimize the risks of loss and mutation.

2. Maintain large RIL populations. For the purposes of genotyping and phenotyping as well as for species that cannot be stored, it is very important to maintain large populations of each RIL to minimize the chance of fixing new mutations.

3. Notes

1. Selecting parent strains based on significant phenotypic divergence is typical, though there are exceptions. RIL panels might be constructed as a general resource, not meant for any specific trait (e.g., the Collaborative Cross of *Mus musculus* (12)). Additionally, parents with similar phenotypes may be chosen in cases where transgressive trait variation (offspring trait variation exceeds parental extremes) might be sought or expected (such as cases of compensatory evolution or canalization).
2. The equation listed in Subheading 2.1, step 1 assumes a circular genome, which will result in an underestimation of the required number of markers for linear chromosomes due to loss of information at chromosome ends. See Lynch and Walsh (4) for a correction for linear genomes.
3. High genotypic divergence is important for providing sufficient densities of markers for high-resolution QTL mapping. However, polymorphism levels greatly exceeding that needed for markers can result in inefficiencies in identifying causal variants within QTL harboring a great many polymorphisms, as there may be too many candidates.
4. At small population sizes (<32), Rockman and Kruglyak (7) found that random mating with variance in offspring number can actually decrease mapping resolution relative to RILs with no advanced intercrossing. This is due to the high degree of drift and fixation of recombinant chromosomes during the advanced intercross in this small population.
5. It is sometimes desirable to perform reciprocal crosses of the parent lines to get equal contributions of cytoplasm, mitochondrial DNA, and other sex-specific DNA to the RIL population.
6. Over the course of many generations of intercrossing and inbreeding, it is quite straightforward to inadvertently impose selection on life history traits, like growth rate. Even if parent strains show little divergence in a life history trait, segregating alleles can lead to transgressive phenotypes. Selection on traits during RIL construction causes departures from balanced allele frequencies near any genes associated with the traits, potentially affecting QTL mapping power and resolution for your traits of interest. To avoid imposing selection, attempt to implement a

procedure for picking progeny for subsequent generations in as unbiased and random a way as possible. In nematode worms, researchers have attempted to avoid selection on life history traits by using a bleaching technique on gravid adults to extract a population of fertilized embryos from which to select random individuals for the next generation (13).

7. When crosses fail, your intercross design cannot be implemented as planned. Unless you are depending on your intercross design to be perfectly implemented, it may be more desirable to violate the design and keep more lines going than to strictly maintain the design and lose lines. Therefore, one might set up the wrong crosses for a generation just to keep as many lines going as one can, make note of the change, and then adjust the plan for the next generation.

References

1. Bailey DW (1971) Recombinant-inbred strains. An aid to finding identity, linkage, and function of histocompatibility and other genes. Transplantation 11:325–327
2. Haldane JB, Waddington CH (1931) Inbreeding and linkage. Genetics 16:357–374
3. Teuscher F, Guiard V, Rudolph PE, Brockmann GA (2005) The map expansion obtained with recombinant inbred strains and intermated recombinant inbred populations for finite generation designs. Genetics 170:875–879
4. Lynch M, Walsh B (1998) Genetics and analysis of quantitative traits. Sinauer, Sunderland
5. Seidel HS, Rockman MV, Kruglyak L (2008) Widespread genetic incompatibility in *C. elegans* maintained by balancing selection. Science 319:589–594
6. Felix MA (2008) RNA interference in nematodes and the chance that favored Sydney Brenner. J Biol 7:34
7. Rockman MV, Kruglyak L (2008) Breeding designs for recombinant inbred advanced intercross lines. Genetics 179:1069–1078
8. Nagylaki T (1992) Introduction to theoretical population genetics. Springer, Berlin, New York
9. Kimura M, Crow JF (1963) On maximum avoidance of inbreeding. Genet Res 4:399–415
10. Wright S (1921) Systems of mating. II. The effects of inbreeding on the genetic composition of a population. Genetics 6:124–143
11. Crow JF, Kimura M (1970) An introduction to population genetics theory. Harper and Row, New York
12. Churchill GA, Airey DC, Allayee H, Angel JM, Attie AD, Beatty J et al (2004) The collaborative cross, a community resource for the genetic analysis of complex traits. Nat Genet 36:1133–1137
13. Ebert RH 2nd, Cherkasova VA, Dennis RA, Wu JH, Ruggles S, Perrin TE et al (1993) Longevity-determining genes in *Caenorhabditis elegans*: chromosomal mapping of multiple noninteractive loci. Genetics 135: 1003–1010

Chapter 4

Two Flavors of Bulk Segregant Analysis in Yeast

Maitreya J. Dunham

Abstract

Genetic mapping methods typically rely upon genotyping many individuals in a mapping population. In contrast, bulk segregant analysis looks for biases in genotype in phenotyped pools of segregants. For relatively strong and genetically simple traits, it can be a fast, inexpensive approach. Although it is technically possible to use many genotyping platforms, microarray-based methods are convenient for their genome-wide coverage, ease of use, and quantitative output. Also, precise knowledge of polymorphic sites is not required. I present two methods for bulk segregant analysis using microarrays, one based on hybridization differences between polymorphisms, and the other using an enzymatic method for enriching identical by descent segments of the genome. The first method requires specialized array platforms, while the second, genomic mismatch scanning (GMS), is compatible with any microarray. Although the methods presented are with yeast, most steps are equivalent for other organisms.

Key words: Bulk segregant analysis, Genomic mismatch scanning, Pooled mapping

1. Introduction

Bulk segregant analysis is a pool-based mapping approach that was first developed (1) and implemented using modern genomic technologies (2, 3) in plant systems and later in yeast (4, 5). Segregants from a mapping cross are binned into phenotype pools. These entire pools are then genotyped en masse. Regions of the genome that segregate independently will maintain a 50% allele frequency in all pools. DNA linked to the trait of interest will show a bias towards one parental genotype in one phenotype pool and the other parental genotype in the other pool. Pool genotype frequencies can be obtained genome-wide in several ways, including SNP detection arrays, genomic mismatch scanning (GMS), array-based RAD tags, and deep sequencing.

Because bulk segregant analysis examines the average allele frequency of a pool of individuals, the resolution typically does

Scott A. Rifkin (ed.), *Quantitative Trait Loci (QTL): Methods and Protocols*, Methods in Molecular Biology, vol. 871, DOI 10.1007/978-1-61779-785-9_4, © Springer Science+Business Media New York 2012

not match individual genotyping approaches where every additional recombination breakpoint is informative. However, considerably less genotyping is required, making bulk segregant analysis attractive for quickly and cheaply locating strong QTLs or Mendelian traits. In many cases, the resolution is adequate for prioritization of obvious candidate loci. At a minimum, a single cross and a single array can generate quality mapping data.

Two genotyping strategies are presented here, in parts 3.3/3.4 and 3.5/3.6. The genetic manipulations (Subheading 3.1) and DNA preparations (Subheading 3.2) are the same for both protocols.

Subheadings 3.3 and 3.4 describe genotyping and analysis using Affymetrix tiling microarrays (see Fig. 1 for procedure outline), which contain overlapping 25-mers at a four or eight base tile across the yeast genome. Polymorphisms that generate a mismatch at the complementary 25 base sequences in the mapping strains lead to decreases in hybridization at so-called Single Feature Polymorphisms (SFPs). Affymetrix yeast expression arrays are also adequate for bulk segregant analysis and follow the same procedure. Recent reports (6, 7) describe custom Agilent microarrays targeted to specific segregating polymorphic sequence that can also be used similarly (though, obviously, with Agilent-specific hybridization procedures). Calibration hybridizations using the parental strain backgrounds are recommended for this approach.

Subheadings 3.5 and 3.6 use GMS (8–10). DNA from each pool is hybridized to DNA from each parental strain, and a series of enzymatic manipulations remove heterohybrid DNA molecules that are not perfectly matched. This identity by descent fraction is then hybridized to an array. This approach is compatible with any microarray, including home-printed PCR products, and does not require initial calibration hybridizations.

For both methods, prior knowledge of polymorphism location and identity are not required, though sufficient polymorphism distribution and density are important. For tiling microarrays, these can easily be discovered de novo or borrowed from prior results. GMS relies on polymorphisms in large PstI fragments as opposed to individually queried SNPs.

Next-generation sequencing approaches have also been developed for bulk segregant analysis (6, 11–13), although these are beyond the scope of this. Subheadings 3.1 and 3.2 would still be applicable to the new methods, as would the post-data-processing analytical methods in Subheadings 3.4 and 3.6. Sequencing holds the promise of allowing both linkage and detection of mutations or polymorphisms simultaneously (11, 13), making it an attractive route for further investigation.

Choices for data analysis methodology are varied and not well explored in the literature. They will also differ markedly depending on the computational resources available. For simplicity, I have included straightforward methods for analyzing and

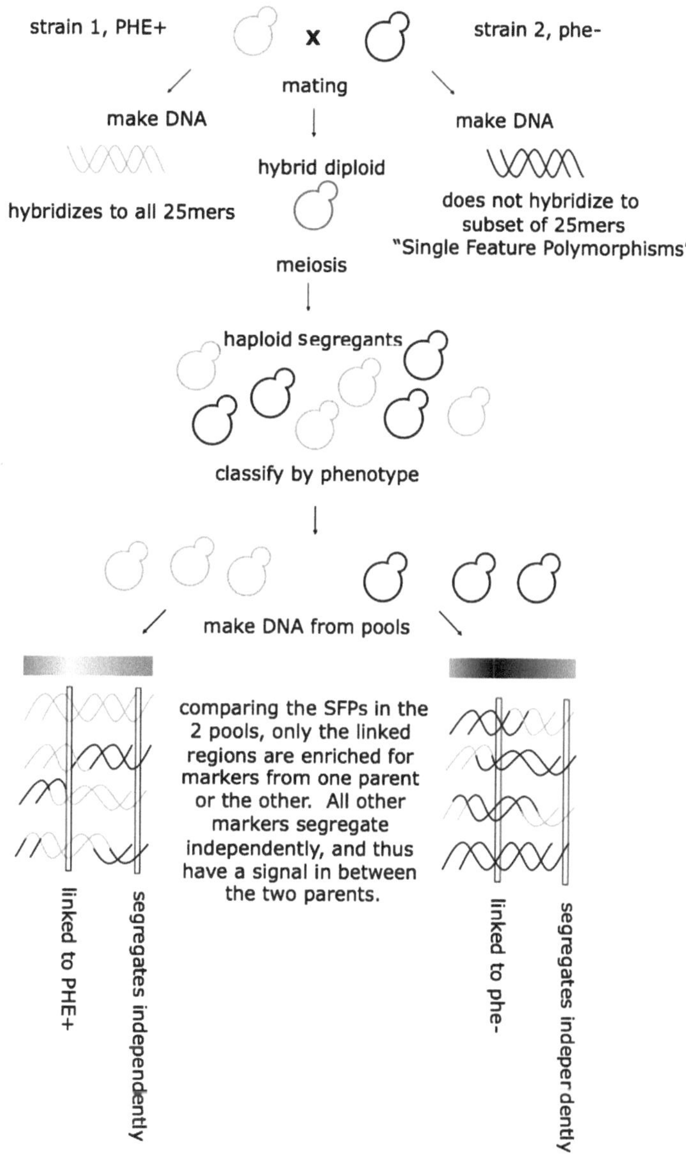

Fig. 1. Overview of bulk segregant using a Mendelian trait PHE+/phe– and Affymetrix array genotyping.

visualizing the data. Because fine-scale mapping will generally be required to confirm results anyway, this reflects a typical use of bulk segregant analysis as a gross mapping method to be coupled with targeted follow-up. For this reason, I recommend performing a positive control mapping cross when first learning the methods, both to ensure the many steps have worked properly and to see what a true positive result looks like amid a somewhat user-specific noise term. I have included several examples of mapping datasets throughout.

2. Materials

2.1. Genetic Cross

1. Standard yeast growth and sporulation media. These should be tailored to the exact strain backgrounds utilized in order to equalize growth and maximize sporulation efficiency.

2.2. DNA Preparation

1. Genomic DNA buffer set (Qiagen).
2. Lyticase (Sigma) or zymolyase (Seikagaku Corporation): 1,000 U/mL in water. Make day of use.
3. Proteinase K (Roche): 20 mg/mL in water. Make day of use.
4. RNase A (Sigma): 100 mg/mL in water.
5. Midi or maxi genomic columns depending on desired yield (Qiagen).

2.3. Genotyping Pools Using Affymetrix Tiling Microarrays

1. 10× one-phor-all buffer: 100 mM Tris-acetate pH 7.5, 100 mM magnesium acetate, 500 mM potassium acetate.
2. DNase I (Invitrogen): diluted to 0.15 U/μL in 1× one-phor-all buffer.
3. 2% agarose gel in 1× TAE.
4. DNA ladder spanning 50 bp range (NEB).
5. BioArray Terminal labeling kit (Enzo).
6. 12× MES: 1.22 M MES hydrate, 0.89 MES sodium salt in water. Filter sterilize. pH should be between 6.5 and 6.7. Store 4°C in dark. If solution discolors yellow, discard.
7. 2× hybe buffer: 200 mM MES, 2 M NaCl, 40 mM EDTA, 0.02% Tween-20 in water. Store at 4°C in dark.
8. 10 mg/mL salmon sperm DNA (Invitrogen), control oligo B2 (Affymetrix).
9. Affymetrix Yeast tiling array. Arrays intended for expression analysis are also adequate.
10. Wash buffer A: 0.9 M NaCl, 60 mM NaH_2PO_4, 6 mM EDTA, 0.01% Tween-20 in water. Filter sterilize. May be reused if filtered after each use.
11. Wash buffer B: 100 mM MES, 0.1 M NaCl, 0.01% Tween-20 in water. Filter sterilize. Store 4°C in dark. May be reused if filtered after each use.
12. 2× stain buffer: 200 mM MES, 2 M NaCl, 0.1% Tween-20 in water. Filter sterilize. Store 4°C in dark.
13. Streptavidin, R-phycoerythrin conjugate solution (SAPE): 10 μg/mL R-streptavidin (Invitrogen), 2 mg/mL BSA, 1× stain buffer in water. Make day of use. Store 4°C in dark until needed.

14. Antibody solution: 0.1 mg/mL goat IgG (Sigma), 2 mg/mL BSA, 3 μg/mL biotinylated anti-streptavidin antibody from goat (Vector Labs), 1× stain buffer in water. Make day of use. Store 4°C in dark until needed.

2.4. Genotyping Pools Using Genomic Mismatch Scanning

1. PstI, 10× buffer 3, and 100× BSA (NEB).
2. For DNA extraction and precipitation: phenol/chloroform 50/50 mix, using buffer-saturated pH 7–8 phenol, chloroform, 3 M NaOAc, and 100% ethanol. Take appropriate precautions using phenol/chloroform.
3. TE pH 8.
4. Dam methylase, 10× dam methylase buffer, and SAM (NEB).
5. MboI, DpnI, and Sau3A (NEB).
6. 5 N NaOH, 3 M MOPS buffer, formamide.
7. 2× FPERT buffer: 4 M sodium thiocyanate, 20 mM Tris–HCl pH 7.9, 0.2 mM EDTA.
8. Exonuclease III and 10× Exo III buffer (Promega).
9. 0.5 M EDTA, 8 M LiCl.
10. Single Stranded Affinity Matrix (SSAM, see Note 1 for more information), 0.45 μm filter cartridges (Millipore).
11. Linear acrylamide (Ambion).
12. 10× ENH: 500 mM Hepes pH 8, 200 mM KCl, 40 mM $MgCl_2$, 10 mM DTT.
13. PPD: 20 mM KPi pH 7.4, 50 mM KCl, 0.1 mM EDTA pH 8. Divide into 225 mL aliquots and freeze. Before use, add 2.5 μL 0.1 M DTT and 25 μL 10 mg/mL BSA (nonacetylated) to a 225 μL aliquot of PPD.
14. MutH, MutL, MutS (USB).

3. Methods

3.1. Genetic Cross

1. Identify two strains with the following characteristics: (a) can be crossed, (b) the cross results in reasonable spore viability, (c) the trait of interest segregates, and (d) the strains are divergent at the nucleotide level throughout the genome. See Note 2 for further information on good strain choices.
2. Cross the strains and isolate segregants by tetrad analysis or random spore analysis. I prefer tetrad analysis for the increased information about the underlying genetic architecture. Because bulk segregant analysis relies on the average genotype of pooled

segregants, increasing pool size offers diminishing returns. Modeling pools of different sizes (data not shown) indicates that simple traits can be reliably mapped with 30 segregants in each phenotype class, and we have obtained reasonable results with as few as 23 in a pool (4). I typically use 50–100. Independent segregants (i.e., not from the same tetrad) are preferred, but not required. It should be noted that other applications of this technique use much larger pool sizes, which may be required for very complex traits. These large populations of segregants may be generated by FACS or counterselection of appropriate traits (5, 6).

3. Phenotype the segregants for the trait of interest and pool them accordingly. In the simplest case of a Mendelian trait, this would generate two pools. Quantitative traits may be mapped using the high and low tails of the phenotype distribution.

3.2. DNA Preparation

1. Equal representation of each segregant is important for accurate genotype frequencies. Grow each segregant in a separate overnight culture, typically individual 18 mM test tubes containing 2.5 mL YPD, though 96-well plates may also be used. Culture conditions should be chosen to ensure approximately equal saturation densities among the segregants.
2. Combine all the segregants with a shared phenotype into a single flask to create each pool.
3. Prepare DNA from each pool and each parental strain. At least 20–40 μg high molecular weight DNA of high purity is desired. I have gotten the most consistent results using spooled DNA made with the Qiagen genomic DNA preparation kit (see Note 3 for further tips).

3.3. Genotyping Pools Using Affymetrix Tiling Microarrays

See Fig. 1 for overview. Before beginning, preheat hybridization oven to 45°C. Prepare heat blocks at 37 and 99°C. I prefer to perform all steps in 1 day, though possible pause points are indicated.

1. Bring 10 μg DNA to 15.8 μL total volume in 10 mM Tris pH 8. Add 2 μL 10× one-phor-all buffer and 1.2 μL 25 mM $CoCl_2$. Mix and spin down.
2. Quickly add 1 μL (0.15 U) DNase I. Flick to mix, touch spin to collect volume, and incubate at 37°C for exactly 5 min. Move to 99°C for 15 min.
3. Run 1 μL on a 2% gel for 50 min at 50 V. Also run a similar amount of undigested DNA to check quality. The remaining reaction may be stored at 4°C, while the gel is run or frozen indefinitely. The DNA should be all in a smear ~50 bp. This result is crucial for the success of the protocol. If the digestion

has not proceeded appropriately, see Note 4 for advice on optimizing this step.

4. Perform end-labeling reaction as directed by the Enzo labeling kit: to the entire volume of fragmented DNA, add 20 μL 5× reaction buffer, 10 μL 10× $CoCl_2$, 1 μL biotin-ddUTP, 2 μL terminal deoxynucleotide transferase, and 48 μL water to a total of 100 μL. Incubate 37°C 15 min to 1 h. Ice. Add 5 μL 0.2 M EDTA to stop reaction.
5. Once labeling reaction is stopped, add 27 μL water, 150 μL 2× hybe buffer, 15 μL 10 mg/mL BSA, 3 μL 10 mg/mL salmon sperm DNA, and 5 μL 3 nM control oligo B2. Incubate 99°C 5 min.
6. During incubation, load array with 200 μL 1× hybe buffer: first, place a 200-μL filter pipette tip in one septum of the array. Holding the array vertically with the vent pipette tip towards the top, slowly pipette in the solution through the other septum. Remove tips. An air bubble should be present in the chamber, and no solution should be present in the vent tip. Place array in holder and load into hybridization oven. Rotate at 60 rpm for 10 min.
7. Returning to probe solution, incubate at 45°C for 5 min. Spin at max speed in a microcentrifuge for 5 min to pellet debris.
8. Remove buffer from array using a similar strategy as described above. Load 200 μL hybridization mixture, avoiding volume at bottom of tube. Seal septa using tape or stickers.
9. Place array in holder and load in hybridization oven. Incubate at 45°C and 60 rpm for 20 h.
10. Prepare wash buffers A and B. For each array, prepare two fresh aliquots of 600 μL SAPE and one 600 μL aliquot antibody solution.
11. Ensure fluidics have been appropriately washed and primed. Perform washes as directed by your particular Affymetrix wash station. In my setup, this is the EukGE-WS2v4 protocol. Once complete, seal septa with correction fluid.
12. Scan array as directed by your Affymetrix scanner setup.

3.4. Analysis of Affymetrix Data

1. Using Affymetrix software, process data from each array to generate CEL files. Extract the normalized intensity data at each feature (see Note 5 for a special caution about array geometry which may affect normalization).
2. If you have run calibration arrays with each parental strain, use the SNP Scanner package (14) or another method to identify polymorphisms between the two strains (SFPs) which show distinct differences in hybridization intensity. This may not be necessary if the linkage signal is strong enough.

3. Recover the intensity data from features covering the polymorphic locations between the strains.
4. Calculate the $\log_2$ratio comparing the data from each pool. This value may have some noise in it as the differential hybridization at each SFP varies. If more resolution is required, it may be useful to scale the data at each SFP such that one parental intensity value equals −1 and the other parental intensity equals 1. This scaling also gives an intuitive view of genotype frequency.
5. Plot genotype frequency data in chromosomal order. This is conveniently done using the Integrated Genome Browser available from Affymetrix. IGB can also generate ratios from intensity tracks if desired.
6. Scan chromosome plots for deviations in genotype frequency. Unlinked regions of the genome will segregate independently and be present at 50% representation from each parent in both pools. Therefore, these regions of the genome will have a $\log_2$-ratio or scaled genotype frequency of 0. Regions linked to the phenotype will show biased inheritance and will deviate from 0. See Fig. 2 for an example. In general, the highest portion of the peak is the best indicator of the QTL. See Note 6 for anecdotes otherwise.
7. Follow-up gross linkage data with fine mapping methodology of your choice. I have had success using strains from the yeast deletion collection as a source of mapping markers.

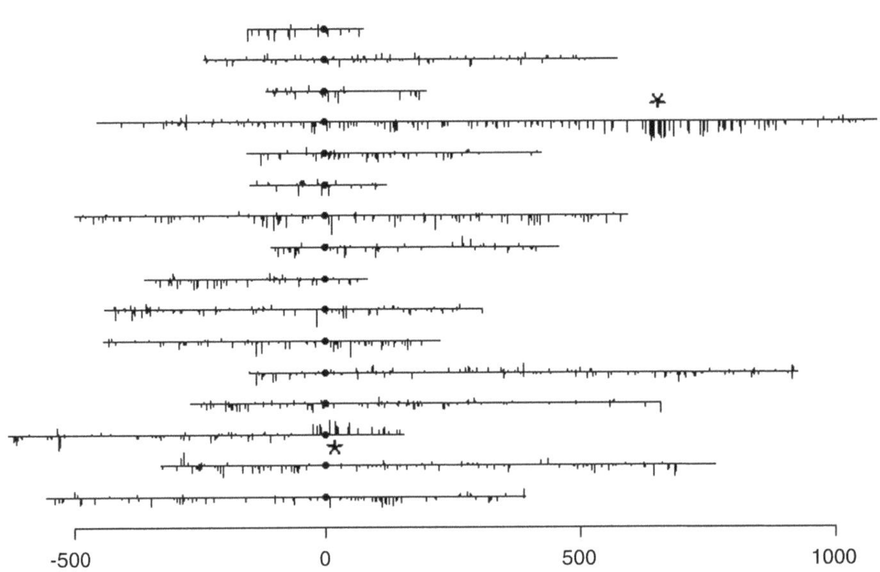

Fig. 2. Example mapping result using Affymetrix microarrays showing a primary locus on chromosome 14 and a modifier locus from the other parent on chromosome 4 (marked with stars). *Small circles* represent centromeres. Figure modified from Chiang (21).

3.5. Genotyping Pools Using Genomic Mismatch Scanning

The GMS protocol consists of many steps which span several days. First, DNA from the parent strains and pools is digested with PstI. Parental DNA is methylated. Methylated parental DNA is hybridized to each pool DNA in a controlled reaction, then digested with methylation-sensitive restriction enzymes to generate hemimethylated heterohybrid DNA. Bacterial mismatch repair enzymes nick this DNA at sites of mismatches, and this nicked DNA is digested with exonuclease and removed from the reactions. The resulting pool DNAs are identical by descent with the matched parent strain and can be competitively hybridized to a microarray to determine the genotype ratio at each PstI fragment.

1. PstI digest a minimum of 40 μg DNA from each parent strain and from each pool: bring DNA to 200 ng/μL in a reaction with 5 U/μg PstI, 1× NEB Buffer 1, and 1× BSA. Incubate 37°C for 2 h. Add 2.5 U/μg PstI and allow reaction to proceed another 2 h. Digested DNA may be stored at −20°C indefinitely.
2. Check 2 μL digested DNA and a similar mass undigested DNA on a 0.8% gel to ensure complete digestion.
3. Extract DNA with phenol/chloroform, followed by chloroform alone. Precipitate DNA using sodium acetate and ethanol precipitation. Dissolve lightly dried pellet in 100 μL TE. Digested DNA may be stored at −20°C indefinitely.
4. Methylate parental DNAs: to 20 μg DNA, add 10 μL 10× dam methylase buffer, 0.25 μL SAM (may be diluted 10× if preferred), and 10 μL dam methylase in a total volume of 100 μL. Incubate at 37°C for 4 h, spiking reaction with an additional 0.25 μL SAM every hour. This step may be scaled up if many samples from the same parents will be processed.
5. Extract and precipitate DNA as above.
6. Determine the quality of the methylation by digesting 1 μL pre- and postmethylated DNA with MboI, DpnI, and Sau3A in separate reactions. Sau3A should cut all species; MboI will cut only unmethylated DNA; DpnI will cut only methylated DNA.
7. In this step, DNA from each pool and each parent is hybridized using a controlled method called formamide phenol emulsion reassociation technique (FPERT). Mix 20 μg methylated parent DNA with 20 μg pool DNA in a total volume of 200 μL. This leads to four reactions total for a two-pool mapping population. Add 14 μL 5 N NaOH to denature the DNA. Mix every 5 min for 15 min at room temperature. Neutralize reaction with 29 μL 3 M MOPS buffer. Check that pH is close to 8.5 by pipetting a small drop onto pH paper. If not, adjust pH. The next steps are most easily performed in 1.5 mL screw-cap tubes. Split each reaction between two tubes. To each, add 32 μL formamide, 45 μL water, and 200 μL 2× FPERT buffer.

Mix well. Add 150 μL phenol to each tube. If the solution is clear, continue to add phenol in 25 μL increments until solution becomes cloudy. Agitate solution for 24 h at room temperature. Agitation must be sufficient to maintain the emulsion. Extract each tube with 150 μL chloroform followed by extraction with 400 μL chloroform. Add 1 mL ethanol to each tube. Incubate −80°C for 30 min. Spin at 4°C in a microfuge at max speed for 30 min. Carefully remove the supernatant, wash the pellet with 70% ethanol, and allow to air dry briefly. Pellet may be a clear, viscous liquid. If so, dissolve pellet in 0.5 mL 70% EtOH and spin at max speed 10 min. Repeat until viscous pellet is fully dissolved after spin, and all that remains is "typical" salt/DNA precipitate. Dissolve each pellet in 45 μL TE and recombine split reactions. Quantify DNA by measuring A260 of a 1:25 dilution. The spectrum may have a peak at 230 nm and a shift upwards of the 260 nm peak.

8. To select for just the hemimethylated heterohybrid DNA, digest with DpnI and MboI, which will digest the methylated and unmethylated homohybrids: mix 20 μg DNA, 20 μL 10× NEB buffer 3, 40 U DpnI, and 40 U MboI in 1× TE to 195 μL. Incubate 37°C for 1 h. Ice reaction while preparing the ExoIII mix. For each reaction, add 60 μL 10× ExoIII buffer and 60 U ExoIII to water for a total volume of 600 μL. Add one 600 μL aliquot ExoIII mix to each digestion reaction, working as quickly as possible. Incubate 15 min at 37 C. Stop reaction with 8 μL 0.5 M EDTA and 80 μL 8 M LiCl. Add 30 μL SSAM that has been well resuspended before use. Incubate at room temperature for 10 min, mixing every 2 min. Spin down the SSAM using gentle centrifugation in a benchtop minicentrifuge for 1 min. Divide the supernatant between two 0.45 μm filter cartridges. Spin at 2,000 × *g* for 3 min. Add 1 μL linear acrylamide and mix well. Add 900 μL ethanol to each tube. Incubate −80°C for 30 min. Spin at maximum RPM at 4°C for 30 min. Wash pellet with 70% ethanol and briefly airdry pellet. Resuspend each pellet in 26 μL TE. Measure DNA concentration.

9. Nick mismatch DNA: bring 1 μg DNA to 25 μL with TE. Add 5 μL 10× ENH, 3 μL PPD, 0.5 μL 100 mM ATP, 10 ng MutH, 100 ng MutL, and 2.5 μg MutS in a total volume of 50 μL. (See Note 7 for more information about enzyme amounts.). Incubate at room temperature for 20 min. Stop reaction by heating to 80°C for 5 min and then placing on ice.

10. Deplete nicked DNA: mix 5 μL 10× ExoIII buffer, 45 μL water, 20 U ExoIII. Add to nicked DNA. Incubate at 37°C for 10 min. Stop reaction with 1 μL 0.5 M EDTA and 5 μL 8 M LiCl. Add 5 μL SSAM and incubate for 10 min at room temperature, mixing every 2 min. Spin down SSAM for 1 min

in a benchtop centrifuge at 2,000 × *g*. Transfer supernatant to a 0.45-μm filter cartridge and spin through at 2,000 × *g* for 3 min. Add 1 μL linear acrylamide. Add 240 μL ethanol and incubate at −80°C for 30 min. Spin at maximum g force at 4°C for 30 min. Wash pellet with 70% ethanol and airdry pellet. Resuspend DNA in 15 μL TE. Check concentration.

11. Hybridize DNA to preferred microarray. See Note 5 for advice on array configuration. Although single color microarrays will likely work, the methods described in Subheadings 3.3 and 3.4 are more amenable to that platform. Two-color platforms such as spotted arrays or Agilent arrays allow direct comparison of the parental representation in each pool. For example, assuming a Mendelian trait, the class of segregants with one parental phenotype will have the linked region enriched in the reaction using that parent and depleted in the reaction vs. the other parent, leading to a clear representational difference. Amplification is not typically required if sufficient yield is obtained.

3.6. Analysis of GMS Data

1. If a two-color platform was used, genotype ratio data are obtained directly. For single color arrays, preprocessing may be required to generate equivalent ratio representation of the data.
2. Plot $\log_2$ratio data in genome order. I like the Karyoscope function of Java Treeview (15) for this application. Custom coordinates files can be created for any array platform. Deviations in each pool will be accentuated by subtracting the data from the two pools from one another.
3. Scan the genome for imbalances in genotype frequency. See Fig. 3 for an example.

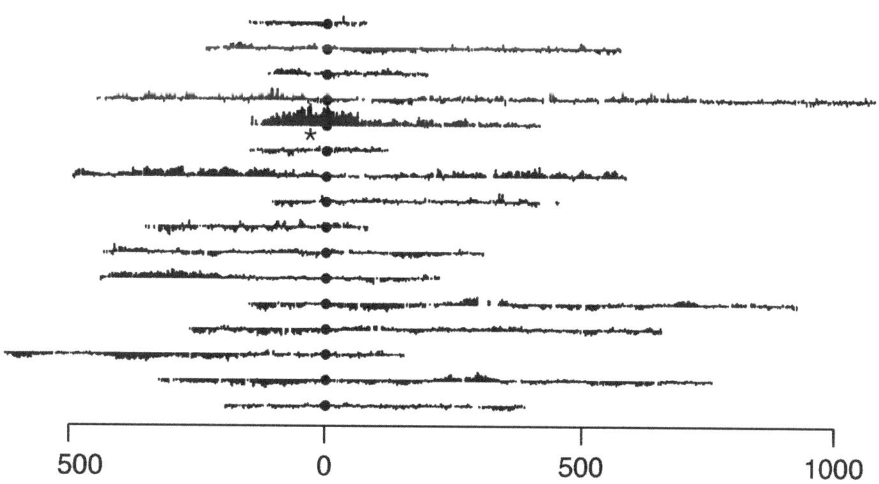

Fig. 3. Example mapping result using GMS and spotted PCR product arrays. Data are graphed across chromosomes using the karyoscope function of Java Treeview (15). *Small circles* represent centromeres. The primary locus is marked with a star.

4. Follow-up gross linkage data with fine mapping methodology of your choice. I have had success using strains from the yeast deletion collection as a source of mapping markers.

4. Notes

1. SSAM, which was once produced by Clontech and may still be found in some labs, may be substituted with any appropriate ssDNA-specific agent such as BNDC.
2. Validated pairs of strains include S288C derivatives (including true S288C strains as well as patchwork genotypes like W303 and CEN.PK) vs. SK1 (4, 5, 16), Y55 (4), D273-10B (17), RM11 (6, 18), and a variety of wine strains (12). Many other combinations are possible. Though all published examples so far seem to use one S288C-related parent (as illustrated in Fig. 1), pairs where neither strain is of the S288C background would likely perform better with tiling array approaches given the additional informative sites. Strain compatibility can be checked computationally for divergence by comparing genome sequences (e.g., (19)) or tiling microarray-based SNP profiles (e.g., (20)) Note that pairs of strains that share ancestry are not good choices unless there is reason to think the trait lies in a divergent segment of the genome. For example, W303, Σ1278b, and CEN.PK contain large patches of the S288C genome. For mutation mapping, a control cross using the wt strain is first required to determine the background segregation of the trait of interest. For example, if a mutation causes altered growth on a particular substrate, it could not be mapped using a pair of strain backgrounds in which that trait already segregates strongly. In some cases, the phenotype caused by the mutation can be discerned even in the presence of background variation, but in my experience this can lead to inadvertent mapping of modifier loci (see Fig. 2 for an example).
3. The Qiagen Genomic DNA kit performs more consistently on divergent strain backgrounds with a couple of modifications. The enzyme used for digestion may perform differently on strains with varying cell wall content and flocculation features. Experimenting with lyticate vs. zymolyase may help, as does gentle agitation during the incubation. Also, we double the incubation time for all enzymatic digestion steps.
4. DNase I digestion is a critical step and tends to be a main source of variations between people and labs. Handle a small number of samples to allow for precise timing. Some researchers may find it convenient to digest several samples for 5–15 min and choose the best sample.

5. One caution about array layout: special considerations may be required for platforms in which features are spatially placed on the array in a nonrandom way with respect to chromosome location. For example, the Affymetrix yeast expression array is largely in genome order, as are early layouts of the Agilent yeast expression array. If a spatial smoothing normalization is used, this may incorrectly dilute linkage signals, and, conversely, hybridization artifacts may create false signals. If designing a custom array for bulk segregant analysis, it is highly recommended to place the features randomly on the surface.
6. I have published one example in which linkage fell towards the shoulder of a peak as opposed to the center (17). Additional unpublished work from my lab contains at least two other examples of this phenomenon. With the increased resolution of recombination maps, and better appreciation for related strain background dependencies, perhaps some reason will eventually present itself. Also, in at least one published case (12), the causative variant was carried in a large DNA insertion not present in the other strain, leading to a somewhat confusing pattern.
7. Mismatch repair enzyme concentration may benefit from further optimization as unit activities may be variable. See ref. (10) for optimization options.

Acknowledgments

The author would like to thank Matthew Brauer for joint development of these methods. Appreciation also goes to Mark Rose and Elbert Chiang for collaboration on mapping data shown in Fig. 2. Caroline McCoach, Pat Brown, and David Botstein contributed to development of GMS protocols, and USB provided preproduction MutHLS enzymes. This work was supported in part by P50 GM071508 to the Lewis-Sigler Institute at Princeton University.

References

1. Michelmore R, Paran I, Kesseli R (1991) Identification of markers linked to disease-resistance genes by bulked segregant analysis: a rapid method to detect markers in specific genomic regions by using segregating populations. Proc Natl Acad Sci U S A 88:9828–9832
2. Borevitz J, Liang D, Plouffe D, Chang H, Zhu T, Weigel D, Berry C, Winzeler E, Chory J (2003) Large-scale identification of single-feature polymorphisms in complex genomes. Genome Res 13:513–523
3. Hazen S, Borevitz J, Harmon F, Pruneda-Paz J, Schultz T, Yanovsky M, Liljegren S, Ecker J, Kay S (2005) Rapid array mapping of circadian clock and developmental mutations in Arabidopsis. Plant Physiol 138:990–997
4. Brauer MJ, Christianson CM, Pai DA, Dunham MJ (2006) Mapping novel traits by array-

assisted bulk segregant analysis in *Saccharomyces cerevisiae*. Genetics 173:1813–1816

5. Segre A, Murray A, Leu J (2006) High-resolution mutation mapping reveals parallel experimental evolution in yeast. PLoS Biol 4:e256
6. Ehrenreich IM, Torabi N, Jia Y, Kent J, Martis S, Shapiro JA, Gresham D, Caudy AA, Kruglyak L (2010) Dissection of genetically complex traits with extremely large pools of yeast segregants. Nature 464:1039–1042
7. Gresham D, Curry B, Ward A, Gordon DB, Brizuela L, Kruglyak L, Botstein D (2010) Optimized detection of sequence variation in heterozygous genomes using DNA microarrays with isothermal-melting probes. Proc Natl Acad Sci U S A 107:1482–1487
8. McAllister L, Penland L, Brown P (1998) Enrichment for loci identical-by-descent between pairs of mouse or human genomes by genomic mismatch scanning. Genomics 47:7–11
9. Nelson S, McCusker J, Sander M, Kee Y, Modrich P, Brown P (1993) Genomic mismatch scanning: a new approach to genetic linkage mapping. Nat Genet 4:11–18
10. Smirnov D, Bruzel A, Morley M, Cheung V (2004) Direct IBD mapping: identical-by-descent mapping without genotyping. Genomics 83:335–345
11. Schneeberger K, Ossowski S, Lanz C, Juul T, Petersen AH, Nielsen KL, Jorgensen J-E, Weigel D, Andersen SU (2009) SHOREmap: simultaneous mapping and mutation identification by deep sequencing. Nat Methods 6:550–551
12. Wenger JW, Schwartz K, Sherlock G (2010) Bulk segregant analysis by high throughput sequencing reveals a novel xylose utilization gene from *Saccharomyces cerevisiae*. PLoS Genet 6:e1000942
13. Birkeland SR, Jin N, Ozdemir AC, Lyons RH, Weisman LS, Wilson TE (2010) Discovery of mutations in *Saccharomyces cerevisiae* by pooled linkage analysis and whole genome sequencing. Genetics 186(4):1127–1137
14. Gresham D, Ruderfer DM, Pratt SC, Schacherer J, Dunham MJ, Botstein D, Kruglyak L (2006) Genome-wide detection of polymorphisms at nucleotide resolution with a single DNA microarray. Science 311:1932–1936
15. Saldanha AJ (2004) Java Treeview—extensible visualization of microarray data. Bioinformatics 20:3246–3248
16. Boer VM, Amini S, Botstein D (2008) Influence of genotype and nutrition on survival and metabolism of starving yeast. Proc Natl Acad Sci U S A 105:6930–6935
17. Fiumera H, Dunham M, Saracco S, Butler C, Kelly J, Fox T (2009) Translocation and assembly of mitochondrially coded *Saccharomyces cerevisiae* cytochrome c oxidase subunit Cox2 by Oxa1 and Yme1, in the absence of Cox18. Genetics 182:519–528
18. Demogines A, Smith E, Kruglyak L, Alani E (2008) Identification and dissection of a complex DNA repair sensitivity phenotype in baker's yeast. PLoS Genet 4:e1000123
19. Liti G, Carter DM, Moses AM, Warringer J, Parts L, James SA, Davey RP, Roberts IN, Burt A, Koufopanou V, Tsai IJ, Bergman CM, Bensasson D, O'Kelly MJT, van Oudenaarden A, Barton DBH, Bailes E, Nguyen AN, Jones M, Quail MA, Goodhead I, Sims S, Smith F, Blomberg A, Durbin R, Louis EJ (2009) Population genomics of domestic and wild yeasts. Nature 458:337–341
20. Schacherer J, Shapiro JA, Ruderfer DM, Kruglyak L (2009) Comprehensive polymorphism survey elucidates population structure of *Saccharomyces cerevisiae*. Nature 458:342–345
21. Chiang EC (2005) Transcriptional regulation of cdc31-30::kanMX as mechanism for its suppression. Princeton University, Princeton

Chapter 5

Selecting Markers and Evaluating Coverage

Matthew A. Cleveland and Nader Deeb

Abstract

The availability of genetic markers in many species has enabled the analysis of marker-trait associations ranging from small genomic regions to genome-wide scale. An appropriate set of markers must be identified to meet the objectives of any research, using a custom discovery and selection approach or by using a commercial product. The key considerations in selecting markers are the quantity and the distribution across the genome. Though decisions about how many markers to use are often pragmatic, influenced by costs and available technology, an evaluation of the marker coverage is important in understanding how to design an effective genomic research study with reasonable expectations about the power to obtain desired results. An important parameter to evaluate coverage is linkage disequilibrium, which can be used to determine the appropriate number of markers for a particular analysis and is related to the proportion of variance that can be explained by a given marker, or power. Finally, the type of analysis used to identify marker-trait associations may depend on marker coverage as the optimal approach, from a statistical or computational standpoint, may differ with changes in marker number and distribution.

Key words: Genome-wide association study, Linkage disequilibrium, Marker density, Minor allele frequency, Quantitative trait loci, Single nucleotide polymorphism

1. Introduction

A key research tool in genetics is the ability to associate sequence variation with variation in a phenotype. Sequence variants are responsible for genetic variation in a population and contribute to individual phenotypic characteristics. Single nucleotide polymorphisms (SNPs) are the most common sequence variants and one of the most common research tools in molecular genetics. A SNP is a difference in a single nucleotide (A, T, C or G) within a specific DNA fragment between two or more individuals. The identification, mapping, and annotation of SNPs make fine-scaled genetic studies possible.

Mapped SNPs can be used to target a specific gene or genomic region based on preexisting knowledge about gene location and/or

Scott A. Rifkin (ed.), *Quantitative Trait Loci (QTL): Methods and Protocols*, Methods in Molecular Biology, vol. 871,
DOI 10.1007/978-1-61779-785-9_5,

function for what has been generally called the candidate gene approach. SNPs can also be selected at random to cover the entire genome for what has become known as a genome-wide association study (GWAS). Today the two approaches have converged as the abundance of known SNPs allows researchers to select SNPs within coding regions of genes and to cover the entire genome simultaneously. We can select SNPs in multiple regions of the genome to ensure targeted genes are captured through direct association or through proxy by a SNP that is in linkage disequilibrium (LD) with the causative mutation. Targeting specific genomic regions vs. model-free random SNPs depends largely on the objective of the research, but both require a large number of SNPs.

Public databases harbor tens of millions of SNPs for a variety of species (1). Although the number of available SNPs varies dramatically by species, these numbers are continuously growing due to the development of new sequencing technologies that make sequencing affordable. For many species today the limiting factor is how best to select a subset of SNPs that meet our needs rather than discovering new SNPs. The cost of genotyping continues to decline, though, making it possible to genotype for all available SNPs rather than tailoring the SNPs to a specific research question. Regardless of the source and number of SNPs, however, the marker density/coverage will impact study design and expectations about power, and thus must be considered.

The purpose of this chapter is to describe options for discovering and selecting SNPs for GWAS-type analyses and to outline the approach for evaluating subsequent marker coverage especially in light of its relationship to the power to detect quantitative trait loci (QTLs), sample size, and considerations for analysis.

2. SNP Discovery

2.1. Review Available SNPs

The most important repository for SNPs is dbSNP from the National Center for Biotechnology Information (NCBI) ((1); e.g., see http://www.ncbi.nlm.nih.gov/projects/SNP/snp_summary.cgi). For example, Build 132, released on September 23, 2010, includes about 231 million SNPs from 100 organisms. The top ten species, in descending order (using number of submitted SNPs (ss#)), are Human, House mouse, Chicken, Norway rat, Soybean, Rice, Cattle, Maize, Dog, and Platypus. Figure 1 shows the ss# by species. Human is leading with 143.4 million SNPs; however, other species such as chickens, cattle, and pigs are quickly catching up due to the recent sequencing projects in these species and the following deep sequencing projects carried out by public institutions (USDA and universities) and industry (livestock

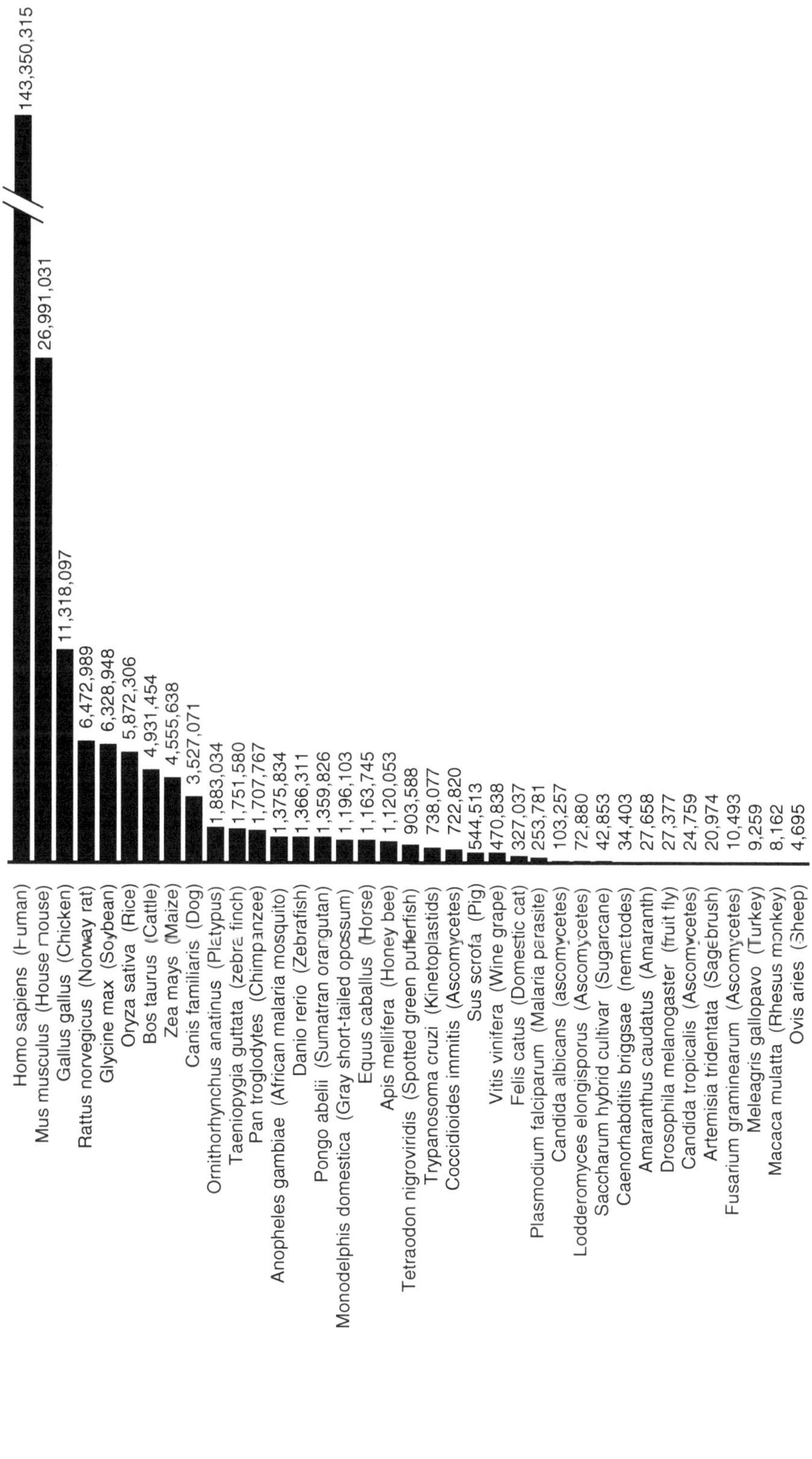

Fig. 1. Number of submitted SNPs (ss#'s) by species (dbSNP summary Build 132).

breeding companies). Available sequences in these species provide a good resource for within species genomic research, but also can be used for across species comparative genomics and to help develop model species.

SNPs in the database are usually identified by the polymorphism (e.g., C/T) and a flanking sequence of 30 bp or more from each side of the polymorphism. Map information is not available for all SNPs in the database; however, it is relatively easy to use flanking sequences to align the sequence against genomic sequence using BLAST (see Note 1). SNPs in dbSNP can be viewed individually or downloaded through an ftp site.

2.2. De Novo Sequencing

Next-generation sequencing or high-throughput sequencing techniques have dramatically reduced the cost of sequencing in recent years. Some of the main commercial products include 454-Pyrosequencing (Roche Diagnostics), Solexa (Illumina), and SOLiD (Applied Biosystems). These platforms, combined with publicly funded genome sequence projects, technology to sequence pools of individuals, and free bioinformatic tools for sequence analysis (e.g., BLAST), have made de novo sequencing a very powerful option for SNP discovery. Moreover, the NIH has promoted the development of such technology through its $1,000 genome grant (see http://grants.nih.gov/grants/guide/rfa-files/RFA-HG-10-013.html). The goal of this initiative is to reduce the cost of sequencing a mammalian-sized genome to approximately $1,000.

2.3. Comparison of Discovery Approaches

In most cases, and for most species, the SNPs available in the public repositories will be suitable for GWAS (and other genome-wide approaches), where large numbers of "random" markers are desired, and will likely be preferable in terms of time and money. One exception is for species that have limited sequence and therefore likely have few SNPs already available. The only choice in these cases is to initiate "in-house" sequencing to obtain a large pool of SNPs to choose from. Additionally, there may be cases where large numbers of SNPs are generally available (e.g., humans), but not for a target population in a specific genomic region. By directly sequencing this region, researchers may attain the desired localized density in the population and answer questions that were not accessible using previously discovered SNPs.

3. SNP Selection

3.1. Number of SNPs

The basic idea of GWAS is that by testing many SNPs (or any other form of sequence variation) there is a greater probability of capturing true associations (compared to testing few SNPs), but it is not the case that a study with a higher number of SNPs must have higher chance of success. The absolute count of SNPs used in a study, in most cases, is meaningless. For example, if the research includes ten SNPs that are all known to be within a strong candidate gene for the trait of interest, this might be a much better approach than genotyping for 100 times more SNPs where the original ten are not part of the genome scan. Additionally, if a study included tagging SNPs, where individual SNPs provide complete information for a segment of the genome containing multiple SNPs, then adding more SNPs within these segments will not improve the amount of available information. More consideration is needed than to just evaluate the number of SNPs. Two important factors that often are a direct function of number of SNPs are cost and genotyping platform. For a fixed number of samples to be genotyped, the cost is positively associated with the number of SNPs used, and number of SNPs can also affect the available technology that can be used (see Note 2).

3.2. SNP Distribution

One of the most important aspects of SNP selection, beyond availability and cost, is their distribution across the genome. In a well-annotated species, it is possible to select SNPs that are within known genomic regions (QTLs), in genes within known QTLs, and in coding sequence within a gene. It is even possible to choose a nonsynonymous rather than synonymous mutation where it is more likely that any detected association is due to the direct effect of a causative mutation rather than due to LD with the mutation (see Subheading 4 for more on LD). However, for most species, the genomes are not well annotated and SNP selection will be generally considered random. In these cases, there are two things to consider: distance between adjacent SNPs and pair-wise LD between them. In the simplest approach, SNPs (with known map position) are selected to be evenly spaced and to cover the entire genome. This selection is based on the required number of SNPs, which is often driven by cost and available technology, but also has a theoretical basis as described in Subheading 4. When selection is focused on a specific trait, knowledge concerning inheritance patterns of the trait can be used for more specific spacing of SNPs, e.g., sex chromosomes could be excluded to increase the density on autosomal chromosomes when there is a clear evidence of an autosomal trait or the opposite for sex-linked traits. The disadvantage of this approach is that while the physical distance between SNPs is constant, the genetic distance can vary based on the average LD across the entire genome and within some specific regions due to recombination rate variation, for example. Thus, it may be sensible to increase the SNP density (number of SNPs per cM or bp) in some regions and reduce the density in others.

Figure 2 illustrates different SNP selection options based on knowledge of the trait and of the population. With no additional

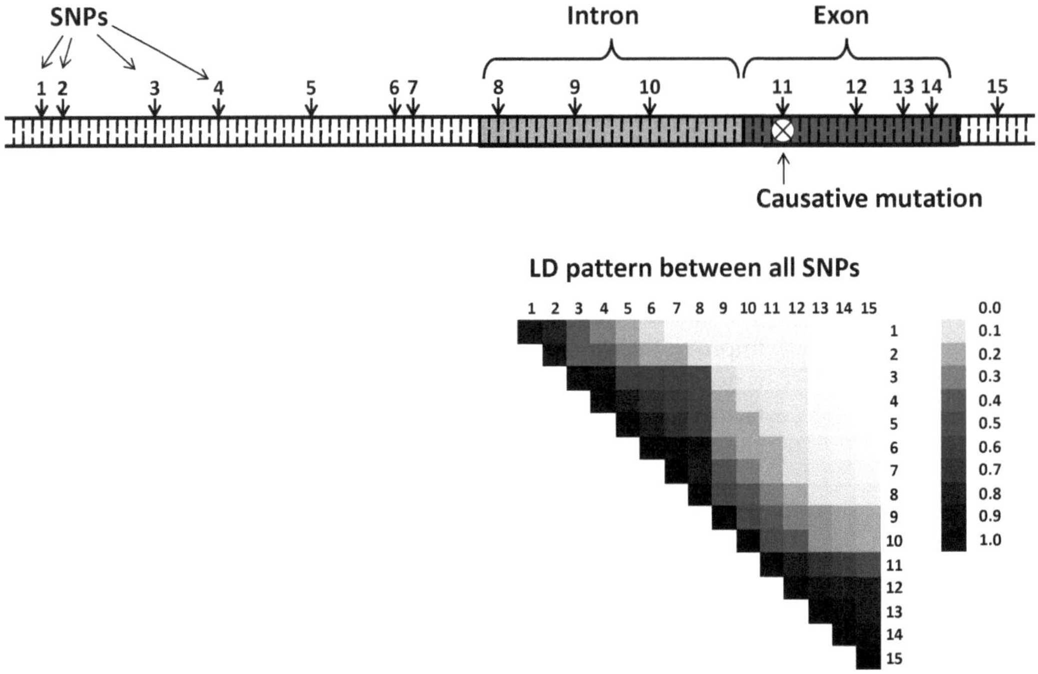

Fig. 2. Illustration of the different SNP selection options based on relationship between SNPs and known exon–intron boundaries.

information, selecting SNPs between SNP1 and SNP15 would be difficult. When the LD pattern is known, tagging SNPs based on the pair-wise LD between each pair allows us select one SNP from each group (LD block) reducing the number of SNPs to 5 without reducing the power of the experiment: e.g., [1-2]-[3-4-5-6-7-8]-9-10-[11-12-13-14-15]. If the boundaries of genes in the region are known and/or exon–intron boundaries are known, one could select SNP8 from the second LD block and SNP11 from the third LD block (instead of random selection within block) increasing the chance of identifying the causative mutation.

3.3. Minor Allele Frequency

Minor allele frequency (MAF) is the frequency of the rare allele in a population and ranges from 0.0 to 0.5. MAF is an important measure of SNP usefulness; however, there is no consensus about the threshold for which markers should be excluded. Excluding markers with very low MAF reduces the numbers of false positive results, but, by definition, rare mutations, which are often of interest, are rare and markers associated with these mutations are expected to have low frequencies (2). Although one is a function of the other, the number of observations within each genotype category is more important than MAF to decide what SNPs should be excluded from the study. For a study that consists of $N = 100$ individuals, excluding markers with MAF < 0.05 (expected counts of the genotypes: $N_{11} = 0$, $N_{12} = 10$, $N_{22} = 90$) may be

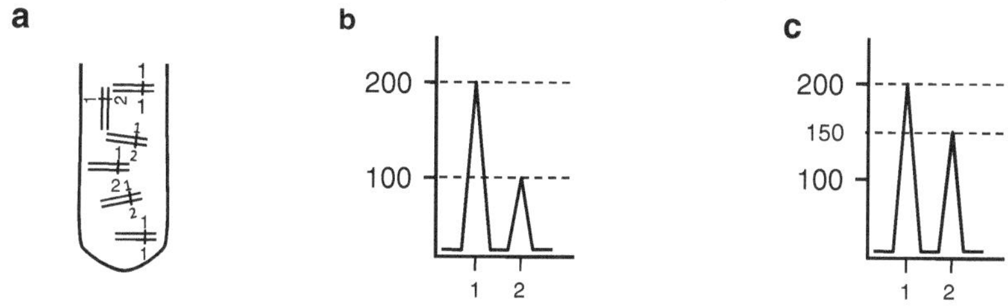

$$f(1) = \frac{8}{8+4} = 0.66 \qquad f(1) = \frac{200}{200+100} = 0.66 \qquad f(1) = \frac{200}{200+(0.66\mathrm{x}150)} = 0.66$$

$$f(2) = \frac{4}{8+4} = 0.33 \qquad f(2) = \frac{100}{200+100} = 0.33 \qquad f(2) = \frac{100}{200+(0.66\mathrm{x}150)} = 0.33$$

Fig. 3. (**a**) Estimating allele frequency from real counts of alleles of all individuals in the pool. (**b**) Example of estimating allele frequencies in a pool from peak intensities. (**c**) Estimating allele frequencies in a pool using peak intensities and *k*-correction.

acceptable. In the case of a study with a 1,000 samples, using the same threshold to exclude markers might be considered too harsh as "enough" samples exist in each genotype category to provide an accurate estimate of the marker effect and least squares means (LSMs) (see Note 3). Therefore, any threshold should be a function of the minimal number of observations that the researcher feels comfortable with rather than a general MAF threshold that fits all studies (see Note 4). For a pregenotyping MAF threshold, one should also take into account the prevalence of the disease/disorder/phenotype in the resource population (in case/control studies) when deciding about a threshold to use.

MAF can be calculated based on the number of observed genotypes as:

$$\mathrm{Min}\left[\frac{2N_{11} + N_{12}}{2(N_{11} + N_{12} + N_{22})}, \frac{2N_{22} + N_{12}}{2(N_{11} + N_{12} + N_{22})}\right]$$

or can be estimated from DNA pools (see Fig. 3). Pooling of DNA has been used as a cost-effective approach to many types of genetic investigations, including identifying ancestral origin, variant detection, allele frequency estimation, QTL mapping, and genome-wide association studies (e.g., see refs. (3–7)). In DNA pooling, equal amounts of DNA of several individuals representing the targeted population(s) is pooled together and genotyped as if it was a single individual. The relative difference between intensity of the two alleles gives a very accurate estimate of allele frequency. However, unequal amplification (differential hybridization or differences in sensitivity of reading the two alleles) can lead to bias in estimating allele frequency from the pool. Allele frequency, however, can be adjusted by using the *k*-correction factor. For each SNP marker, *k* is estimated by the ratio of *A* to *B* from a number of independent heterozygote individuals ($n_{\mathrm{het.}}$) (8)

$$k = \frac{1}{n_{\text{het.}}} \sum \frac{A}{B}$$

where A and B are the signal intensities of alleles A and B, respectively. In the second step, the allele frequency estimates are corrected with the estimated k-correction factor applied,

$$p = \frac{A}{A + k \cdot B}$$

where A and B are the observed peak heights of alleles A and B from a DNA pool.

3.4. Custom Versus Commercial Panels

Advances in genome sequencing have led to the discovery of tens of thousands of SNPs in many genomes which has led to the development of SNP-chip panels (see Table 1) by a unique collaboration between the private sector and universities across the globe. Panels were developed to be as general as possible by mainly selecting SNPs that had even coverage across the entire genome, but were also segregating in a maximum number of breeds (ancestries) within the targeted species. However, this strong selling point of the panels can also be their weakness, as many SNPs were found to be fixed (not segregating) in a specific line/breed/population for which it was used (e.g., it is not unusual for up to 30% of the PorcineSNP60 to be fixed, unpublished data). Nevertheless, unless a large quantity of samples are genotyped, the cost of building a custom SNP panel optimized for the targeted population that exhibits similar numbers of SNPs as the commercial products can

Table 1
Examples of commercial SNP chips offered by Illumina, for illustration purposes only

Product	Number of SNPs
Human1M-Duo	>1 million
Human660W-Quad	>660,000
BovineSNP50	>54,000
BovineHD	>770,000
CanineSNP20	>22,000
EquineSNP50	>54,000
OvineSNP50	>50,000
PorcineSNP60	>60,000

Additional details and products can be found at http://www.illumina.com/support/literature.ilmn

easily cost several times the price of the commercial panels. The choice between a custom and commercial panel may depend both on cost and on the research objective if specific SNPs or genomics regions are desired. Both approaches might be used with a commercially available SNP chip for the initial evaluation followed by small custom panels.

4. Evaluating SNP Coverage

Selection of SNPs for a particular project is often a pragmatic decision based on budgetary constraints and/or available technology, but the evaluation of marker coverage is useful both in designing panels (which may also be subsets of larger panels) or when using existing commercial panels (e.g., SNP chips in many species). This evaluation can provide insight into the number of SNPs required for a particular analysis (generally in reference to GWAS as SNP coverage is mostly an issue for genome-wide approaches) or, in the case of a preexisting SNP panel, the appropriate study design and expected power for a given population. In a genome-wide context, power is a function of LD and the proportion of variance explained by a QTL.

4.1. Defining Linkage Disequilibrium

Linkage disequilibrium is the nonrandom association of alleles at different loci that may or may not be physically linked. LD can result from selection, migration, drift, mutation, etc. (9) and therefore can differ considerably between populations, particularly between species which may have large differences in history (i.e., differences in effective population size (N_e)). Population-wide LD is a function of effective population size as $(1/(1+4N_e c))$, where c is the recombination fraction (10). A measure of LD is an important parameter when determining the power of genomic analyses using SNPs.

Many approaches to genomic analysis, especially those using outbred populations, take advantage of the LD that exists across families (exploiting historical recombination events) to make inferences about effects on a population, as opposed to linkage analysis approaches that require specific family structures. The assumption of these approaches is that there is at least one SNP in LD with each putative QTL (otherwise the QTL would be undetectable) and that the variance explained by the SNP is proportional to the variance explained by the QTL as a function of LD. Characterization of LD, then, can provide some guidance about the marker density needed to mark all putative QTL (or more specifically to capture all/part of the variance explained by the QTL). The average LD over a given genomic distance is a specific measure that can be used to evaluate marker spacing.

The first step is to calculate pair-wise LD between each SNP and all other SNPs for a specific population (see Note 5). A number of LD measures have been published, but r^2 is easy to interpret and has been shown to be less biased than other measures (11). r^2 can be calculated for a single SNP pair using the following formulae (12):

$$D = \left(\frac{N}{N-1}\right) \times \left(\frac{4N_{11\cdot 11} + 2(N_{11\cdot 12} + N_{12\cdot 11}) + N_{12\cdot 12}}{2N}\right) - 2p_1p_2$$

$$D_a = \left(2p_1q_1 - \left(\frac{N_{12\cdot 11} + N_{12\cdot 12} + N_{12\cdot 22}}{N}\right)\right) \times 0.5$$

$$D_b = \left(2p_2q_2 - \left(\frac{N_{11\cdot 12} + N_{12\cdot 12} + N_{22\cdot 12}}{N}\right)\right) \times 0.5$$

$$r^2 = \frac{D^2}{(p_1q_1 + D_a) \times (p_2q_2 + D_b)}$$

where N is the sample size, the subscript on N refers to the genotypes of SNP1 and SNP2 (e.g., $N_{11\cdot 11}$ is the number of samples with the first homozygous genotype for each SNP), and p and q are the allele frequencies for the SNP designated by the subscript. The advantage of this formulation for r^2 is that the usually unknown haplotype frequencies are not required. Generally, some quality control is performed to exclude SNPs that may give spurious results. This might include the exclusion of SNPs with low MAF, large numbers of missing values, and extreme values for the Pearson χ^2 statistic, which is a test of Hardy–Weinberg equilibrium (9) and often indicates technical issues with the genotyping. The specific values to use are fairly subjective, but in general excluding the most extreme observations should be sufficient (see Note 6).

4.2. Using LD to Evaluate Density

The r^2 calculated for each SNP pair can be easily visualized for specific regions of the genome (e.g., by chromosome) by ordering the SNPs based on their map position and shading the intersection of two SNPs based on the magnitude of the r^2, in a so-called heat map. This can be done using general statistical software with graphing capabilities or more specific software such as Haploview (see http://www.broadinstitute.org/haploview), among others. As marker density increases, however, the number of SNP pairs increases exponentially, and calculating and plotting r^2 becomes computationally demanding such that smaller genomic regions may need to be used. (The number of unique SNP pairs can be calculated from the number of SNPs as $(m^2 - m)/2$.) Figure 4 shows an example of a heat map for the first ten million bases of chromosome 1 in a Large White pig population. These maps can be used to identify regions or blocks with relatively high levels of LD compared to regions where the LD is much lower, which may influence selection of SNP subsets as discussed in the previous section.

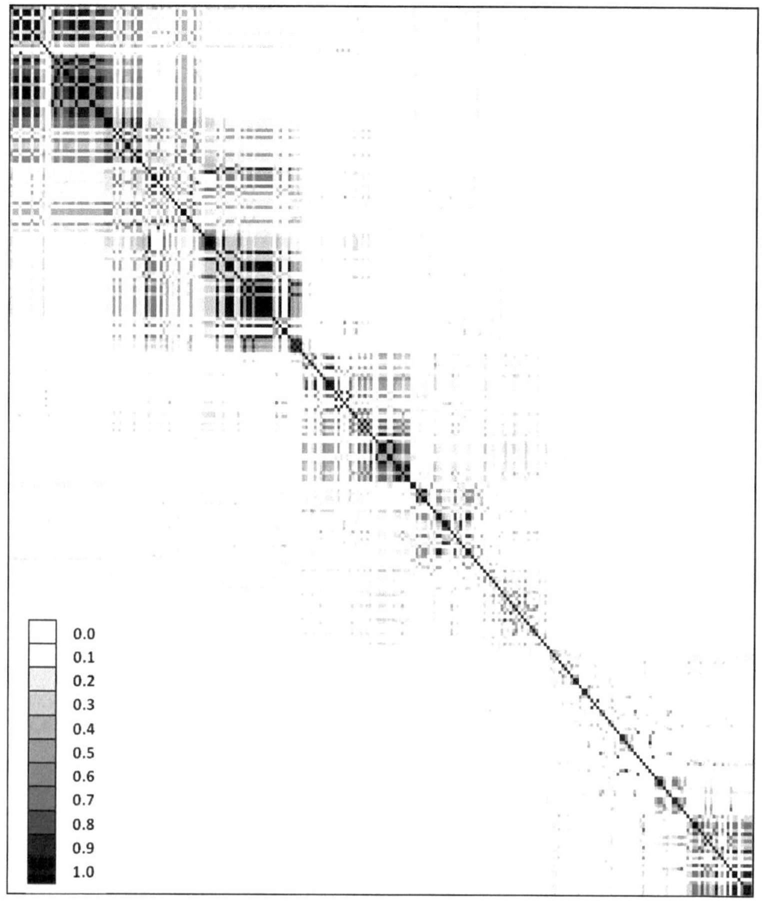

Fig. 4. Heat map of pair-wise LD (r^2) for SNPs in the first ten million bases of chromosome 1 in a Large White pig population.

The next step in assessing the SNP density is the evaluation of r^2 based on genomic map distances. This can show the maximum distance between two SNPs that will maintain a certain level of LD (discussed further below), where any QTL between the two SNPs will have an r^2 of at least that same level, with one or both of the SNPs (see Note 7). The distance between SNPs in each pair should be calculated and then placed into predetermined bins (say 0–1 million base pairs (mbp), 1–2 mbp, etc.). The r^2 by map distance can then be plotted as in Fig. 5, showing the level of r^2 at increasingly larger distances between SNPs. In general, we can see that the LD level decreases when SNPs are farther apart, which we expect, as greater distances increase the chance of recombination events between the SNPs. However, the relationship between distance and r^2 is not always straightforward. There are some SNP pairs that are quite distant from one another yet have high r^2 and pairs that are very close, but have an r^2 near zero.

To better evaluate the level of r^2 at particular map distances, the average r^2 in each bin can be used. The plots can then be more

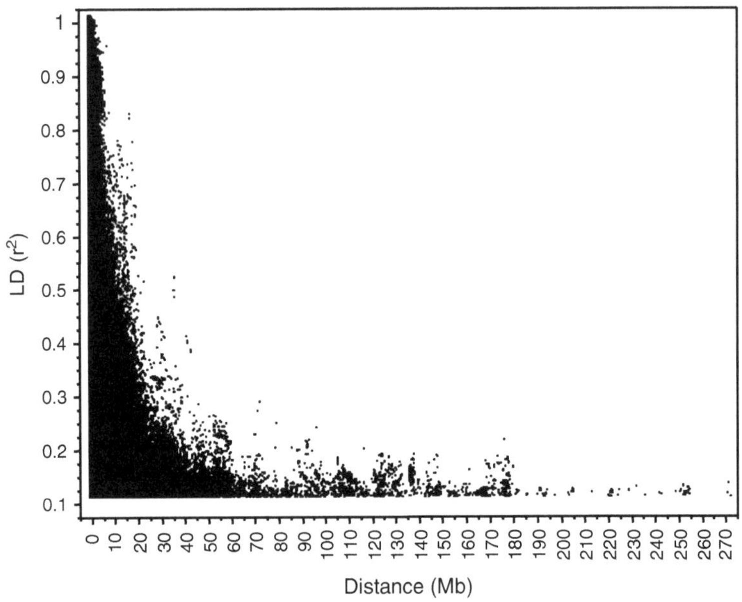

Fig. 5. LD (r^2) level by genome map distance for chromosome 1 in a pig population.

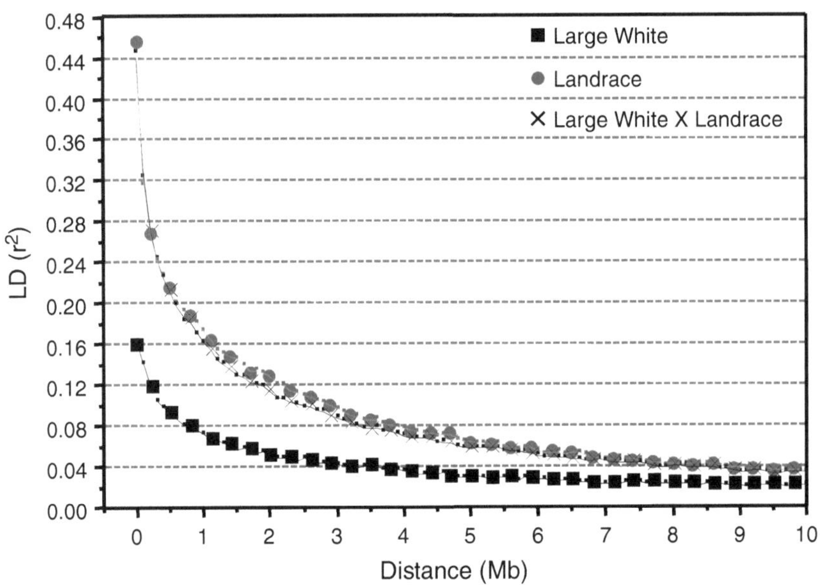

Fig. 6. Average LD (r^2) by genome map distance for three commercial pig populations.

easily interpreted as the LD decay for average map distances and general conclusions about a population can be made. Figure 6 illustrates this concept using average r^2 for chromosome 1 of three commercial pig populations. These results can then be extrapolated for the rest of the genome and the total marker density required for a specified level of LD estimated. For example, in the Landrace population depicted in Fig. 6, an r^2 of 0.2 occurs at an average map distance of ~1 Mb. Using a genome length of 2,800 Mb in pigs, a minimum of 2,800 markers would be needed to have an average genome-wide LD level of at least 0.2. For the Large White population, the average map distance at an LD level of 0.2 can be extrapolated to be near 0 Mb and thus many more markers would be needed. The desired level of LD is likely larger than 0.2, and combined with the differences in average LD across the genome and the fact that markers are not distributed in equal distances, the number of markers required will likely be much larger for these populations. This sort of analysis generally gives minimum numbers of markers.

4.3. Analysis Power and LD

In association mapping approaches, the threshold for useful LD is related to the power of detecting QTLs between a given set of markers. Power is dependent on the size of the QTL effect to be detected (or more appropriately the proportion of variance explained by the QTL) and the sample size used in the analysis, which is inversely proportional to r^2. In other words, the sample size would need to be increased by $1/r^2$ to have the same power using a SNP in LD with a QTL (or causal mutation) as when evaluating the QTL itself (13). Several authors have suggested values for this LD threshold that generally range between 0.2 and 0.3 for detecting moderately sized QTL effects in livestock (11, 14, 15). A simple estimation of the number of markers required would then be a function of the average spacing at an r^2 of 0.2–0.3 and the length of the genome, assuming sample size is sufficient (see Note 8).

A theoretical approach to determine an appropriate LD threshold can be obtained by rearranging equations described by Goddard and Hayes (16), with specific expectations about the data. This approach accounts for the proportion of variance explained by a SNP (QTL). An approximation for the average LD threshold is:

$$\frac{(1/(r^2(q,g) \times h^2))}{\mathrm{SE}^2 \times N}$$

where $r^2(q, p)$ is the proportion of variance explained by the marker, h^2 is the trait heritability, SE is the expected standard error of the correlation between the marker and the trait, and N is the sample size. For example, for a dataset with 1,000 records, a trait heritability of 0.25, an expected proportion of variance explained by any one marker (QTL) of 4%, and a standard error of 0.55, the LD level would be 0.33. In practice, the standard error may not be obvious, and thus simulations using the original Goddard and Hayes equations with different sample sizes to determine appropriate levels of SE may be useful. Once an LD threshold has been identified, the number of markers can simply be calculated then as the total genome length (in Mb, for example) divided by the average spacing at that threshold. Alternatively, the equation can be rearranged to approximate the sample size needed, or proportion of variance explained, for a particular level of LD.

A potential difficulty in marker selection is the fact that LD is not uniformly distributed across the genome (14, 15). In theory, marker selection would account for the regional patterns of LD, but in practice this is difficult and markers are often selected to have generally even coverage across the genome. The calculations above for required marker density assume average levels of LD and may therefore underestimate marker numbers, and a higher density may be needed. When smaller panels of SNPs are selected from large commercial panels, it may be useful to account for the regional LD differences, which can be evaluated as in Fig. 4, and increase density in regions where the LD is low and reduce the number of SNPs in high LD regions.

5. Analysis Considerations

There are a number of approaches that can be used to evaluate marker-trait associations, and the desired outcome of the study will mostly determine the appropriate analysis method (e.g., QTL mapping, genome-wide association, genomic selection in livestock, etc.), but in general the size, density, and SNP distribution of the panel should be considered before choosing a methodology.

The number of markers has implications for computational efficiency. As the complexity of the analysis increases, the computational burden can increase (exponentially in some cases) such that the computing time needed becomes unreasonable. For example, an evaluation of all two-way interactions for a GWAS using a one million SNP chip would involve nearly 500 billion analyses, compared to the one million analyses in the standard single SNP GWAS. While this may be an extreme example, it illustrates the potential computational issues that exist for large-scale SNP data. Advances in computing technology (e.g., distributed high performance computing clusters) can significantly reduce the computation time as can statistical approaches to reduce the data dimensionality (e.g., ref. (17)). While single SNP approaches as described above can be distributed across computing nodes, thus saving real time, approaches involving simultaneous estimation of marker effects often cannot (e.g., ref. (18)).

Marker density and distribution may dictate analyses that are more localized vs. genome-wide. True genome-wide approaches (e.g., GWAS) assume that all QTLs or even causal mutations are associated with at least one marker, and thus density and distribution are critical in explaining a large proportion of variation for a given trait (as described above). Lower-density approaches are often targeted to specific genomic regions where sequence variation is expected to exist, for example as the result of previous GWAS-type analyses, in order to identify specific QTLs. The design of these low-density studies will likely differ from studies with higher densities (i.e., family-based vs. population-based). In other cases, the low-density evaluation is an extension of the high-density approach where the same population is used, but analysis methods differ. A genome-wide method may be initially employed for the full marker set, but an alternative method used for a subset of the markers. The key consideration is to use methodology that is computationally tractable and makes optimal use of information available in the marker data.

6. Notes

1. In many cases due to the short sequence available and the quality of the sequence assembly of the species in question, the BLAST result can produce multiple hits of similar scores to multiple positions. If genotypes are available, it is possible to improve the chance of mapping the SNPs by using LD information between unmapped SNPs and mapped SNPs.
2. While it is quite acceptable to start with a large number of SNPs in a GWAS experiment and use only a small subset of the SNPs in a second scan or in a validation exercise, changing technologies is not always straightforward. One obvious example is the interaction between primers in a multiplexing assay. While SNPs have been optimized to work best on an Illumina SNP chip assay for example, putting them together in a multiplex for a Sequenom assay is complex and difficult, and in many cases, can lead to the loss of several SNPs that would not work in a mix. Of course, it is always possible to isolate these SNPs in an individual assay, but that would increase the complexity and the cost.
3. The LSMs of each genotype (11, 12, 22) fit as a class effect can be used in addition to the additive and/or dominance effects (often fit as covariates) to evaluate the association of the trait with the marker. The LSMs for each genotype are expressed in the measurement unit rather than as a function of number of alleles which makes it easier to understand and capture possible errors.
4. For a general rule about MAF across a large number of SNPs, excluding SNPs with MAF less than 1% is probably appropriate when comfortable with the quality of the genotyping and a reasonably large number of samples have been genotyped.
5. In practice, LD between SNPs on different chromosomes is not really useful and so LD for these pairs is generally not calculated

to save computational resources. SNPs should then be grouped by chromosome (where map position is known) and all pair-wise LD calculated within the group.

6. In practice, the quality control performed on the SNPs may depend on the analysis approach used. In a single SNP approach, one could analyze all SNPs and then evaluate the quality of only the SNPs that are of interest post analysis. In a simultaneous evaluation using all SNPs, if the SNP numbers and sample size are large enough, then even moderately extreme SNPs (in terms of MAF, coverage, Hardy–Weinberg equilibrium) have little impact on the outcome of the analysis. In general, though, SNPs that are called for less than 90% of the sample or have most heterozygous genotypes (usually identified by extreme values for the Pearson χ^2 statistic) are excluded.
7. The proportion of variance that can be explained by a SNP is proportional to the LD between the SNP and the QTL. The QTL may only explain a small proportion of the variance itself and so a marker in low LD with that QTL will not explain any of the variance.
8. Sample sizes in livestock studies have tended to be 1,000–2,000 for mostly pragmatic reasons. However, the dependent trait in the analysis is often a progeny deviation (of some sort), which serves to increase the information in the "phenotype." Therefore, the effective heritability of the trait can approach one, significantly increasing the power of the analysis to a level that would normally require many more thousands of samples to be genotyped.

References

1. Sherry ST, Ward MH, Kholodov M, Baker J, Phan L, Smigielski EM et al (2001) dbSNP: the NCBI database of genetic variation. Nucleic Acids Res 29:308–311
2. Tabangin ME, Woo JG, Martin LJ (2009) The effect of minor allele frequency on the likelihood of obtaining false positives. BMC Proc 3 (suppl 7):S41
3. Craig JE, Hewitt AW, McMellon AE, Henders AK, Ma L, Wallace L et al (2009) Rapid inexpensive genome-wide association using pooled whole blood. Genome Res 19:2075–2080
4. Abraham R, Moskvina V, Sims R, Hollingworth P, Morgan A, Georgieva L et al (2008) A genome-wide association study for late-onset Alzheimer's disease using DNA pooling. BMC Med Genomics 1:44
5. Zhao Y, Wang S (2008) Optimal DNA pooling-based two-stage designs in case-control association studies. Hum Hered 67:46–56
6. Chiang CWK, Gajdos ZKZ, Korn JM, Kuruvilla FG, Butler JL, Hackett R et al (2010) Rapid assessment of genetic ancestry in populations of unknown origin by genome-wide genotyping of pooled samples. PLoS Genet 6: E1000866
7. Ronald A, Butcher LM, Docherty S, Davis OSP, Schalkwyk LC, Craig IW et al (2010) A genome-wide association study of social and non-social autistic-like traits in the general population using pooled DNA, 500 K SNP microarrays and both community and diagnosed autism replication samples. Behav Genet 40:31–45
8. Sham P, Bader JS, Craig I, O'Donovan M, Owen M (2002) DNA pooling: a tool for large-scale association studies. Nat Rev Genet 3:862–871
9. Falconer DS, MacKay TFC (1996) Introduction to quantitative genetics, 4th edn. Longmans Green, Harlow

10. Sved JA (1971) Linkage disequilibrium and homozygosity of chromosome segments in finite populations. Theor Popul Biol 2:125–141
11. Du FX, Clutter AC, Lohuis MM (2007) Characterizing linkage disequilibrium in pig populations. Int J Biol Sci 3:166–178
12. Zaykin DV, Meng Z, Ehm MG (2006) Contrasting linkage-disequilibrium patterns between cases and controls as a novel association-mapping method. Am J Hum Genet 78:737–746
13. Pritchard JK, Przeworski K (2001) Linkage disequilibrium in humans: models and data. Am J Hum Genet 69:1–14
14. Amaral AJ, Megens HJ, Crooijmans RPMA, Heuven HCM, Groenen MAM (2008) Linkage disequilibrium decay and haplotype block structure in the pig. Genetics 179:569–579
15. Sargolzaei M, Schenkel FS, Jansen GB, Schaeffer LR (2008) Extent of linkage disequilibrium in Holstein cattle in North America. J Dairy Sci 91:2106–2117
16. Goddard ME, Hayes BJ (2009) Mapping genes for complex traits in domestic animals and their use in breeding programmes. Nat Rev Genet 10:381–391
17. Long N, Gianola D, Rosa GJM, Weigel K, Avendano S (2007) Machine learning classification procedure for selecting SNPs in genomic selection: application to early mortality in broilers. J Anim Breed Genet 124:377–389
18. Meuwissen THE, Hayes BJ, Goddard ME (2001) Prediction of total genetic value using genome-wide dense marker maps. Genetics 157:1819–1829

Part II

Identifying Quantitative Trait Loci

Chapter 6

Composite Interval Mapping and Multiple Interval Mapping: Procedures and Guidelines for Using Windows QTL Cartographer

Luciano Da Costa E. Silva, Shengchu Wang, and Zhao-Bang Zeng

Abstract

Tremendous progress has been made in recent years on developing statistical methods for mapping quantitative trait loci (QTL) from crosses of inbred lines. In this chapter, we provide an introduction of composite interval mapping and multiple interval mapping methods for mapping QTL from inbred line crosses and also detailed instructions to perform the analyses in Windows QTL Cartographer. For each method, we discuss the meaning of each option in the analysis procedures and how to understand and interpret the mapping results through a work-out example.

Key words: CIM, Inbred lines, MIM, QTL mapping, Windows QTL Cartographer

1. Introduction

Many traits that are important to agriculture, human health, and evolutionary biology are quantitative in nature, influenced by multiple genes. Efficient and robust identification and mapping of the genomic positions of those genes are very important goals in quantitative genetics. The availability of genome-wide molecular markers provides the means to locate and map such quantitative trait loci (QTL) in a systematic way.

The identification of QTL effects associated with genetic markers dates back to Sax (1). While earlier methods simply tested for differences between means of a phenotype that was associated with marker genotypes by a *t*-test (2–4), more elaborate methods such as interval mapping (IM) (5) use information from more than one genetic marker at a time and give relatively more power for identifying QTL and for estimating their effects. Because IM assumes a single QTL in the model, the effects of unaccounted QTL remain in the model

Scott A. Rifkin (ed.), *Quantitative Trait Loci (QTL): Methods and Protocols*, Methods in Molecular Biology, vol. 871,
DOI 10.1007/978-1-61779-785-9_6, © Springer Science+Business Media New York 2012

residual sum of squares. In addition, the estimate of a QTL effect by IM is biased if there are multiple linked QTL. Zeng (6, 7) proposed a method based on a multiple regression that fits both the effects of a QTL as well as the effects of covariates, which are a subset of selected genetic markers. The method is a combination of interval mapping and multiple regression. Interval mapping is used to fit a linear model at every position for the genome scan, and multiple regression is used to fit covariates to control linked and unlinked QTL effects and reduce the model residual. When well chosen, covariates can reduce the model residual sum of squares, enhancing the power of identifying QTL and controlling linked QTL effects thus effectively resolving issues with linkage. The multiple regression method proposed by Zeng is known in the literature as composite interval mapping (CIM).

Multiple intervals mapping (MIM) (8–10) is similar to CIM in concept but quite different in procedure. The rationale of CIM is to fit genetic markers closely linked to other QTL across the genome as covariates when searching for a putative QTL. The rationale of MIM is to fit estimated positions of other QTL rather than their closely linked genetic markers, thereby delivering more power as well as better parameter estimates. Furthermore, since MIM can fit multiple QTL, it allows analyses of QTL interaction (epistasis).

Our goal in this chapter is to provide readers with the rationale behind both CIM and MIM methods of QTL mapping and also the step-by-step procedures on how to perform these analyses in Windows QTL Cartographer software.

2. Materials

2.1. Windows QTL Cartographer Software

CIM, MIM, and other commonly used methods for mapping QTL have been implemented in Windows QTL Cartographer 2.51 (11). Windows QTL Cartographer also includes several other functions, such as those for computing the score- and the permutation-based thresholds, for importing and exporting data in a variety of formats, and for genome-wide scanning, and graphical tools for presenting and summarizing results. Windows QTL Cartographer is freely available for download at http://statgen.ncsu.edu/qtlcart/WQTLCart.htm.

2.1.1. Windows QTL Cartographer Source File

Windows QTL Cartographer requires a source data file with a list of user-defined fields describing the data for analysis. This source data file must have extension *mcd*, for instance *mydata.mcd*. In what follows, we first describe the list of fields that must be in the *mcd* file as well as their meaning, and then we provide a series of steps to create the *mcd* file using a built-in tool in Windows QTL Cartographer. The fields that must appear in the *mcd* file are:

`#FileID`: a string of numeric values indicating the file's identification, usually a 10-digit number.

#bychromosome: a void field indicating that the information about chromosomes is about to begin.

-type: a character string that indicates how marker positions are numbered along the chromosome; it can be either position or interval. Position indicates that the numbers listed are positions of markers from the leftmost marker in the current chromosome, so numbers should be in increasing order. Interval indicates that the numbers listed are distances between two consecutive markers. If Interval is chosen, then an extra number zero must be included at the end of the list of distances.

-function: a numeric value indicating which map function is used to transform recombination frequency between markers and genetic distance in Morgans. The most common values that it takes are 1, 2, and 3, for Haldane, Kosambi, and Morgan, respectively.

-Units: a character value that indicates the unit of marker positions. The choices are cM (*centiMorgan*), M (*Morgan*), and r (*recombination*). If recombination is chosen, then the field -function should be 3.

-chromosome: a numeric value indicating the total number of chromosomes in the data file.

-maximum: a numeric value indicating the number of markers in the chromosome that has the largest number of markers in the data.

-named: it takes value yes if markers have names, no otherwise.

-start: a void field indicating that information of marker positions in all chromosomes is about to begin.

-Chromosome: a character value indicating the chromosome's name. The position of markers in that chromosome will start in the next line. The field -Chromosome is used as many times as the number of chromosomes in the data, and the position of markers are entered in the following lines immediately after the field -Chromosome.

-stop: a void field indicating that information of marker positions in all chromosomes has ended.

#bycross: a void field indicating that cross information is about to begin.

-SampleSize: a numeric value indicating the sample size.

-Cross: a code indicating the type of mating design (see Note 1).

-traits: a numeric value indicating the number of continuous traits in the data.

-otraits: a numeric value indicating the number of categorical traits in the data (see Note 2). The field -otraits is optional, in the sense that if the data has no categorical traits this field should not appear in the source file.

`-missingtrait`: a symbol indicating missing values of traits, for instance, a dot.

`-TranslationTable`: a table with six rows and three columns defining how marker genotypes are translated (see Note 3).

`-start markers`: a void field indicating that information on marker genotypes is about to begin. The information about marker genotypes will start in the next line immediately after the field `-start markers`. There are two options: one marker per line or one subject per line. In the one subject per line option, each line contains the genotypes of all markers for a subject. The order of markers must be the same for all subjects. In the one marker per line option, each line contains the genotypes of all subjects for a marker. The order of subjects must be the same for all markers.

`-stop markers`: a void field indicating that information on all markers has ended.

`-start traits`: a void field indicating that information on continuous traits is about to begin. The information of traits values will start in the next line immediately after the field `-start traits`. Each line contains the trait values for all subjects. The order of subjects must be the same for all traits and in the same order as they appear in the information on marker genotypes. There would be as many lines of trait values as the number of traits in the data, one line per trait.

`-stop traits`: a void field indicating that information on continuous traits has ended.

`-start otraits`: a void field indicating that information on categorical traits is about to begin. The information of trait values will start in the next line immediately after `-start otraits`. Each line contains the trait values for all subjects. The order of subjects must be the same for all traits and in the same order as they appear in the information on marker genotypes. There would be as many lines of trait values as the number of categorical traits in the data, one line per trait. The field `-start otraits` is optional, in the sense that if the data has no categorical traits this field should not appear in the source file.

`-stop otraits`: a void field indicating that information on continuous traits has ended. The field `-stop otraits` is optional, in the sense that if the data has no categorical traits this field should not appear in the source file.

`-quit`: a void field telling Windows QTL Cartographer to stop inputting of data.

`-end`: a void field indicating the end of the source data file.

2.1.2. Creating an mcd Source Data File Using Windows QTL Cartographer

Remember that Windows QTL Cartographer can run analysis only on *mcd* source files, and the software has several functions that help create them. Windows QTL Cartographer can easily convert a comma-separated values (*csv*) file of raw data (including map, cross information, marker scores, and trait values; see Fig. 1), into a formatted *mcd* source file. Figure 1 illustrates a *csv* file of data from a hypothetical population (`Populations`) with sample size ten

#START#								
Populations	1							
Samples	10							
Traits	1							
Chromosomes	2							
Markers	3	2						
MapFunction	Haldane							
CrossType	SF2							
MisTraitValue	.							
TranslationTable	2	1	0	12	10	-1		
Other Traits	2							
#END#								
MkID (Pop=1)	C1Mk1	C1Mk2	C1Mk3	C2Mk1	C2Mk2	Trait1	OTrait1	OTrait2
Position	0	9.3	16.2	0	15.5	1	1	2
Chromosome	1	1	1	2	2	1	1	2
Chr Label	C11	C11	C11	C12	C12	1	1	2
IND-01	2	0	-1	1	0	.	M	1
IND-02	0	1	1	2	2	40.1	F	2
IND-03	1	1	1	0	1	39.81	M	1
IND-04	2	0	2	1	1	41.02	M	1
IND-05	0	1	2	0	1	35.5	F	2
IND-06	1	2	0	1	0	41.43	F	3
IND-07	2	1	2	2	2	34.92	F	3
IND-08	2	2	0	1	1	38.2	M	2
IND-09	1	1	1	2	0	37.56	F	3
IND-10	1	2	1	1	1	36.24	F	2

Fig. 1. An illustrative hypothetical comma-separated values (*csv*) file. Line `MkID` specifies the labels for markers (C1Mk1 through C2Mk2), continuous traits (Trait1), and categorical traits (OTrait1 and OTrait2). Line `Position` specifies marker positions from left end to right end of each chromosome. Line `Chromosome` identifies chromosomes. Line `Chr Label` specifies chromosome labels. In this example, minus one (−1) specifies missing marker genotype, and dot (.) specifies missing trait value.

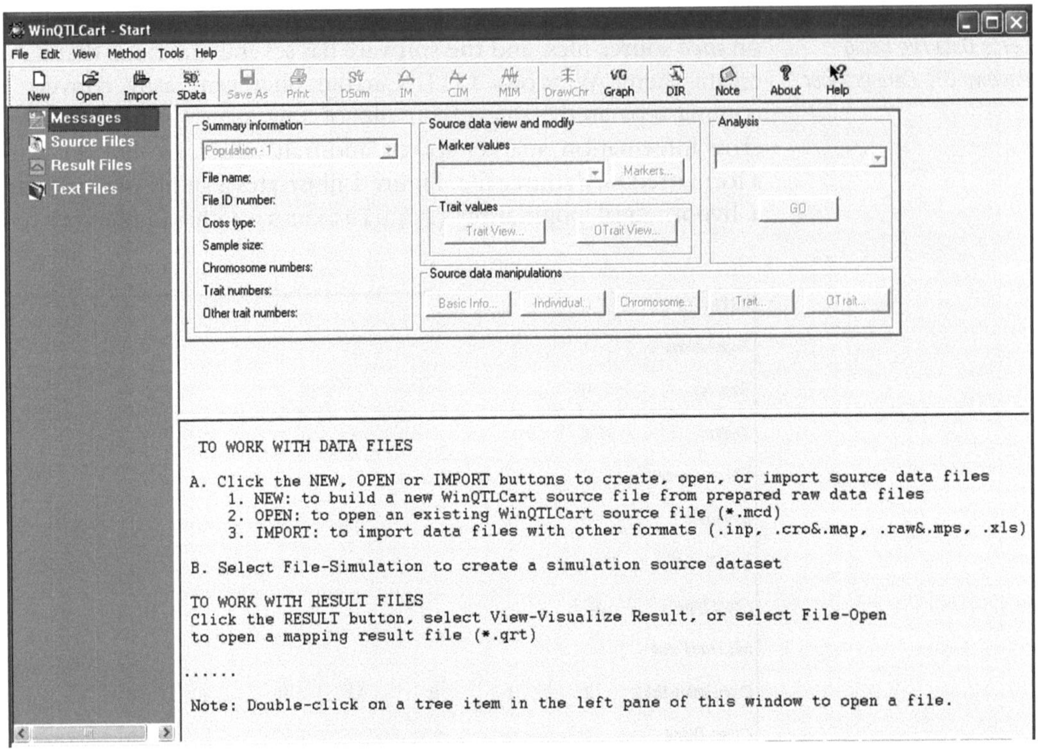

Fig. 2. Windows QTL Cartographer main window.

(`Samples`) and two chromosomes (`Chromosomes`), first and second chromosomes contain three and two markers (`Markers`), respectively (see Note 4 for more details on other example files available for Windows QTL Cartographer's users). The unit of distance between markers is in Haldanes (`MapFunction`), and the hypothetical population is intercross F_2 (coded as SF2 in `Cross-Type`; see Note 1). There is one continuous trait (`Traits`) and two categorical traits (`Other traits`). Markers have been coded as 2 for **HH**, 1 for **Hh**, 0 for **hh**, and "−1" for missing genotype (`TranslationTable`; see Note 3). Notice that the first subject has missing genotype (coded as −1) for the third marker in the first chromosome, as well as a missing trait value for `Trait1` (coded as dot in `MisTraitValue`).

Save the *csv* file within a folder of your choice, say `C:\Example`. A working directory can be set by clicking on `Tools` in the menu of the Windows QTL Cartographer main window (Fig. 2), and then by clicking on `Set Working Directory` in the drop-down list.

With the *csv* file on hand, the process of creating an *mcd* source file is straightforward. There are five steps to follow:

1. Start Windows QTL Cartographer (Fig. 2) and click on `Import` icon. In the newly opened window, select `Microsoft CSV format (*.csv)`, then click on `Next`

2. Load the *csv* file into Windows QTL Cartographer by clicking on `CSV File`
3. Enter a name for the *mcd* source file into the blank box
4. Select a directory to save the *mcd* file by clicking on `Directory`
5. Create the *mcd* file by clicking on `Finish`. Windows QTL Cartographer shows a small window with a message of either success or failure in creating the *mcd* data file, click on `OK` to exit the procedure

The *mcd* populated/generated with the information in the *csv* file (Fig. 1) is shown in Fig. 3. Windows QTL Cartographer allows editing entries in the *mcd* file using the options in fields `Trait values` and `Source data manipulations` (Fig. 2). Alternatively, one can open the *mcd* file with a text editing tool, such as *WordPad* or *Notepad*, and make the desired modifications.

By selecting `View` in the menu and clicking on `Data Summary`, Windows QTL Cartographer can compute a variety of summary statistics from the source data, such as averages, variances, coefficient of variation, kurtosis, test of normality, histogram, and marker segregation, among others.

2.2. Data from an Experiment with Fruit Flies

In this section, we describe data obtained from an experiment with *Drosophila melanogaster* (12). The data will be used later on to illustrate both CIM and MIM analyses. It is worth mentioning that our major goal in using real data is to provide readers with some insights in the CIM and MIM analyses, and, when necessary, also to provide some rationale on how to perform the analyses. Information on chromosome, marker genotypes, and trait values have been put together in the source file named *Genetics-01-WZ-Data.mcd*, freely available for download at http://statgen.ncsu.edu/zeng/Genetics-01-WZ-Data.htm. This source data file contains the genotypes of 48 markers on chromosome 2 of *D. melanogaster* and phenotypic values of one trait, wing size index, for 701 recombinant inbred lines (Chap. 3). Coded genotypes are 1, 0, or −1 for homozygotes AA, aa, and missing values, respectively. This *Drosophila* experiment has a somewhat unique design similar to a backcross in terms of recombination process, so we treat it as backcross mating design in both CIM and MIM analyses.

3. Methods

3.1. CIM Procedure

3.1.1. CIM Statistical Model

As mentioned in the introduction, CIM is an extension of IM. The extension consists of fitting some selected markers as cofactors (covariates) in the model to control for the genetic variation in

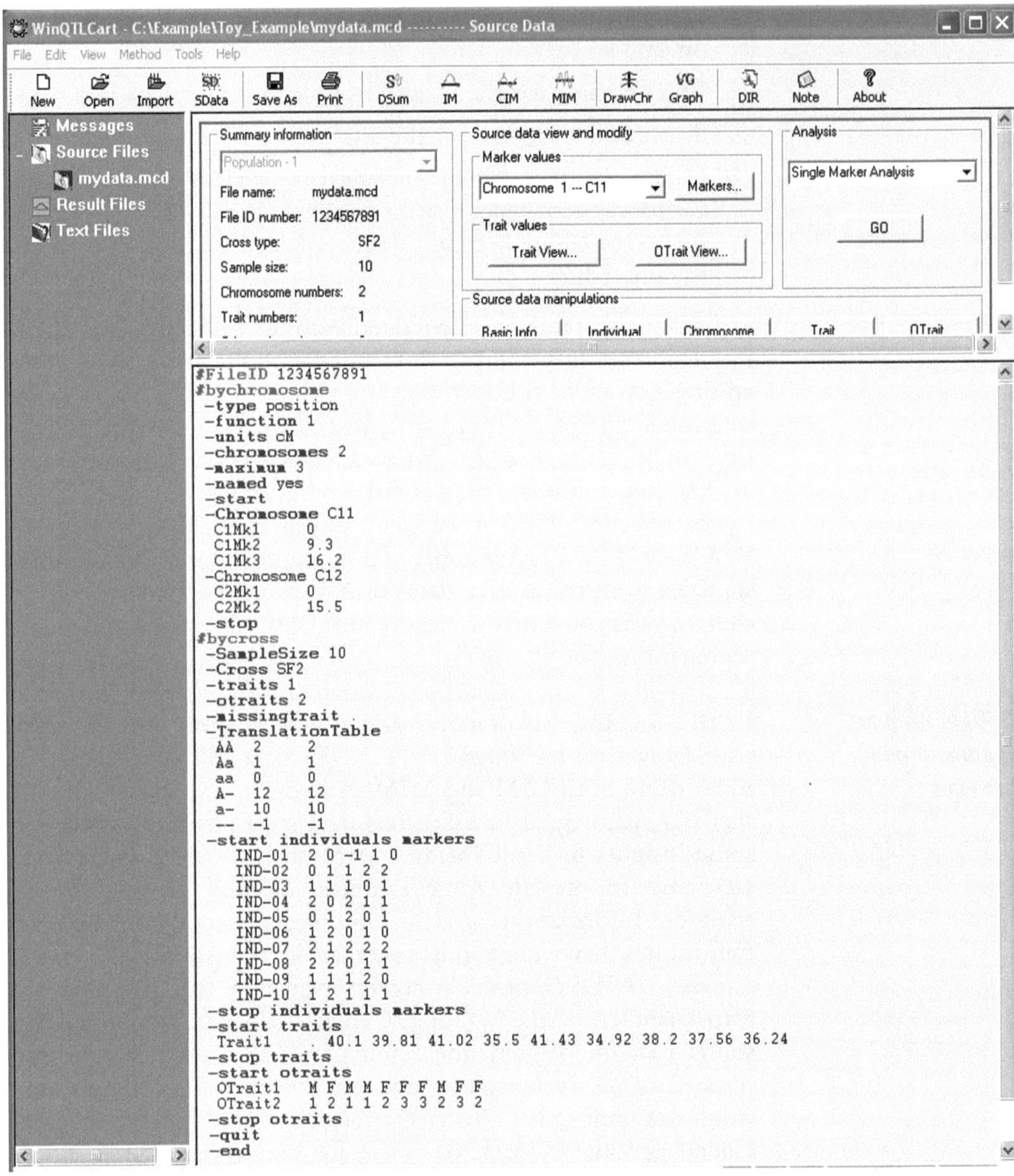

Fig. 3. View of an *mcd* source file created by Windows QTL Cartographer with the information available in the *csv* file displayed in Fig. 1.

other possibly linked and unlinked QTL. The general CIM statistical model can be written as:

$$y_i = \mu + Z_i B + \sum_{r=1}^{m} X_{ir}\beta_r + e_i$$

where y_i is the phenotypic trait value of subject i; μ is the overall mean; B is a column vector for the effects of a putative QTL, which depends on the mating design; Z_i is a row vector of predictor variables corresponding to the effects of the putative QTL; X_{ir} is a row vector of predictor variables corresponding to the rth cofactor marker; β_r is a column vector with the coefficient of the rth cofactor marker; and e_i is the random error that is assumed to follow a normal distribution with mean zero and variance σ^2. As an example, consider an intercross F_2 population where subject i could have either genotype QQ, Qq or qq for a putative QTL. Similarly, subject i could have either genotype MM, Mm or mm for cofactor marker r. Also consider a parameterization of additive and dominance effects of the QTL as a and d, respectively (13). Therefore, $B = (a, d)^{\mathrm{T}}$, $\beta_r = (\beta_{r1}, \beta_{r2})^{\mathrm{T}}$ (the superscript "T" stands for transpose),

$$Z_i = (z_{i1}, z_{i2}) = \begin{cases} (1, -0.5) & \text{if subject } i \text{ has genotype QQ for QTL} \\ (0, 1) & \text{if subject } i \text{ has genotype Qq for QTL} \\ (-1, -0.5) & \text{if subject } i \text{ has genotype qq for QTL} \end{cases}$$

and

$$X_{ir} = (x_{ir1}, x_{ir2}) = \begin{cases} (1, -0.5) & \text{if subject } i \text{ has genotype MM for cofactor marker } r \\ (0, 0.5) & \text{if subject } i \text{ has genotype Mm for cofactor marker } r \\ (-1, -0.5) & \text{if subject } i \text{ has genotype mm for cofactor marker } r \end{cases}$$

Hypotheses regarding parameters in the CIM model can be formulated and tested with the logarithm of the likelihood ratio test (LRT) statistic, which has a one-to-one mathematical correspondence with the logarithm of odds (LOD), LRT $= 2\log_e(10)$LOD $\approx$4.6 LOD (see Note 5).

3.1.2. CIM Cofactors

Perhaps, the most crucial step in the CIM procedure is the choice of cofactor markers. Selecting too few cofactor markers would not reduce most of the residual genetic variation of other QTL. On the other hand, selecting too many cofactor markers would reduce the residual genetic variation of other QTL, but at a cost of decreasing the residual degrees of freedom, therefore, possibly diminishing the power to identify QTL.

The distance of cofactors from the testing position of a putative QTL is as important as the number of cofactor markers. The neighboring regions on the left and right sides of the closest left and right markers enclosing a putative QTL are known as `window size`. Therefore, a putative QTL has two `window sizes`, unless it is located either within the first or last interval in a chromosome, in which cases the putative QTL has one `window size` only. Any cofactor marker located within the `window size` (left or right) of a putative QTL is excluded from the set of cofactors as it is considered to be too tightly linked to the putative QTL and could decrease the power of the test statistic due to strong correlation (collinearity). A rule of thumb is to set `window size` wider to start with and gradually reduce it if there is evidence of linked QTL (see Note 6 for more details on cofactors).

3.1.3. CIM Genome-Wide Threshold

The CIM procedure uses a genome-wide threshold to determine the statistical significance of effects of putative QTL. Generally, there are two options to determine the threshold: (1) a user-defined threshold in the case that the user knows the threshold a priori and (2) an empirically estimated threshold (the permutation method (14, 15)). The genome-wide threshold controls the amount of false positives, which is known as Type I error. While using a lower threshold could produce more false positives, using a higher threshold could potentially miss more QTL.

3.1.4. CIM Procedure in Windows QTL Cartographer

Windows QTL Cartographer contains a comprehensive implementation of the CIM procedure. In what follows, we split the CIM procedure into two parts. In the first part we describe the CIM procedure step-by-step. In the second part (in Subheading 3.1.5), we discuss the implications of using each option in the analysis and how to understand and interpret results properly through a worked-out example.

It is worth emphasizing again that all statistical analyses in Windows QTL Cartographer must be run on an *mcd* source data file. Windows QTL Cartographer provides default values for all user-defined options in the CIM procedure; but keep in mind that these default values are meant only to provide the best all-around parameter settings to begin with. In what follows, we will go through the CIM procedure step-by-step.

1. Open the *mcd* source data file into Windows QTL Cartographer main window.
2. Start the CIM procedure by electing `Method` in the menu and then `Composite Interval Mapping`. Windows QTL Cartographer will display the CIM analysis window (Fig. 4).
3. Name a file to store QTL mapping results by clicking on `Result File`. This file must have the extension *qrt* (*mydata-C.qrt* in our example).
4. Select the grid of positions to be tested for putative QTL in `The Walk speed (cM)` box. The default value is 1.0 cM. Click the spin dial beside `The Walk speed (cM)` box to increase or decrease the walk speed by 0.5 cM increments. There is a tradeoff between walk speed and time for running the analysis. Increasing the walk speed (greater than 1.0) means less precision but the analysis takes less time. Decreasing the walk speed (less than 1.0) yields a more precise result but will take more time (see Note 7).

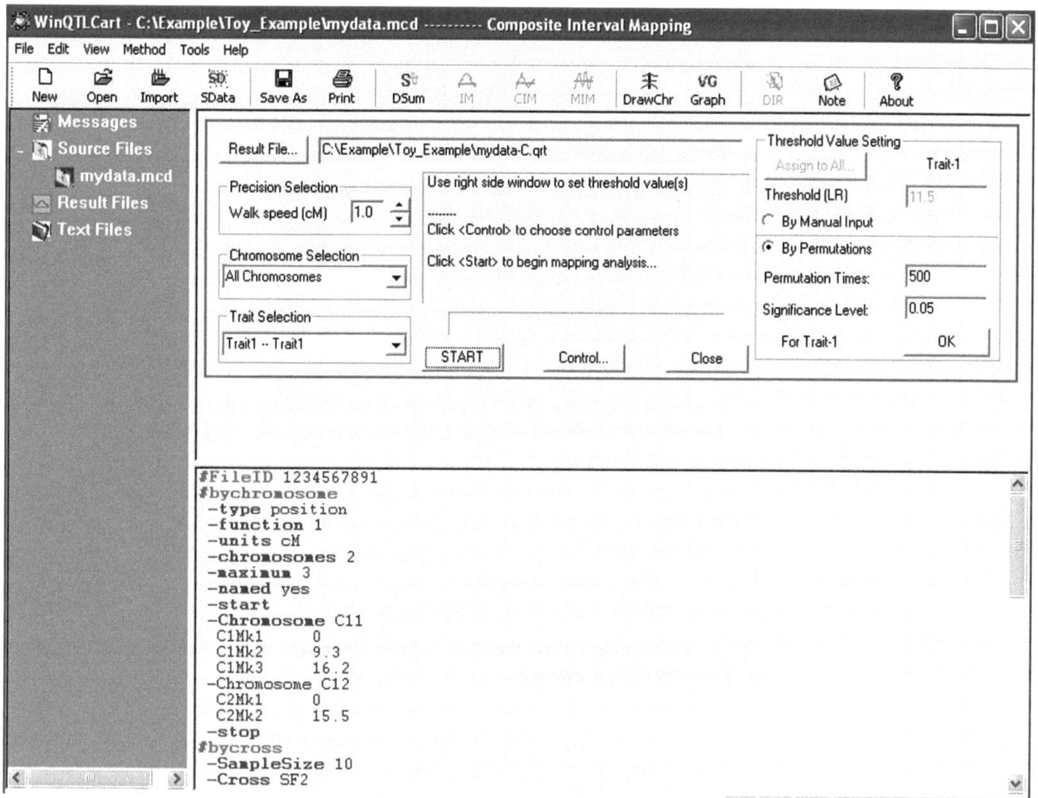

Fig. 4. Composite interval mapping (CIM) procedure window. Buttons and boxes in this window are user-defined options with default values.

5. Select either one or all chromosomes for analysis in the `Chromosome Selection` drop-down list. The analysis can be performed either for one chromosome at a time or all together. But if one chromosome is analyzed at a time, be sure to keep the same threshold value across all chromosomes, unless there is some reason why a chromosome may require a different threshold (e.g., chromosomes with a significant amount of segregation distortion).

6. Select one or all traits for analysis in the `Trait Selection` drop-down list. Be aware that the threshold value in the `Threshold Value Setting` box may change depending on the traits being selected.

7. Select cofactor markers by clicking on `Control`. In the newly opened `Set CIM Control Parameters` dialog window (Fig. 5), one can select markers cofactors through statistical selection and/or manually, as follows.

   7.1 Statistical marker selection. This step allows the user to specify certain models and statistical procedures for automatic selection of cofactor markers. In `CIM Model` box,

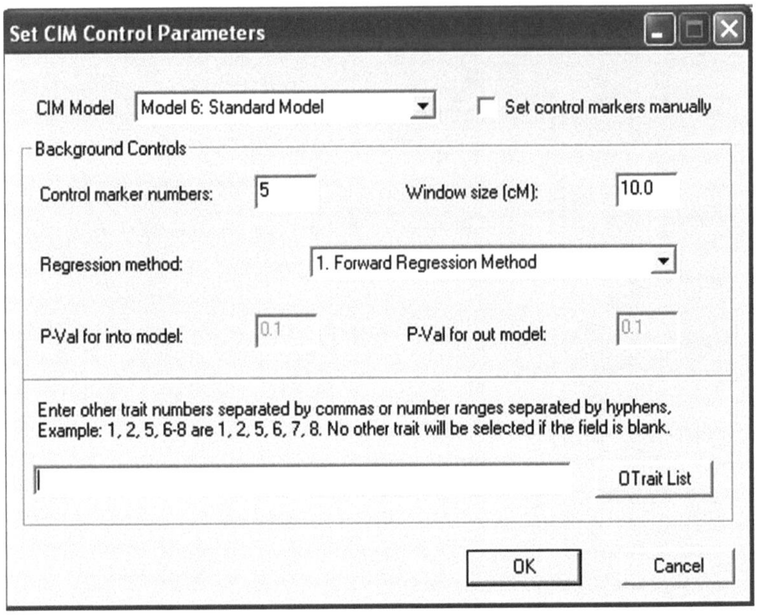

Fig. 5. CIM cofactor control window. Buttons and boxes in this window are user-defined options with default values.

one must specify the type of cofactors to be used in the CIM analysis: `Model 1- All Marker Control` uses all markers in the data as cofactors; `Model 2- Unlinked Marker Control` uses all markers that are unlinked to the putative QTL as cofactors; and `Model 6- Standard Model` is the default model that selects certain markers as cofactors by defining three additional user-defined options: number of cofactor marker, `window size`, and cofactor selection method (see Note 8). Number of cofactors is defined in `Control marker numbers` box, `window size` in `Window size (cM)` box, and cofactor selection method in `Regression method` box. Number of cofactor markers only sets the maximum number of markers that can be selected as cofactor by a selection method; therefore, fewer markers than the number of cofactors could be selected. Cofactor selection method is either `Forward Regression Method`, `Backward Regression Method` or `Forward & Backward Method`. If `Forward & Backward Method` is chosen, then two additional user-defined options are required, *p*-value used for a statistical test to add a marker (`P-Val for into model`) and to remove a marker (`P-Val for out model`) to the set of cofactors (see Note 9).

7.2 Manual marker selection. This step allows the user to exclude certain undesirable cofactor markers that may have been selected automatically in step 7.1. Check the box near `Set control markers manually` to prevent Windows QTL Cartographer from entering the CIM analysis without asking for a final manual selection.

7.3 Select categorical traits as covariates. If the data file contains any categorical traits and some of these traits could serve as covariates in the CIM analysis, these traits can be listed in `OTrait List` box. Enter their identifying numbers separated by commas in the blank box.

7.4 Return to the CIM analysis window by clicking on `OK`.

8. Set the genome-wide threshold via either manual input or via permutation test in `ThresholdValueSetting` box. The value of threshold to appear in the graph window is the value given in the box beside `Threshold (LR)`, by default it is 11.5 units of the LRT.

9. Start the CIM analysis by clicking on `START`. If manual selection is not chosen (step 7.2), CIM analysis will start immediately; otherwise a dialog window will be displayed. In this dialog window, cofactor markers can be chosen manually by entering into the blank box a list of numbers identifying cofactor markers. Be sure to separate the numbers identifying cofactor markers in the list with a space. Clicking over markers in the dialog window also allows editing the list of cofactor markers.

10. As soon as the CIM analysis is complete, Windows QTL Cartographer will open a graph window and create some output files (see Note 10 for more details about the graph window). The relevant files are (1) a file with *qrt* extension containing QTL mapping results (this file is named on step 3); (2) a text file with summary of cofactor markers, *Cofactor.txt* file; and (3) a text file with results of the permutation test, if the permutation test is chosen. This file is named **-C-all-pm.txt* file, where "*" is the name of the *mcd* source data file. For instance, if the source data file is *mydata.mcd*, then it would be named *mydata-C-all-pm.txt*. Once created, these three files will be listed in the left side of the Windows QTL Cartographer main window, and their content can be viewed at any time by clicking over the file name. In the next section, we explain the meaning of results stored in each of these files.

11. Exit the CIM procedure by clicking on `Close`.

3.1.5. A Worked-Out CIM Analysis in Windows QTL Cartographer

In this section, we run CIM analysis on data from an experiment with *D. melanogaster* (12) described in Subheading 2.2. In what follows, first we carefully detail the reasons why each user-defined option was chosen, and then we explain with details the outputs. User-defined options are shown in Table 1, and results are shown thereafter.

Table 1
User-defined options used in CIM analysis for *Genetics-01-WZ-Data.mcd* source data file

User-defined option	Value	Reasons
`Walk speed (cM)`	`1`	The data contains information only on chromosome 2 of *D. melanogaster.* Therefore, the grid of positions every 1 cM produces a QTL map with good resolution, while still allowing for fast analysis. For long genomes, higher grid values are recommended if the speed of the analysis is an issue
`Chromosome Selection`	No need to define because our data has only one chromosome	Unless a dataset contains too many chromosomes which would slow down the analysis dramatically, we recommend the analysis be performed on all chromosomes at once. This will create a single QTL mapping data file thereby allowing graphical visualization of the QTL mapping on all chromosomes at once in the Graph tool of Windows QTL Cartographer. Moreover, since the genome-wide threshold depends on the whole length of the genome under analysis, even if the analysis is performed on subsets of chromosomes each time, the threshold must be based on all chromosomes. If a chromosome has significant amount of segregation distortion, it is better to have this chromosome analyzed separately with a different threshold evaluated specifically for this chromosome
`Trait Selection`	No need to define because our data has only one trait	Unless a dataset contains too many traits, we recommend the analysis be performed on all traits at once. This will create a single QTL mapping data, thereby allowing for graphical visualization of QTL mapping on all traits in the Graph tool of Windows QTL Cartographer
`CIM Model`	`Model 6: Standard Model`	The Standard model (`Model 6`) is statistically more appealing than both `Model 1` and `Model 2` because of its flexibility. `Model 1` and `Model 2` are inflexible models in the sense that either all markers or all unlinked markers are used as cofactors, respectively (see Note 11)
`Window size (cM)`	`2`	The chromosome analyzed here has regions with tightly linked markers. When testing for a putative QTL in these regions, tightly linked cofactor markers to the putative QTL must be avoided; otherwise, the power of test statistic will decrease; hence the `window size` should not be too narrow. On the other hand, the analysis shows evidence of multiple close linked QTL in the chromosome; hence the `window size` should not be too wide. Therefore, a wide enough window, 2 cM, was chosen. But keep in mind that final choice of `window size` should also depend on how QTL are distributed across the chromosomes as indicated by analysis

Regression method	Forward & Backward Method P-Val for into model=0.10 P-Val for out model=0.10 The option set control markers manually was not selected	The stepwise forward and backward method of variable selection was chosen because it can select a better set of cofactor markers as compared to the forward and backward variable selection methods (see Note 9 for more details) The *p*-values for a marker entering and leaving a model, P-Val for into and out, respectively, were set to 0.10 and 0.10. With these somewhat liberal values, markers can enter the set of cofactors more easily and stay in it (see Note 9) allowing the set of cofactors to be larger. This setup is appropriate when there is evidence of many linked and unlinked QTL
Control marker numbers	No need to define because we chose Forward & Backward Method	Control marker numbers needs to be chosen if we select either forward or backward methods. By choosing combined forward and backward with defined P-Val for into and out, the number of cofactor markers will be determined automatically
Threshold	By Permutations was selected Permutation Times=1000 Significance Level=0.10	The permutation test was chosen because there is no knowledge a priori regarding the chromosome (in this case) threshold. The permutation test was set to run 1,000 times, which provides sufficient samples to have a good estimate of the threshold of null distribution in the tail (10%). Recent results (Laurie, Wang, Carlini-Garcia, and Zeng, unpublished data; (18)) suggest that more liberal genome-wide significance levels may be used for detecting QTL without compromising the number of false positives. Therefore, the genome-wide significance of 10% was chosen rather than the usual 1 or 5%

```
1    #=# Graphic Format of Mapping Result #=# #=# Used by Windows QTL Cartographer V2.5 #=#
2    -tnum 1  Trait_1  0.016470
3    -cnum 1

4    C1 48 22A2 2.2000 22B2 2.4000 23B1 6.6000 23C3 7.5000 24C1 10.3000 24D4 11.2000 24E5 12.0000 25A1 13.0000 25A3 13.5000 27B1 19.8000 29F1 30.4000 32C1

5    -threshold 11.50
6    -mtraits -1
7    -otrait 0
8    -cross B2

9    #The position is from the left telomere on the chromosome
10   -window        2.00      Window size for models 5 and 6
11   -background       5      Background parameters in model 6
12   -Model            6      Model number
13   -trait            1      Analyzed trait [Trait_1]
14   -cross           B2      Cross
15   #
16   #  Note that our Likelihood ratio test statistic compares two nested hypotheses
17   #  and is two times the negative natural log of the ratio of the likelihoods.  For example,
18   #  assume that  hypothesis H0 is nested within H1 and that they have likelihoods L0 and L1 respectively.
19   #  Then, the "Likelihood Ratio Test Statistic" is -2ln(L0/L1).
20   #
21   #  Test Site    * Like. Ratio Test Statistics    *     Additive        *     Dominance        * Misc. HT
22   c  m position    H0:H1     R2(0:1)   TR2(0:1) H1:a     S1      ....  ....  ....  ....  ....       ....   ....  .....      ....  ....  ....  ....  ....
23   -s
24   1  1  0.0001     902.474  0.259     0.901     0.01876  11.630  0.00  0.00  0.00  0.00  0.0000268  0.00   0.00  0.0000268  0.00  0.00  0.00  0.00  0.00
25   1  2  0.0021     875.461  0.255     0.897     0.01854   9.004  0.00  0.00  0.00  0.00  0.0000278  0.00   0.00  0.0000278  0.00  0.00  0.00  0.00  0.00
26   1  2  0.0121     881.254  0.258     0.900     0.01873   1.691  0.00  0.00  0.00  0.00  0.0000269  0.00   0.00  0.0000269  0.00  0.00  0.00  0.00  0.00
27   1  2  0.0221     880.579  0.259     0.901     0.01875   2.030  0.00  0.00  0.00  0.00  0.0000268  0.00   0.00  0.0000268  0.00  0.00  0.00  0.00  0.00

132  1 47  1.0411     162.722  0.028     0.902     0.00778  10.127  0.00  0.00  0.00  0.00  0.0000264  0.00   0.00  0.0000264  0.00  0.00  0.00  0.00  0.00
133  1 47  1.0511     151.254  0.026     0.900     0.00736   9.632  0.00  0.00  0.00  0.00  0.0000270  0.00   0.00  0.0000270  0.00  0.00  0.00  0.00  0.00
134  -e
```

Fig. 6. Partial view of quantitative trait loci (QTL) mapping results stored in *Genetics-01-WZ-Data.qrt* file created in the CIM analysis for *Genetics-01-WZ-Data.mcd* source data file. The *left column* of *numbers* shown here does not belong to the output file created by Windows QTL Cartographer. This column was included here only to facilitate referring to each line's explanations in the text.

The results of CIM analysis are stored in *Genetics-01-WZ-Data-C.qrt* (partially shown in Fig. 6). All lines starting with the symbol "#" provide explanatory comments. All lines starting with the symbol "–" provide information about the user-defined values chosen for the CIM analysis. The meaning of each line (Fig. 6), ignoring blank lines, from top to bottom is:

Line 1: gives the version of Windows QTL Cartographer software.

Line 2: shows the number of traits, their names and average values. In our example, we analyzed one trait (`tnum`= 1) whose name is `Trait_1` and it has mean 0.016470. If more than one trait is analyzed together, their names and means will appear in this line.

Line 3: shows the total number of chromosomes analyzed (`cnum`= 1 in our example).

Line 4: shows the name of the chromosome (`C1`), the total of markers in `C1`, and the name of each marker immediately followed by its map position in centiMorgan. If more than one chromosome is analyzed together, their names, number of markers, names of markers, and their positions will be all shown.

Line 5: shows the genome-wide threshold entered in the `Threshold (LR)` box. If the permutation test is used to compute the empirical threshold, the estimated threshold will be shown here (see Note 12).

Line 6: shows the number of continuous traits (`mtraits`=−1 in our example).

Line 7: shows the number of categorical traits in the source data file (`otraits`= 0 in our example).

Line 8: shows the mating design. The *Drosophila* experiment has a somewhat unique design similar to a backcross in terms of recombination process, so `cross`= B2 is chosen (see Note 1).

Line 9: shows an explanation regarding the manner in which the QTL mapping is carried out. Windows QTL Cartographer carries out the analysis from the left end to the right end of the chromosome. This line also defines the beginning of results for each trait. Had we analyzed more than one trait together, line 9 through line "`-e`" would have contained the results of the first trait, followed by results of other traits one-by-one.

Line 10: shows `window size` to block out cofactors. In our analysis, `window size`= 2 cM.

Line 11: shows the number of control markers according to Subheading 3.1.4, step 7.1. In our analysis, we accepted the default number of control markers, which is five, so `background`= 5. Notice that since we chose `Forward & Backward Method` of automatic selection of cofactor markers, this information is meaningless.

Line 12: shows the procedure that was chosen for automatic selection of cofactor markers according to step 7.1 of the CIM procedure. The possibilities are `Model 1`, `2`, and `6`, for `forward`, `backward`, and `forward & backward` (stepwise), respectively. In our example, we chose `forward & backward model` method, so `Model`= 6.

Line 13: indicates the trait for which the results are shown bellow. In our example, the following lines of results refer to `Trait_1`, so `trait`= 1.

Line 14: shows the mating design from which the data were collected.

Lines 15–21: provide explanatory comments of the test statistic. Windows QTL Cartographer uses the LRT statistic to assess the strength of competing hypotheses.

Line 22: specifies the headers of all columns in the output of QTL mapping displayed from line 23 (start "`-s`") through line 134 (end "`-e`"). Before describing the meaning of each header (Table 2), we will briefly comment on the statistical models evaluated in the CIM analysis. Depending on the mating design, CIM evaluates and tests up to four models (Table 3). `Model 0` is the model without QTL effects, `Model 1` has only the additive effect of a putative QTL, `Model 2` has only the dominance effect of a putative QTL, and `Model 3` has both the additive and dominance effects of a putative QTL.

Table 2
Description of headers shown in the output file (file with *qrt* extension) of the CIM analysis in Windows QTL Cartographer for F_2 design

Header	Description
`c`	Displays the chromosome
`m`	Displays the marker
`position`	Displays the testing position of the putative QTL
`H0:H3`	Displays the LRT statistic from the test of H0: `Model 0` vs. H3: `Model 3`
`H1:H3`	Displays the LRT statistic from the test of H1: `Model 1` vs. H3: `Model 3`
`H2:H3`	Displays the LRT statistic from the test of H2: `Model 2` vs. H3: `Model 3`
`H1:a`	Displays the estimated value of the parameter *a* in `Model 1`
`H3:a`	Displays the estimated value of the parameter *a* in `Model 3`
`H2:d`	Displays the estimated value of the parameter *d* in `Model 2`
`H3:d`	Displays the estimated value of the parameter *d* in `Model 3`
`H0:H1`	Displays the LRT statistic from the test of H0: `Model 0` vs. H1: `Model 1`
`H0:H2`	Displays the LRT statistic from the test of H0: `Model 0` vs. H2: `Model 2`
`R2(0:1)`	Displays the partial R^2 statistic of `Model 1` due to parameter *a*
`R2(0:2)`	Displays the partial R^2 statistic of `Model 2` due to parameter *d*
`R2(0:3)`	Displays the partial R^2 statistic of `Model 3` due to parameters *a* and *d*
`TR2(0:1)`	Displays the total R^2 statistic of `Model 1`
`TR2(0:2)`	Displays the total R^2 statistic of `Model 2`
`TR2(0:3)`	Displays the total R^2 statistic of `Model 3`
`S1`	Test statistic for the normality of residuals under H1
`S2`	Test statistic for the normality of residuals under H2
`S3`	Test statistic for the normality of residuals under H3

For backcross, recombinant inbred lines, and double haploids, some headers are omitted, because only Model 0 and Model 1 are generated and compared

Table 3
Set of statistical models evaluated in the CIM analysis for F_2 design

Model 0	$y_i = \mu + \sum_{r=1}^{m} \beta_r x_{ir} + e_i$	Model 2	$y_i = \mu + z_{i2} d + \sum_{r=1}^{m} x_{ir} \beta_r + e_i$
Model 1	$y_i = \mu + z_{i1} a + \sum_{r=1}^{m} x_{ir} \beta_r + e_i$	Model 3	$y_i = \mu + z_{i1} a + z_{i2} d + \sum_{r=1}^{m} x_{ir} \beta_r + e_i$

For backcross, recombinant inbred lines, and double haploids, only Model 0 and Model 1 are generated and compared

```
#       634333548    -filetype SRmapqtl.out
# # QTL Cartographer v. 1.17e, 27 August 2003
# This output file (tmp.00r) was created by SRmapqtl...
# # It is 11:31:37 on Monday, 15 March 2010
# # # -FB Stepwise regression analysis for -trait 1
# 1 DOF in the numerator: The given DOF is for the denominator...
-----------------------------------------------------
-----------------------------------------------------
Chromosome    Marker      Rank          F-Stat      DOF
-----------------------------------------------------
-start
         1         1          5       130.12862          694
         1         7          8        37.17713          691
         1         9         15         3.31632          684
         1        10          6        95.32538          693
         1        11         12         8.65186          687
         1        13         14         3.66299          685
         1        14          1       741.53049          699
         1        17         11         8.03209          688
         1        27          3       283.05222          696
         1        31         10        11.34360          689
         1        38          7        44.78586          692
         1        40         16         3.09561          683
         1        42          2       640.96327          697
         1        45         13         7.07641          686
         1        46          4       183.14817          695
         1        48          9        16.63661          690
-end
-----------------------------------------------------
-----------------------------------------------------
```

Fig. 7. View of cofactor selection results stored in *Cofactor.txt* file created in the CIM analysis of *Genetics-01-WZ-Data.mcd* source data file. From *left* to *right*, the first column identifies the chromosomes in which the selected cofactor markers shown in the second column are located. The third column shows the rank of each cofactor marker according to the order of the marker picked up in the forward regression analysis. The fourth column shows the *F*-statistic for the test of markers. The last column shows the degrees of freedom in the denominator of the *F*-statistic.

Notice that some of the headers described in Table 2 do not appear on line 22 of the result file from the analysis of *Genetics-01-WZ-Data.mcd* source data file (Fig. 6) as the data are from recombinant inbred lines (modeled as a backcross population). Therefore, only the estimate of additive effect is feasible. If the data were from an intercross F_2, both additive and dominance effects would have been estimated, and all headers would have been shown in the result file.

The results of cofactor selection through `Forward & Backward Method` (Subheading 3.1.4, step 7) are shown in Fig. 7.

A partial view of results from the empirical estimation of the genome-wide threshold through the permeation method is shown in Fig. 8. The permutation test is carried out as follows: check `By Permutations`, enter the total number of permutations (`N`) in the `Permutation Times` box, leave the `Significance Level` box with its default value of 0.05, and click `OK`. The program will store results in a file named **-C-all-pm.txt*, in which "*" represents the name of the *mcd* file. For instance, for *mydata.mcd*, "*" is *mydata*, and the results are stored in *mydata-C-all-pm.txt*. The output file has two columns and `N` rows. The first column shows the number

1	17.36
2	16.77
3	14.87
4	14.59
5	13.35
6	12.93
7	12.70
8	12.56
9	12.24
10	12.21
⋮	⋮
99	7.04
100	7.03
101	7.02
⋮	⋮
999	0.53
1000	0.52

Fig. 8. Partial view of results from empirical estimation of genome-wide threshold through permutation method in the CIM analysis of *Genetics-01-WZ-Data.mcd* source data file. The *left column* identifies the number of permutation tests and the *right column* shows the maximum of the logarithm likelihood ratio test (LRT) statistic in decreasing order.

of permutation tests (1, 2,. . ., `N`) and the second column shows the ordered values of the maximum LRT statistic for each permutation test. The threshold for a given genome-wide significance level α is the value in the second column for which the value in the first column closely matches the value $p = N\alpha$. For $N = 1{,}000$ and $\alpha = 0.1$, $p = 100$, and the estimated threshold is 7.03 in LRT units (Fig. 8).

In Fig. 9, we show the linkage map representing chromosome 2 of *D. melanogaster*. This linkage map was built with the data of distance between markers available in the *Genetics-01-WZ-Data.mcd* source data file. In the linkage map, we identified (vertical arrows) the position of all cofactor markers automatically selected in the `Forward and Backward` method. In order to fix ideas on how cofactors and `window size` are interrelated to each other in the CIM analysis, we also show (horizontal arrows) the `window size` in the left and right sides of a hypothetical putative QTL (indicated by a star). All selected cofactor markers, except cofactor markers *50D1*, *52A1*, and *56B7* within either the left or right `window size` of the putative QTL, will be included in the CIM model of the putative QTL identified by the star. It is important to

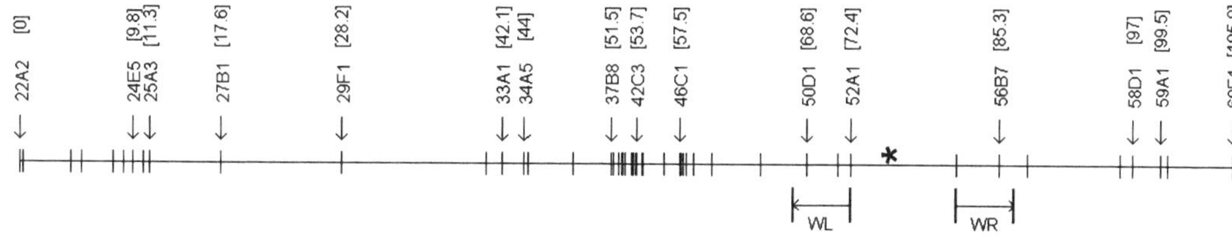

Fig. 9. Linkage map of chromosome 2 of *Drosophila melanogaster*. This linkage map was built with data of distance between markers available in the *Genetics-01-WZ-Data.mcd* source data file. Tight linkage between some markers (ticks in the *horizontal line*) in the chromosome limits graphing their names and positions in a readable manner. Therefore, we indicate only the cofactor markers (selected from our analysis and indicated by *vertical arrows*) with their respective names and positions (in *square brackets*). A hypothetical putative QTL is indicated by a *star* above the *horizontal line*. `Window size` on both *left* (WL) and *right* (WR) sides of the markers flanking the putative QTL is shown. Cofactor markers *50D1*, *52A1*, and *56B7* are located within the `window size` of the hypothetical putative QTL.

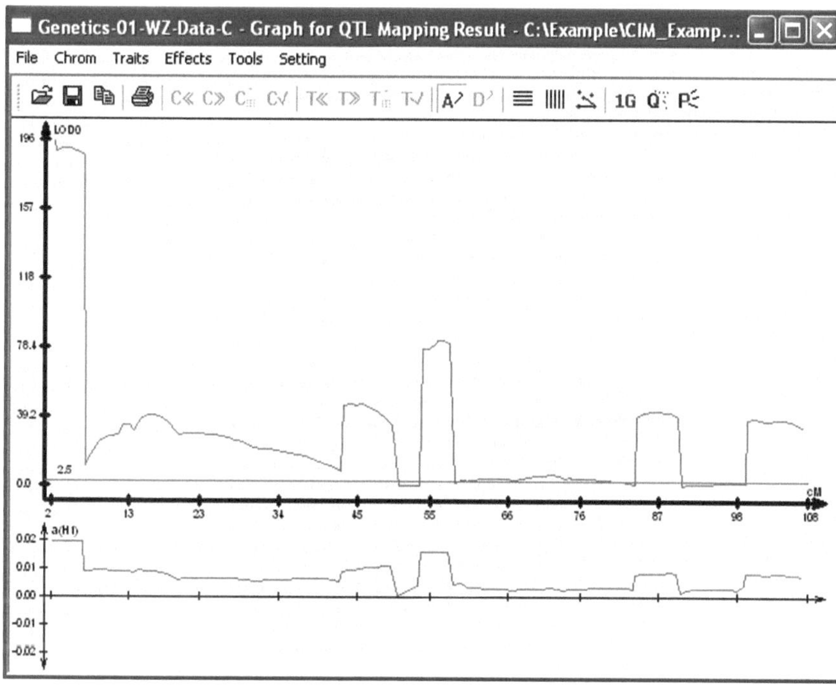

Fig. 10. View of default graph window displaying QTL mapping results from CIM analysis of *Genetics-01-WZ-Data.mcd* source data file. This graph shows logarithm of odds (LOD) profile along the chromosome (*upper panel*) and estimated effects of putative QTL (*lower panel*). The *horizontal line* running across the LOD profile in the *upper panel* represents the threshold computed by the permutation method (see Note 12 for details on how to plot the correct threshold). In the menu of this graph window, there are several user-defined options that enable the user to redefine the displaying of QTL mapping.

understand that all putative QTL within the same marker interval have the same cofactor markers in their CIM models, while putative QTL in distinct intervals may or may not have the same cofactor markers in their CIM models.

Figure 10 shows the default graph window displaying the LOD profile from the CIM analysis of the *Genetics-01-WZ-Data.mcd*

Table 4
Estimated positions, effects, LOD, and LOD-1.5 support interval of QTL mapped in the CIM analysis of *Genetics-01-WZ-Data.mcd* source data file

QTL	Position[a]	Additive effect[b] (100×)	LOD[c]	LOD-1.5 support interval[d] (cM)
1	0	1.88	195.97	0–0.2
2	14.3	0.87	40.40	12.3–16.3
3	43.1	0.99	46.82	40.2–44.3
4	54.2	1.52	82.62	53.5–56.1
5	84.6	0.84	42.72	81.6–87.3
6	98.0	0.82	38.56	96.9–105.1

Numeric values shown in this table were retrieved from the *Genetics-01-WZ-Data.qrt* file
[a] Distance (cM) from the QTL to the left end of chromosome. Results were collected from third column of the *Genetics-01-WZ-Data.qrt* file
[b] Results were collected from seventh column of the *Genetics-01-WZ-Data.qrt* file and multiplied by 10^2
[c] LRT values in forth column of the *Genetics-01-WZ-Data.qrt* file were converted to LOD (see Note 5)
[d] LOD-1.5 support interval for QTL position (see Note 13)

source data file. Peaks in the graph above the threshold (horizontal line running across the graph of LOD) give good evidence of the presence of QTLs. The threshold controls how high or low the horizontal line sits on the graph. If it is too high, no QTL may be found; if it is too low, many QTL may be found, a portion of which may be false QTL. As already mentioned (Table 1), the 10% significance level threshold (7.03 in LRT scale or equivalently 1.5 in LOD scale) was computed by the permutation method. Figure 10 clearly shows that almost every position in the chromosome has LOD larger than the threshold at significance level of 10%. However, six regions in the chromosome stand out with higher LOD peaks. Therefore, we have stronger statistical evidence for QTL affecting the wing size index of *D. melanogaster* in these six regions. Upon having identified these regions harboring QTL, we summarize (Table 4) estimates of QTL positions, effects, and LOD-1.5 support interval for QTL position, which has a confidence level close to 95% (5) (see Note 13 for more details on LOD support interval).

3.2. MIM Procedure

3.2.1. MIM Statistical Model

As previously mentioned in the introduction, the rationale of MIM is to fit estimated positions of other QTL as covariates in the model when testing for a putative QTL, thereby delivering more power as well as better parameter estimates when compared to CIM, which fits closely linked markers to other QTL as covariates. Furthermore, since MIM can fit multiple QTL, it allows for modeling interaction (epistasis). The general MIM statistical model can be written as:

$$y_i = \mu + \sum_{r=1}^{m} Z_{ir} B_r + \sum_{r<k}^{p} x_{irk} w_{rk} + e_i$$

where y_i is the phenotypic trait value of subject i; μ is the overall mean; B_r is a column vector with the effects of putative QTL r, which depends on the mating design; Z_{ir} is a row vector of predictor variables corresponding to the effects of putative QTL r; x_{irk} is a predictor variable referring to the epistatic effect between QTL pair r and k; w_{rk} is the epistatic effect between QTL pair r and k; and e_i is the random error that is assumed to follow a normal distribution with mean zero and variance σ^2. As an example, consider an intercross F_2 population where subject i could have either genotype QQ, Qq or qq for a putative QTL. Also consider a parameterization of additive and dominance effects of QTL r as a_r and d_r, respectively (9, 13, 16). Therefore, $B_r = (a_r, d_r)^{\mathrm{T}}$ (the superscript "T" stands for transpose),

$$Z_{ir} = (z_{ir1}, z_{ir2}) = \begin{cases} (1, -0.5) & \text{if subject } i \text{ has genotype QQ for QTL } r \\ (0, 1) & \text{if subject } i \text{ has genotype Qq for QTL } r \\ (-1, -0.5) & \text{if subject } i \text{ has genotype qq for QTL } r \end{cases}$$

and

$$x_{irk} = \begin{cases} z_{ir1} z_{ik1} & \text{if subject } i \text{ is homozygous for both QTL } r \text{ and } k \\ z_{ir1} z_{ik2} & \text{if subject } i \text{ is homozygous for QTL } r \text{ and heterozygous for } k \\ z_{ir2} z_{ik1} & \text{if subject } i \text{ is heterozygous for QTL } r \text{ and homozygous for } k \\ z_{ir2} z_{ik2} & \text{if subject } i \text{ is heterozygous for both QTL } r \text{ and } k \end{cases}$$

Hypotheses regarding parameters in the MIM model can be formulated and tested with the score statistic or logarithm of LRT, which has a one to one mathematical correspondence with the LOD, which is LRT $= 2 \log_e(10)$LOD $\approx$4.6 LOD.

3.2.2. MIM Genome-Wide Threshold

While the permutation-based threshold (14, 15) is suitable to assess the significance level of the QTL effect in models that fit one QTL only, such as the IM and CIM models, it is not so appropriate to assess significance level of QTL effects in models that fit multiple QTL. On the other hand, the score-based threshold (17) has been shown to be suitable for assessing significance level of QTL effects in models with multiple QTL (Laurie, Wang, Carlini-Garcia, and Zeng, unpublished data; (18)). We can select putative QTL and refine the model, by including or excluding QTL effects, all based on their statistical significances assessed through the score-based method. The MIM procedure in Windows QTL Cartographer 2.51 has the score-based threshold implemented for QTL mapping for the backcross mating design. For other mating designs, the MIM procedure offers Bayesian information criterion (BIC)-based and Akaike's information criterion (AIC)-based criteria of model selection (see Note 14 for more details).

3.2.3. MIM Procedure in Windows QTL Cartographer

Windows QTL Cartographer contains a comprehensive implementation of the MIM procedure. In what follows, we split the MIM procedure into two parts. In the first part we describe the MIM procedure step-by-step. In the second part (in Subheading 3.2.4), we discuss the consequences of each option in the analysis and how to understand and interpret results through a worked-out example.

It is worth emphasizing again that all statistical analyses in Windows QTL Cartographer must be run on an *mcd* source data file. Windows QTL Cartographer provides default values for all user-defined options in the MIM procedure; but keep in mind that these default values are meant only to provide the best all-around parameter settings to begin with. In what follows, we will go through the MIM procedure step-by-step.

1. Open the *mcd* source data file into Windows QTL Cartographer main window.
2. Start the MIM procedure by selecting `Method` in the menu and then `Multiple Interval Mapping`. If the source data file contains more than one continuous trait, then a window will be displayed (Fig. 11), in which the user can choose a trait for analysis. Otherwise, Windows QTL Cartographer will go straight to the MIM analysis window (Fig. 12).

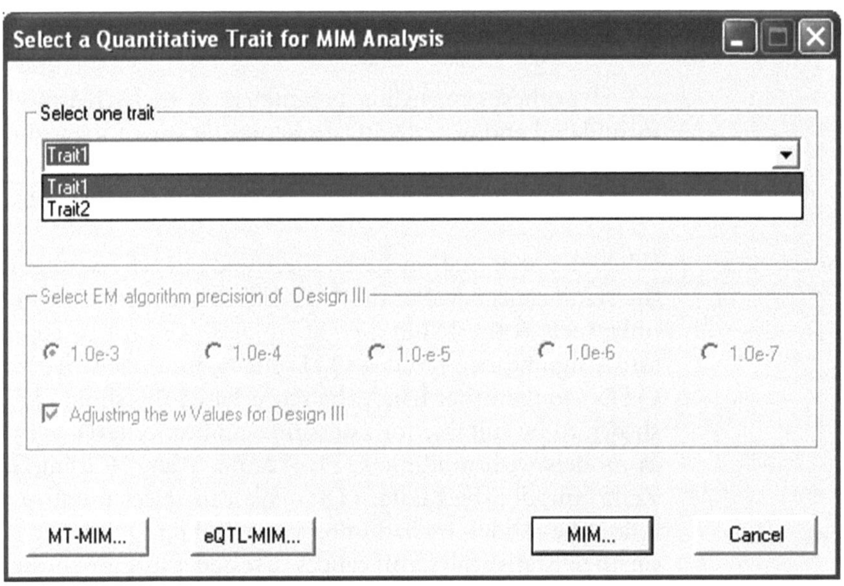

Fig. 11. Window displayed at the beginning of multiple intervals mapping (MIM) analysis if a source data file contains two or more continuous traits. The user chooses a trait in the `Select one trait` drop-down list and clicks on `MIM` to start the analysis.

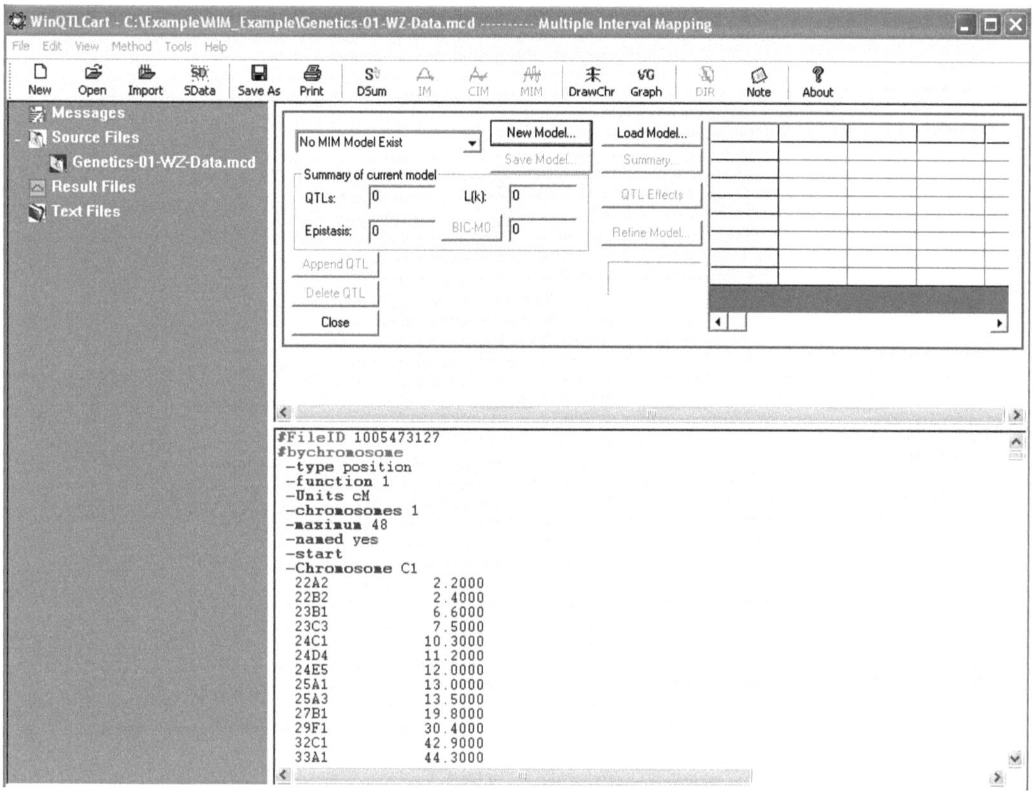

Fig. 12. MIM procedure window. Buttons and boxes in this window are user-defined options.

3. Build an initial MIM model either (1) upon a priori model (e.g., a model from CIM analysis) or (2) from scratch. Click on `New Model` and the `Create New MIM Model` window will appear (Fig. 13), then:
   1. To build an MIM model upon a priori model, check `Scan through QTL mapping result file` option and click on `Criterion`. In the newly opened window, define a set of criteria for uploading QTL from a priori model and click on `Open QTL Result File` to open the priori model saved on a *qrt* file. Finally, the uploaded QTL will be displayed on the `Parameters of the initial MIM model` field.
   2. To build an MIM model from scratch, check one of the four options in the `Initial MIM model selection method` field:

      (i) `Regression forward selection on markers`, (ii) `Regression backward selection on markers`, and (iii) `Forward and Backward selection on markers`, all use regression on markers to create an initial model, and they require additional information passed on through the `Criterion` button (see Table 5); once the additional

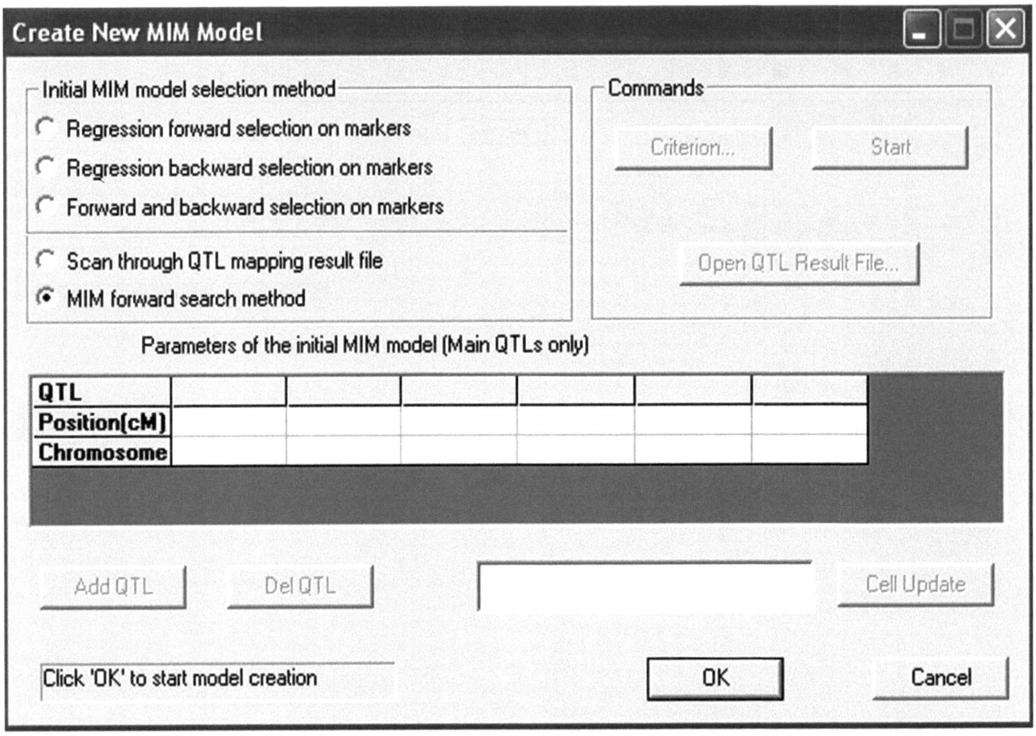

Fig. 13. `Create New MIM Model` window. This window contains three fields: `Initial MIM model selection method`, `Commands`, and `Parameter of the initial MIM model (Main QTLs only)`. Buttons and boxes in this window are user-defined options.

Table 5
Information passed on to options in the `Initial MIM model selection method` field

Options in the `Initial MIM model selection method` field	Information passed on to options `Initial MIM model selection method` field	Information passed on through button
Regression forward selection on markers	Criterion of model selection: BIC related criteria or Probability of partial R^2	Criterion
Regression backward selection on markers	Criterion of model selection: BIC related criteria or Probability of partial R^2	Criterion
Forward and backward selection on markers	Criterion of model selection: BIC related criteria or Probability of partial R^2	Criterion
Scan through QTL mapping result file	A priori QTL mapping results (e.g., a model from CIM analysis)	Open QTL Result File
MIM forward search method	Criterion of model selection and grid of positions (walk speed)	OK

information is declared, click on `Start` to build an initial model; the chromosomes and positions of QTL in the model will be displayed on the `Parameter of the initial MIM model` field.

Once an initial model is loaded on `Parameter of the initial MIM model`, additional QTL can be added by clicking on `Add QTL`. Likewise, undesirable QTL can be excluded by selecting them and clicking on `Del QTL`. Once the initial MIM model has been created, click on `OK` to continue the MIM analysis.

(iv) `MIM forward selection method` builds an initial model using forward selection on a grid of positions. Statistical significance of QTL effects selected on the forward selection is assessed through a model selection criterion (BIC-based, AIC-based, or score-based). Both grid of positions and model selection criterion will be available for choice after clicking on `OK`.

The initial MIM model built in this step (either built from a priori model or from scratch) will be displayed in the upper-right corner of the `MIM procedure` window (see Fig. 14). The user can, at any time, append (by clicking on `Append QTL`), delete (by selecting a QTL and clicking on `Delete QTL`), or edit QTL in the MIM model. To edit a QTL, click over the parameter to be updated in the upper-right corner

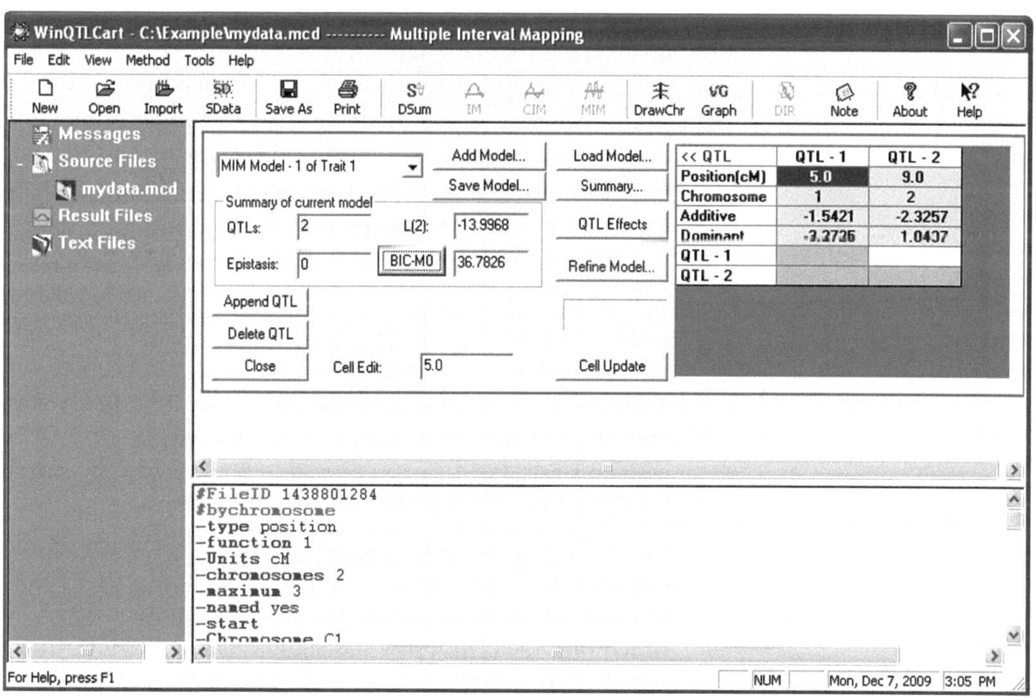

Fig. 14. Illustrative initial MIM model with two QTL (*upper-right corner table*) displayed in the MIM procedure window.

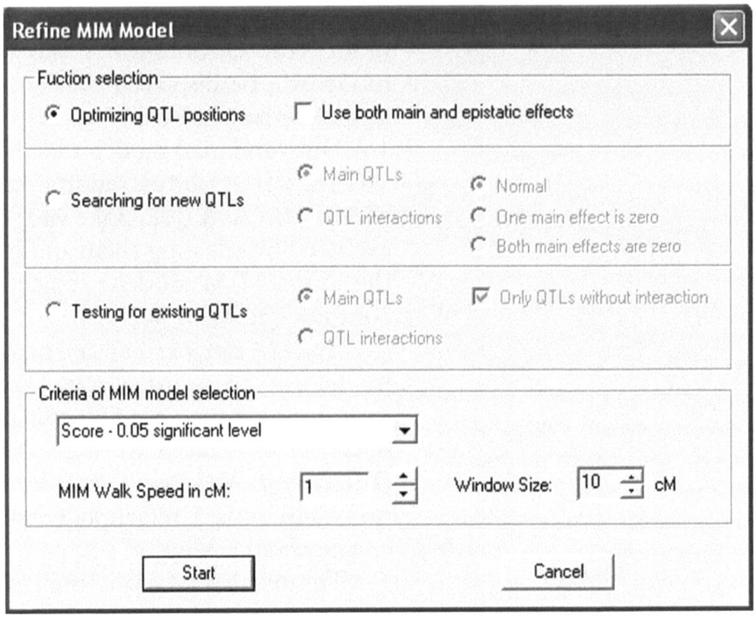

Fig. 15. Refine MIM model window with user-defined options.

table (blue cell indicates a selected parameter), enter the new parameter value in `Cell Edit`, then click `Cell Update`. Lastly, MIM models can be stored in *mds* files (by clicking on `Save Model`) and uploaded at any time (by clicking on `Load Model`).

4. Iterative MIM model refinement. Click on `Refine Model`, and the `Refine MIM model` window of user-defined options will be displayed (Fig. 15). Three main options of model refinement will be available, from which an option is chosen at a time:

   1. `Optimizing QTL positions`: adjusts positions of QTL with either main or epistatic effects if the `Use both main and epistatic effects` option is checked, otherwise only positions of QTL with main effects are adjusted. After all adjustments are made, effects of all QTL are updated accordingly (see Note 15).

   2. `Searching for new QTLs`: searches for new QTL with only main effects if `Main QTLs` is checked, or new QTL with epistasis if `QTL interactions` is checked. The search for QTL interactions has three modalities:

      (i) `Normal` searches for epistasis among QTL with significant main effects already in the model; (ii) `One main effect is zero` searches for pairs of epistatic QTL in which one QTL in a pair has significant main effect and is already in the model (1D search); (iii) `Both main effects are zero` searches for pairs of epistatic QTL in which neither QTL in a pair has significant main effect (2D search).

New QTL from the search are automatically included in the MIM model if they have significant effects assessed by a predefined criterion in the `Criteria of MIM model selection` drop-down list. Otherwise, Windows QTL Cartographer will display a message asking either to confirm or to decline the inclusion of insignificant QTL into the MIM model.

3. `Testing for existing QTLs`: tests the statistical significance of main and epistatic effects of QTL in two manners: (i) if `Main QTLs` and `Only QTLs without interaction` are checked, only main effects of QTL without epistasis are tested, otherwise main effects of QTL with interaction will be tested as well; (ii) if `QTL interaction` is checked, only epistatic effects are tested.

Next, upon having chosen either options (2) or (3), select a criterion of model selection in the `Criteria of MIM model selection` drop-down list, which includes BIC-based, AIC-based, and score-based criteria (see Note 14). Then, choose a grid of positions for search in the `MIM Walk Speed in cM` spin dial box. Finally, use the `Window Size` spin dial box to define a no search region surrounding all estimated QTL already in the model (see Note 16 for more details), and click on `Start` to begin the model refinement. MIM models can be refined many times until a final model is built, usually in the order: (1) search for QTL, (2) test QTL effects, and (3) optimize QTL position; however, some rules may apply (see Table 6).

Table 6
Some rules to follow when refining an MIM model

Refining action	Rule
`Optimizing QTL positions`	`The Use both main and epistatic effects option should always be checked if QTL interactions were included in the model through either One main effect is zero or Both main effects are zero options. This will allow adjustment of positions of all QTL, regardless of their effect type (main or epistatic)`
`Testing for existing QTLs`	`Always test QTL interactions before testing main effects. This will avoid exclusion of QTL with insignificant main effects but with significant interactions`
	The `Only QTL without interaction` option should always be checked when testing for `Main QTLs` if QTL interactions were included in the model through either *One main effect is zero* or `Both main effects are zero` options. This will avoid exclusion of QTL with insignificant main effects but with significant interactions

Statistical significance of QTL effects can be evaluated at any time when performing model refinement, and this is essential because one can make sure all QTL effects included in the model are important. To do that, click on `QTL Effects` to compute and to visualize the LRT for each QTL effect in the model. The results will be displayed in the MIM procedure window as well as stored in the *qtltestall.txt* file within the current working directory. This file will be listed in the left side of the Windows QTL Cartographer main window and its content can be viewed at any time by clicking over the file name.

We want to mention that the search for new epistatic QTL without a statistically significant main effect uses the score-based method, and it is available only for backcross in Windows QTL Cartographer 2.51. Score-based thresholds to assess significance of QTL effects on other mating designs are currently under development. Nevertheless, BIC-based and AIC-based criteria are available for model selection in other mating designs.

5. Create output files with QTL mapping results and summaries. Click on `Summary` to both save the results of MIM analysis (**.qrt* file) and create a summary of mapping analysis (**.txt* file), where "*" is a string concatenation of the name of the *mcd* source data file, and trait in analysis, and current MIM model. For instance, for a source file named *mydata.mcd*, trait *t1* in analysis, and current MIM model *md1*, the *txt* file is named *mydata-sum-t1-md1.txt* and the *qrt* file is named *mydata-mim-t1-md1.qrt*. Once created, these files will be listed in the left side of the Windows QTL Cartographer main window and their content can be viewed at any time by clicking over the file name. In the worked-out example section, we explain the meaning of results in these files.
6. Exit the MIM procedure by clicking on `Close`.

3.2.4. A Worked-Out MIM Analysis in Windows QTL Cartographer

In this section, we run MIM analysis on data from the experiment with *D. melanogaster* (12) described in Subheading 2.2. This *Drosophila* experiment has a somewhat unique design similar to a backcross in terms of recombination process, so we treat it as backcross mating design in the MIM analysis and adopt the score-based threshold to assess significance level of QTL effects.

In what follows, we first carefully detail the reasons why each user-defined option was chosen, and then we explain the outputs of the MIM analysis in detail. User-defined options to create an initial MIM model are shown in Table 7, MIM model refinements to build a final MIM model are shown in Table 8, and results are shown thereafter.

Table 7
User-defined options used to create an initial MIM model for *Genetics-01-WZ-Data.mcd* source data file

User-defined option	Value	Reasons
`Initial MIM model selection method`	`MIM forward search method`	The MIM forward search method is recommended because it can be more powerful than the other counterpart options
`Criteria of MIM model selection`	Score—0.10 genome-wide significance level	Why score? First reason: Desirable model selection criteria are those that can select the best model among their counterparts by assigning a meaningful measure of quality. The score-based threshold (17) has been shown to be suitable for assessing the significance level of QTL effects in models with multiple QTL (Laurie, Wang, Carlini-Garcia, and Zeng, unpublished data; (18)). We can select putative QTL and refine the model by including or excluding QTL effects, all based on their statistical significance assessed through the score-based method. On the other hand, while Akaike's information criterion (AIC)-based and Bayesian information criterion (BIC)-based model selection criteria can also be used to select models with a variety of QTL effects, these criteria provide relative measures of model fit, rather than measures of the significance levels of individual QTL effects in the model. Second reason: The MIM procedure in Windows QTL Cartographer 2.51 has the score-based threshold implemented for QTL mapping for a backcross mating design. This *Drosophila* experiment has a somewhat unique design similar to a backcross in terms of recombination process, so we treat it as backcross mating design in the MIM analysis and adopt the score-based threshold to assess significance level of QTL effects
`Criteria of MIM model selection`	Score—0.10 genome-wide significance level	Why 0.10 (10%) genome-wide significance level? Recent results (Laurie, Wang, Carlini-Garcia, and Zeng, unpublished data; (18)) suggest that more liberal genome-wide significance levels may be used for detecting QTL without compromising the number of false positives. Therefore, the genome-wide significance of 10% was chosen rather than the usual 1 or 5%
`MIM search walk speed in cM`	1	The data contains information only on chromosome 2 of *D. melanogaster*. Therefore, the grid of positions every 1 cM produces a QTL map with good resolution while still allowing for fast analysis. For long genomes, higher grid values are recommended if the speed of the analysis is an issue

Results of QTL mapping are stored in *Genetics-01-WZ-Data-mim-t1-md1.qrt* (partially shown in Fig. 16), results of significance tests for all QTL effects are stored in *qtltestall.txt* (Fig. 17), and QTL mapping summaries (estimates of QTL positions, main and interaction effects, variance–covariance matrix of QTL effects,

Table 8
MIM model refinement rounds to build a final MIM model for *Genetics-01-WZ-Data.mcd* source data file

Rounds	Action[a]	Reason
1	Searching for QTL with main effects (the option `Main QTLs` was checked)	To search for possibly statistically significant main effect QTL not identified in the initial forward selection
2	Searching for QTL with main effects (the option `Main QTLs` was checked)	Since a statistically significant main effect QTL was found in round 1, we proceeded to search for possibly more statistically significant main effect QTL
3	Searching for QTL with main effects (the option `Main QTLs` was checked)	Since a statistically significant main effect QTL was found in round 2, we proceeded to search for possibly more statistically significant main effect QTL
4	Searching for pairs of epistatic QTL among QTL with main effects already in the model (the option `Normal` was checked)	Since no statistically significant main effect QTL was found in round 3, we switched to searching for pairs of interacting QTL among existing QTL in the model
5	Testing epistasis effects (the option `QTL interactions` was checked)	Since a pair of interacting QTL was found in round 4, we tested the interaction effect to guarantee that effects included in the model were all statistically significant
6	Searching for pairs of epistatic QTL in which only one QTL in a pair is already in the model (the option `One main effect is zero` was checked)	Since the pair of interacting QTL found in round 4 and tested in round 5 was statistically significant, we switched to searching for pairs of interacting QTL for which only one QTL in a pair was already in the model (1D search)
7	Testing epistasis effects (the option `QTL interactions` was checked)	Since pairs of interacting QTL were found in round 6, we tested their interaction effects to guarantee that effects included in the model are all statistically significant
8	Testing main effects of QTL without interaction (the option `Only QTLs without interaction` was checked)	Since interaction effects of QTL pairs found in round 6 and tested in round 7 were not statistically significant, we tested their main effects to guarantee that effects included in the model are all statistically significant
9	Searching for pairs of epistatic QTL in which no QTL in a pair is already in the model (the option `Both main effects are zero` was checked)	Since no pairs of interacting QTL found in round 6 (1D search) held significance after testing their interaction effects in round 7, we switched to searching for pairs of interacting QTL in which neither QTL in a pair was already in the model (2D search)
10	Testing epistasis effects (the option `QTL interactions` was checked)	Since pairs of interacting QTL were found in round 9, we tested their interaction effects to guarantee that effects included in the model are all statistically significant
11	Testing main effects of QTL without interaction (the option `Only QTLs without interaction` was checked)	Since interaction effects of QTL pairs found in round 9 and tested in round 10 were not statistically significant, we tested their main effects to guarantee that effects included in the model are all statistically significant

(continued)

Table 8 (continued)

Rounds	Action[a]	Reason
12	Optimizing positions of both main and epistatic QTL (the option `Use both main and epistatic effects` was checked)	Since statistically significant QTL effects could no longer be found using all options of QTL search (QTL with main effect only, pairs of interacting QTL in which only one QTL in a pair has statistically significant main effect, pairs of interacting QTL in which neither QTL in a pair has statistically significant main effect), we stopped the search for QTL and proceeded to optimize QTL positions and to obtain the summary of QTL mapping

After an initial model was created, several model refinements rounds were necessary to build the final model, and in each round an action was taken for a given reason

[a] When searching for main effect QTL and epistatic QTL (1D and 2D searches), we set *window size* of 2 cM. The chromosome analyzed here has regions with tightly linked markers. When testing for a putative QTL in these regions, tightly linked cofactor markers to the putative QTL must be avoided; otherwise, the power of test statistic will decrease; hence the *window size* should not be too narrow. On the other hand, the analysis shows evidence of multiple close linked QTL in the chromosome; hence the *window size* should not be too wide. Therefore, a wide enough window, 2 cM, was chosen. But keep in mind that final choice of *window size* should also depend on how QTL are distributed across the chromosomes as indicated by analysis

and breeding values of subjects (10)) are stored in *Genetics-01-WZ-Data-sum-t1-md1.txt* (partially shown in Fig. 18).

Figure 19 shows the default graph window displaying the LOD profile from the MIM analysis of the *Genetics-01-WZ-Data.mcd* source data file. Nine regions in the chromosome stand out with high LOD peaks. Therefore, there is strong statistical evidence of QTL affecting the wing size index of *D. melanogaster* in these nine regions. Estimates of QTL positions, main and epistatic effects, and LOD-1.5 support interval for QTL position are summarized in Table 9, and variance–covariance matrix of QTL effects in Table 10. Summaries in both tables were retrieved from the *Genetics-01-WZ-Data-sum-t1-md1.txt* file.

4. Final Considerations

In this chapter, we introduced CIM and MIM methods of mapping QTL from inbred line crosses and presented detailed instructions to perform the analyses in Windows QTL Cartographer. Whenever there is evidence of multiple linked or unlinked QTL, either a priori or indicated by analysis, CIM and MIM are preferred over IM. MIM is more powerful than CIM in terms of QTL identification and effect estimation and also allows analysis of QTL interactions (epistasis).

```
#=# Graphic Format of Mapping Result #=#
#=# Used by Windows QTL Cartographer V2.5
#=# -s
====================================== QTL-1 ======================================
  1    2  0.0021     266.1047 0 0     0.011446 0 0 0 0 0 0 0 0 0 0 0 0 0 0 0
  1    2  0.0121     259.7751 0 0     0.011460 0 0 0 0 0 0 0 0 0 0 0 0 0 0 0
  1    2  0.0221     251.5490 0 0     0.011476 0 0 0 0 0 0 0 0 0 0 0 0 0 0 0
  1    2  0.0321     239.0735 0 0     0.011494 0 0 0 0 0 0 0 0 0 0 0 0 0 0 0
  1    4  0.0531     174.9428 0 0     0.011428 0 0 0 0 0 0 0 0 0 0 0 0 0 0 0
  1    4  0.0631     164.3973 0 0     0.011680 0 0 0 0 0 0 0 0 0 0 0 0 0 0 0
====================================== QTL-2 ======================================
  1    2  0.0021      24.4649 0 0     0.002816 0 0 0 0 0 0 0 0 0 0 0 0 0 0 0
  1    2  0.0121      27.4595 0 0     0.003670 0 0 0 0 0 0 0 0 0 0 0 0 0 0 0
  1    2  0.0221      30.1802 0 0     0.004046 0 0 0 0 0 0 0 0 0 0 0 0 0 0 0
  1    2  0.0321      32.5972 0 0     0.004212 0 0 0 0 0 0 0 0 0 0 0 0 0 0 0
  1    4  0.0531      49.7417 0 0     0.005625 0 0 0 0 0 0 0 0 0 0 0 0 0 0 0
  1    4  0.0631      64.3917 0 0     0.006397 0 0 0 0 0 0 0 0 0 0 0 0 0 0 0
  1    9  0.1131      87.5504 0 0     0.006348 0 0 0 0 0 0 0 0 0 0 0 0 0 0 0
  1    9  0.1231     101.8508 0 0     0.007165 0 0 0 0 0 0 0 0 0 0 0 0 0 0 0
  1    9  0.1331     100.7756 0 0     0.007389 0 0 0 0 0 0 0 0 0 0 0 0 0 0 0
  1    9  0.1431      94.0039 0 0     0.007472 0 0 0 0 0 0 0 0 0 0 0 0 0 0 0
  1    9  0.1531      81.5753 0 0     0.007414 0 0 0 0 0 0 0 0 0 0 0 0 0 0 0
  1    9  0.1631      61.9624 0 0     0.007088 0 0 0 0 0 0 0 0 0 0 0 0 0 0 0
====================================== QTL-3 ======================================
  1   10  0.1761      26.5440 0 0     0.003261 0 0 0 0 0 0 0 0 0 0 0 0 0 0 0
  1   10  0.1861      28.2717 0 0     0.003373 0 0 0 0 0 0 0 0 0 0 0 0 0 0 0
  1   10  0.1961      29.8808 0 0     0.003515 0 0 0 0 0 0 0 0 0 0 0 0 0 0 0
  1   10  0.2061      31.0026 0 0     0.003576 0 0 0 0 0 0 0 0 0 0 0 0 0 0 0
  1   10  0.2161      31.7885 0 0     0.003605 0 0 0 0 0 0 0 0 0 0 0 0 0 0 0
  1   10  0.2261      32.2511 0 0     0.003600 0 0 0 0 0 0 0 0 0 0 0 0 0 0 0
  1   10  0.2361      32.3979 0 0     0.003563 0 0 0 0 0 0 0 0 0 0 0 0 0 0 0
  1   10  0.2461      32.2291 0 0     0.003494 0 0 0 0 0 0 0 0 0 0 0 0 0 0 0
  1   10  0.2561      31.7377 0 0     0.003391 0 0 0 0 0 0 0 0 0 0 0 0 0 0 0
  1   10  0.2661      30.8984 0 0     0.003248 0 0 0 0 0 0 0 0 0 0 0 0 0 0 0
  1   11  0.2821      28.8252 0 0     0.002922 0 0 0 0 0 0 0 0 0 0 0 0 0 0 0
  1   11  0.2921      28.6975 0 0     0.003039 0 0 0 0 0 0 0 0 0 0 0 0 0 0 0
  1   11  0.3021      28.4721 0 0     0.003156 0 0 0 0 0 0 0 0 0 0 0 0 0 0 0
```

Fig. 16. Partial view of QTL mapping results stored in *Genetics-01-WZ-Data-mim-t1-md1.qrt* file created in the MIM analysis of *Genetics-01-WZ-Data.mcd* source data file. Descriptions of nonzero columns from left to right are (1) chromosome number; (2) marker interval number (numbers are assigned from left end to right end of each chromosome); (3) grid of positions for each chromosome with increments dictated by the user-defined option of walk speed; (4) Logarithm LRT of the null hypothesis of no QTL effect vs. the alternative of presence of QTL effect; (5) QTL effect estimate, which depends on the mating design (for backcross it is a combined estimative of additive and dominance effects, for recombinant inbred lines or double haploids or intercross F_2 it is the estimative of additive effect).

Num	QTL1	QTL2	LR	Type	Score Statistics	Score Test P-Val
1	1	X	329.0818	Additive	122.1790	0.0000
2	2	X	90.3463	Additive	63.9308	0.0000
3	3	X	32.4319	Additive	35.0691	0.0000
4	4	X	163.8891	Additive	99.8931	0.0000
5	5	X	378.9344	Additive	202.2593	0.0000
6	6	X	33.5715	Additive	26.7850	0.0000
7	7	X	99.9978	Additive	73.1020	0.0000
8	8	X	51.2423	Additive	37.1919	0.0000
9	9	X	20.9776	Additive	17.5717	0.0000
10	2	8	20.5477	AA	21.8822	0.0000

Fig. 17. View of *qtltestall.txt* file with stored statistical tests for all QTL effects in the final model of the MIM analysis of *Genetics-01-WZ-Data.mcd* source data file. The `LR` column shows the logarithm LRT for each type of QTL effect (shown on `Type` column). The `Score Test P-Val` columns show the empirical probability value from the score-based test of the null hypothesis of effect zero vs. the alternative of effect not zero. Smaller values of `Score Test P-Val` give stronger statistical evidences against the null hypothesis.

```
#    Result of MIM analysis for Model 1 of Trait 1
#
#    Windows QTL Cartographer V2.5, March 2010
#
#       It is 14:07:54 on Thursday, 06 May 2010
#
#    Multiple Interval Mapping (MIM) Model
#
#    Y = u + a(1)x(1) + ... + a(m)x(m) + b(1,2)x(1)x(2) + ... + b(m-1,m)x(m-1)x(m) + e
#
#    Y is trait value                      u is model mean
#    m is number of QTL                    a(k) is main effect of QTL k
#    -x(k) is indicate variable            b(i,j) is epistatic effect between QTL i and QTL j
#    e is residual variance
#
##########################################################################################

           Estimates of QTL positions, effects and interactions
----------------------------------------------------------------------------------------
----------------------------------------------------------------------------------------
QTL(pair)     Type     Chrom.  Marker   Position       LOD          Effect           Effect (%)
----------------------------------------------------------------------------------------
1              A        1      1         0.1000       71.41        0.0119             13.8
2              A        1      9        12.3000       19.61        0.0072             11.2
3              A        1     10        23.6000        7.04        0.0036              6.8
4              A        1     14        44.1000       35.56        0.0078             16.9
5              A        1     30        56.2000       82.23        0.0133             27.0
6              A        1     38        69.6000        7.29        0.0033              5.9
7              A        1     41        84.6000       21.70        0.0059              8.4
8              A        1     45        97.1000       11.12        0.0058              3.3
9              A        1     47       105.1000        4.55        0.0033              0.4
2 x8           AA                                       4.459       -0.0031              0.2
----------------------------------------------------------------------------------------

           This is the Variance-Covariance Matrix.

Phenotypic Variance:     0.0002709
Genetic Variance:        0.0002541
Residual Variance:       1.68e-005
-----------------------------------------------------------------------------------------------------------------------
-----------------------------------------------------------------------------------------------------------------------
QTL(s) Type    1          2          3          4          5          6          7          8          9          2x8
-----------------------------------------------------------------------------------------------------------------------
1      A   3.543e-005 3.299e-005 9.687e-006 1.797e-006 -1.163e-005 -3.355e-006 -7.106e-006 -1.124e-005 -7.258e-006 8.169e-008
2      A              1.272e-005 8.618e-006 6.917e-006  1.509e-006 -6.094e-007 -3.071e-006 -6.416e-006 -4.308e-006 -1.345e-007
3      A                         3.172e-006 7.736e-006  7.921e-006  7.875e-007 -2.282e-007  -2.14e-006 -1.581e-006 -1.531e-007
4      A                                    1.504e-005  3.922e-005  5.823e-006  4.417e-006 -1.807e-006 -2.207e-006 -3.267e-007
5      A                                                4.425e-005  1.338e-005  1.096e-005 -6.986e-007 -2.717e-006 -4.411e-007
6      A                                                            2.701e-006  6.312e-006  3.035e-006  1.011e-006 -3.006e-008
7      A                                                                        8.688e-006  1.141e-005  5.207e-006  2.017e-007
8      A                                                                                    8.432e-006  8.273e-006  3.318e-007
9      A                                                                                                 2.71e-006  1.821e-007
2x8    AA                                                                                                           5.556e-007
-----------------------------------------------------------------------------------------------------------------------
Sum        3.742e-005 3.047e-005  1.85e-005 4.582e-005     7.3e-005  1.588e-005  2.274e-005   8.81e-006  1.012e-006 4.115e-007
Total         0.0002541
***********************************************************************************************************************

           Here are the R2 values

Genetic:        0.9380
Residual:       0.0620
-----------------------------------------------------------------------------------------------------------------------
-----------------------------------------------------------------------------------------------------------------------
QTL(s) Type    1          2          3          4          5          6          7          8          9          2x8
-----------------------------------------------------------------------------------------------------------------------
1      A     0.1308     0.1218     0.0358     0.0066    -0.0429    -0.0124    -0.0262    -0.0415    -0.0268     0.0003
2      A                0.0470     0.0318     0.0255     0.0056    -0.0022    -0.0113    -0.0237    -0.0159    -0.0005
3      A                           0.0117     0.0286     0.0292     0.0029    -0.0008    -0.0079    -0.0058    -0.0006
```

Fig. 18. Partial view of QTL mapping summary stored in *Genetics-01-WZ-Data-sum-t1-md1.txt* file created in the MIM analysis of *Genetics-01-WZ-Data.mcd* source data file.

As for now, the MIM procedure in Windows QTL Cartographer allows the identification of epistatic QTL regardless of the statistical significance of their main effects only in a backcross population. Identification of epistasis in other populations is restricted to QTL with statistically significant main effects.

5. Notes

1. *Mating designs*—Examples of crosses and codes indicating the type of mating designs that can be analyzed in Windows QTL Cartographer (Table 11). The field `-Cross` in the *mcd* source file has to be filled out according to the data on hand, for instance, if your data comes from a backcross to parental line 1 (P_1), **B1** must be used.

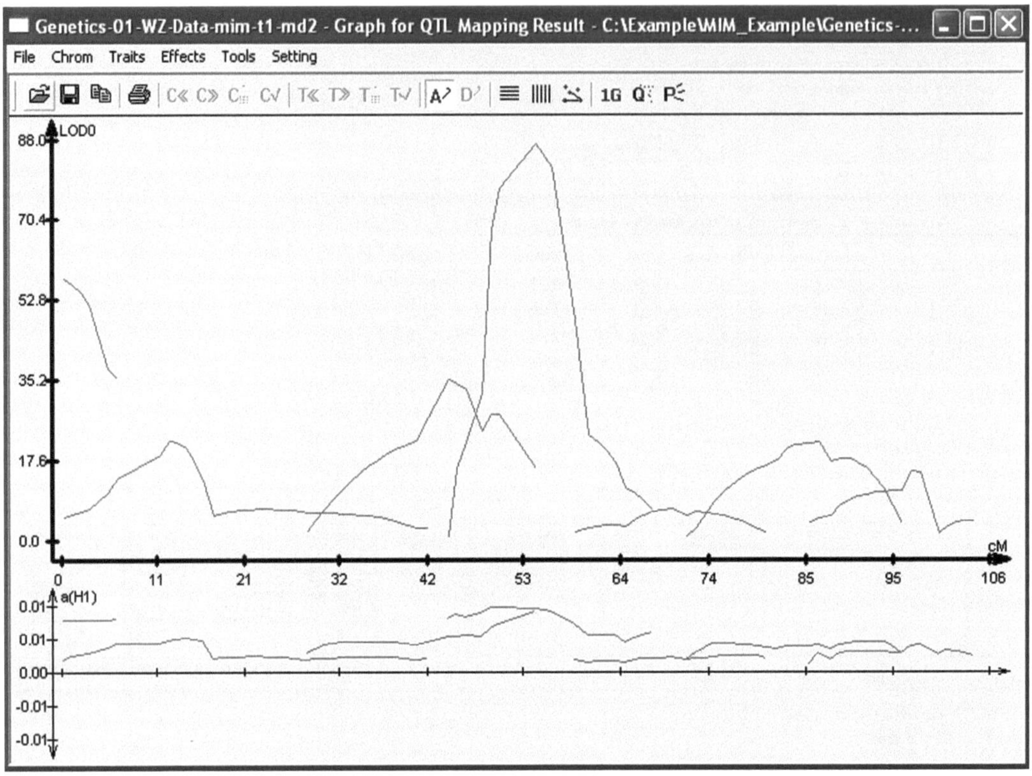

Fig. 19. View of default graph window displaying QTL mapping results from MIM analysis of *Genetics-01-WZ-Data.mcd* source data file. This graph shows LOD profile along the chromosome (*upper*) and estimated effects of putative QTL (*lower*). These results are also stored in the *Genetics-01-WZ-Data-mim-t1-md1.qrt* file. In the menu of this graph window, there are several user-defined options that enable the user to redefine the displaying of QTL mapping.

2. *Categorical traits*—Categorical traits are traits such as sex, color, race, and so on. They are coded with either numerical integer values, for instance 0, 1, 2, and so on, or character values, for instance M and F, for males and females, respectively.
3. *Translation table*—The default and an example of user-defined translation tables are shown below (Table 12). In the default translation table, from left to right, the first column shows the marker genotypes. Windows QTL Cartographer assumes that the ***A*** allele comes from the high line (parental line 1—P_1) and the ***a*** allele comes from the low line (parental line 2—P_2). Minus sign (−) means the allele is unknown (missing information). Dominant as well as codominant markers can be encoded. The second column shows how marker genotypes are output in Windows QTL Cartographer. The third column shows how marker genotypes are coded in the *mcd* source data file. The default translation table maps 2 to 2, 1 to 1, 0 to 0, etc. It is important to notice that just about any set of codes can be used in the third column (corresponding to your data), but

Table 9
Estimated positions, effects, LOD, and LOD-1.5 support interval of QTL mapped in the MIM analysis of *Genetics-01-WZ-Data.mcd* source data file

QTL (pair)	Position[a]	Effect[b] (100×)	LOD[c]	LOD-1.5 support interval[d] (cM)
1	0.1	1.19	57.8	0–2.2
2	12.3	0.70	19.6	11.3–14.3
3	23.6	0.36	7.0	17.6–35.2
4	44.1	0.78	35.6	42.1–46.3
5	56.2	1.33	82.2	50.2–58.7
6	69.6	0.33	7.3	66.5–75.4
7	84.6	0.59	21.7	81.6–87.8
8	97.1	0.58	11.1	95.9–100.1
9	105.1	0.33	4.6	100.1–105.1
(2, 8)		−0.31	4.5	

Numeric values shown in this table were retrieved from the *Genetics-01-WZ-Data-sum-t1-md1.txt* file, except LOD-1.5 support intervals, which were estimated from LRT profile in the *Genetics-01-WZ-Data-mim-t1-md1.qrt* file

[a] Distance (cM) from the QTL to the left end of chromosome

[b] QTL main and epistatic effects multiplied by 10^2

[c] LRT values were converted to LOD

[d] LOD-1.5 support interval for QTL position (see Note 13)

Table 10
Estimated variances and covariances of additive and additive-by-additive effects of QTL mapped in the MIM analysis of *Genetics-01-WZ-Data.mcd* source data file

QTL	1	2	3	4	5	6	7	8	9	(2, 8)
1	35.43	32.99	9.69	1.80	−11.63	−3.36	−7.11	−11.24	−7.26	0.08
2	0	12.72	8.62	6.92	1.51	−0.61	−3.07	−6.42	−4.31	−0.13
3	0	0	3.17	7.74	7.92	0.79	−0.23	−2.14	−1.58	−0.15
4	0	0	0	15.04	39.22	5.82	4.42	−1.81	−2.21	−0.33
5	0	0	0	0	44.25	13.38	10.96	−0.70	−2.72	−0.44
6	0	0	0	0	0	2.70	6.31	3.04	1.01	−0.03
7	0	0	0	0	0	0	8.69	11.41	5.21	0.20
8	0	0	0	0	0	0	0	8.43	8.27	0.33
9	0	0	0	0	0	0	0	0	2.71	0.18
(2, 8)	0	0	0	0	0	0	0	0	0	0.56

Numeric values shown in this table were retrieved from the *Genetics-01-WZ-Data-sum-t1-md1.txt* file and are multiplied by 10^6

Table 11
Examples of crosses and codes indicating mating design types that can be analyzed in Windows QTL Cartographer

General code formula	Mating design	Examples of codes
B_i	Backcross to P_i ($i = 1$ or 2)	$B1 = F_1 \times P_1$, $B2 = F_1 \times P_2$
B_{it}	Repeated backcross i ($i = 1$ or 2) t times to P_i ($i = 1, 2$)	$B12 = B_1 \times P_1$; $B13 = B_{12} \times P_1$; $B13 = P_1 \times B_{13}$;...
SF_t	Advanced intercross by selfing t times ($t = 2, 3,\ldots$)	$SF2 = F_1 \times F_1$; $SF3 = F_2 \times F_2$; $SF4 = F_3 \times F_3$;...
RF_t	Advanced intercross by random mating t times ($t = 2, 3,\ldots$)	RF2, RF3, RF4,...
RI0	Doubled haploid	RI0
RI1	Recombinant inbred lines by selfing	RI1
RI2	Recombinant inbred lines by brother–sister mating	RI2
$T(B_i)SF_t$	Testcross of SF_t to P_j ($t = 2, 3,\ldots$; $i = 1$ or 2)	T(B1)SF3
$T(SF_j)SF_t$	Testcross of SF_t to SF_j ($t = 2, 3,\ldots$; $j = 2, 3,\ldots$)	T(SF4)SF3
$T(B_i)RF_t$	Testcross of RF_t to P_i ($t = 2, 3,\ldots$; $i = 1$ or 2)	T(B1)RF3
$T(D3)SF_t$	Design III. Marker genotype data is collected on SF_t and trait phenotype data is collected on both $SF_t \times P_1$ and $SF_t \times P_2$	T(D3)SF5

Source: Slightly modified from Windows QTL Cartographer manual (24)

Table 12
The default and an example of user-defined translation tables for the genotypes of markers

Default translation table			An example of user-defined translation table		
AA	2	2	AA	2	HH
Aa	1	1	Aa	1	Hh
aa	0	0	aa	0	Hh
A–	12	12	A–	12	H–
a–	10	10	a–	10	h–
–	–1	–1	–	–1	–1

Source: Slightly modified from Windows QTL Cartographer manual (24)

NEVER change the first and second columns. Anything in the data file that is not recognized (does not match something in third column) will become unknown (−1) in the output. We provide an example of a user-defined translation table in which P_1 dominant homozygotes are coded as **HH**, heterozygotes as **Hh**, and recessive homozygotes as **hh**. This user-defined translation table maps **HH** to 2, **Hh** to 1, **hh** to 0, and so on.

4. *Source file*—An example of source file named *NewMcd.mcd* is included as part of the Windows QTL Cartographer distribution. The *NewMcd.mcd* file is automatically downloaded into the folder *Example* in the Windows QTL Cartographer directory, which by default is *C:\NCSU\WinQTLCart2.5\Example*. This source data file may help you better understand how an *mcd* source file should look. Moreover, the availability of the example source file gives you an alternative way to create your own *mcd* file by borrowing the framework in the *NewMcd.mcd* to create your own source file. For that, you could use a text editor, such as *WordPad* or *Notepad*, to open the *NewMcd.mcd* file and to replace the values on all fields by your own values according to the data you have on hand.

   Two *csv* files, *NSimuB1-01-OnePop.csv* and *NSimuB1-01-MulPop.csv*, are also automatically downloaded into the folder *Example*. The *NSimuB1-01-OnePop.csv* is a *csv* file with data from one population, and the *NSimuB1-01-MulPop.csv* is a *csv* file for multiple populations. Similarly, these examples can be used to learn how to create *csv* files, which are easily translated into *mcd* source data files in Windows QTL Cartographer.

5. *Likelihood function and LRT*—The likelihood function of the CIM model is:

$$L(b, \beta, \mu, \sigma^2 | \Upsilon) = \prod_{i=1}^{n} \left[\sum_{j=1}^{K} p_{ij} \phi \left(y_i | \mu + Z_j^* B + \sum_{r=1}^{m} X_{ir} \beta_r \right) \right]$$

   where $\beta = (\beta_1, \beta_2, \ldots, \beta_m)$, $\Upsilon = (y_1, y_2, \ldots, y_n)$, K is the number of possible genotypes (G) of a QTL, M is a matrix of marker genotypes, Z_j^* is a row vector of predictor variables corresponding to genotype G_j ($j = 1, 2, \ldots, K$), p_{ij} is the probability that subject i ($i = 1, 2, \ldots, n$) has QTL genotype G_j conditional on the genotypes of markers on the left (M_i^{L}) and right (M_i^{R}) flanking the QTL located at position λ, i.e., $p_{ij} = P(G_j | M_i^{\mathrm{L}}, M_i^{\mathrm{R}}, \lambda)$. As an example, consider an intercross F_2 population where a subject i could assume either genotype $G_1 = \mathrm{QQ}$, $G_2 = \mathrm{Qq}$ or $G_3 = \mathrm{qq}$. Also consider a parameterization of additive and dominance effects of the QTL as a and d, respectively. Therefore, $K = 3$, $B = (a, d)^{\mathrm{T}}$, $\beta_r = (\beta_{r1}, \beta_{r2})^{\mathrm{T}}$ (the superscript "T" stands for transpose), $p_{i1} = P(G_1 | M_i^{\mathrm{L}}, M_i^{\mathrm{R}}, \lambda)$, $p_{i2} = P(G_2 | M_i^{\mathrm{L}}, M_i^{\mathrm{R}}, \lambda)$, $p_{i3} = P(G_3 | M_i^{\mathrm{L}}, M_i^{\mathrm{R}}, \lambda)$,

$$Z_j^* = (z_{j1}^*, z_{j2}^*) = \begin{cases} (1, -0.5) & \text{if } j = 1 \\ (0, 1) & \text{if } j = 2 \\ (-1, -0.5) & \text{if } j = 3 \end{cases}$$

and

$$X_{ir} = (x_{ir1}, x_{ir2}) = \begin{cases} (1, -0.5) & \text{if subject } i \text{ has genotype MM for cofactor marker } r \\ (0, 0.5) & \text{if subject } i \text{ has genotype Mm for cofactor marker } r \\ (-1, -0.5) & \text{if subject } i \text{ has genotype mm for cofactor marker } r \end{cases}$$

The LRT of hypothesis H0: $B = (a, d) = (0, 0)$ vs. H1: $B = (a, d) \neq (0, 0)$ for a QTL located at position λ is:

$$\text{LRT}(\lambda) = -2 \log_e \left(\frac{L(B = (0, 0), \tilde{\beta}, \tilde{\mu}, \tilde{\sigma}^2 | \Upsilon)}{L(\hat{B}, \hat{\beta}, \hat{\mu}, \hat{\sigma}^2 | \Upsilon)} \right)$$

where $\hat{B}$, $\hat{\beta}$, $\hat{\mu}$, and $\hat{\sigma}^2$ are the maximum likelihood estimates under H1, and $\tilde{\beta}$, $\tilde{\mu}$, and $\tilde{\sigma}^2$ are the maximum likelihood estimates under H0. There is a one-to-one mathematical relationship between LRT and LOD statistics, which is $\text{LRT} = 2 \log_e(10)\text{LOD} \approx 4.6\ \text{LOD}$.

6. *A brief theory on CIM cofactors*—Cofactors are used to block out effects of other QTL located in other regions of the same chromosome that harbors a putative QTL. Consider five genomic locations a, q, b, q_1, and q_2 (where a and b are markers, and q, q_1, and q_2 are QTL) on a chromosome as follows:

$$---q_1 ----a -------q -- ----b ----q_2 ---$$

Let r_{aq}, r_{qb}, and r_{ab} be recombination frequencies between a and q, q and b, and a and b, respectively. For backcross and intercross F_2 populations, the pairwise correlation coefficients between these three locations are as follows: $\gamma_{aq} = 1 - 2r_{aq}$, $\gamma_{qb} = 1 - 2r_{qb}$, and $\gamma_{ab} = 1 - 2r_{ab}$. Then, assuming no crossing-over interference, the recombination frequency between a and b can be written as $r_{ab} = r_{aq}(1 - r_{qb}) + (1 - r_{aq})r_{qb}$. After multiplying both sides of the previous equation by negative two and adding a unit to each side of the equation, and after some algebra, we obtain $(1 - 2r_{ab}) = (1 - 2r_{aq})(1 - 2r_{qb})$, which in terms of correlation coefficients is $\gamma_{ab} = \gamma_{aq}\gamma_{qb}$. Similarly, $\gamma_{q_1 q} = \gamma_{q_1 a}\gamma_{aq}$ and $\gamma_{qq_2} = \gamma_{qb}\gamma_{bq_2}$. Therefore, an unconditional test statistic for the effect of q on a trait will have power diminished by the effects of q_1 and q_2 because q is correlated with both q_1 and q_2.

Nevertheless, the correlation coefficient between a and b conditional on q (i.e., the partial correlation coefficient) is $\gamma_{ab \cdot q} = \gamma_{ab} - \gamma_{aq}\gamma_{qb} / \sqrt{(1 - \gamma_{aq}^2)(1 - \gamma_{qb}^2)} = 0$. Similarly,

$\gamma_{qq_1 \cdot a} = 0$ and $\gamma_{qq_2 \cdot b} = 0$. Therefore, conditional on markers *a* and *b*, a test statistic for the effect of *q* on a trait is independent of the effects of both q_1 and q_2, despite of genetic linkage between *q* and q_1, and *q* and q_2. The conditional test is the basis of the CIM method, and the choice of cofactor markers is the key to the success of the analysis. While conditional on markers *a* and *b*, the test for the effect of *q* on a trait is independent of q_1 and q_2; the test depends on cofactors *a* and *b*, as the test depends on the number of recombinants between *a* and *q*, and *q* and *b*. The closer *q* is to *a* and *b*, the fewer the number of recombinants in the sample and the less statistical power for *q* conditional on *a* and *b*. Moreover, cofactor markers unlinked to *q* but linked to other QTL can potentially reduce the residual variance of the model and thus increase the statistical power to search and test for QTL.

7. *Walk speed*—If there is interest in checking the resolution of different values of walk speed (grid of positions) in the QTL mapping, we recommend that a separate directory be created for each walk speed and the result files be saved in those directories. This helps in keeping track of results and in preventing files from being overwritten by Windows QTL Cartographer.

8. *Relationship between number of control markers, window size, and model selection in CIM procedure.*

Number of control markers	Window size: 0	Window size: Large (such as the size of the largest chromosome)
All markers in the data	`Model 6` reduces to `Model 1`	`Model 6` reduces to `Model 2`

`Model 1- All Marker Control` uses all markers in the data as cofactors; `Model 2- Unlinked Marker Control` uses all markers that are unlinked to the putative QTL as cofactors; `Model 6- Standard Model` is the default model that selects certain markers as cofactors by forward, backward, or forward and backward regression.

9. *CIM cofactor marker selection*—The number of ways in which a set of cofactors can be chosen may be very large; for instance, even with as few as ten markers the number of different ways that a set of cofactors can be chosen is $2^{10} = 1{,}024$. Therefore, some searching technique must be employed in the hope of choosing a good set of cofactors, while searching only a subset of all the possible ways. There are several strategies in the literature ready for use, among them backward, forward, and stepwise selections. Depending on the number of different sets of cofactors, these strategies may reduce tremendously the

Table 13
Relationship between `P-Val for into` and `out model` and degree of difficultly for a marker to enter or exit the group of cofactor markers

`P-Val for into`	`P-Val for out` Smaller	Larger
Smaller	Hard to enter and easy to exit	Hard to enter and hard to exit
Larger	Easy to enter and easy to exit	Easy to enter and hard to exit

burden of computations. However, the savings in computational time may come with the price of possibly missing good sets of cofactors. In backward elimination, in the first step, the full model (model including all markers) is fitted, and in the subsequent steps, one at the time, the marker with smallest regression sum of squares is dropped. In forward selection, from the initial model with no markers, one adds, one at the time, the marker with the largest regression sum of squares into the model. In both methods, a sequence of nested models is created when the algorithm is finished.

The stepwise selection is a general strategy that allows moves in either way, eliminating or adding markers within the same step of search. The backward stepwise selection begins with the full model, and then at each step the least significant marker is dropped and all markers dropped, but the one dropped in the current step, are reconsidered for reentering the model. Two levels of significance are generally used, one for including (`P-Val for into model`) and other for excluding (`P-Val for out model`) a marker. The smaller the `P-Val for into`, the harder is for any marker to enter the group of cofactor markers. The smaller the `P-Val for out`, the easier is for any marker to exit the group of cofactor markers. Table 13 shows the relationship between `P-Val for into` and `out` and degree of difficultly for a marker to enter or exit the group of cofactor markers.

In forward stepwise selection, markers once added to the model may be deleted if they are no longer significant. In backward elimination once a marker is dropped, it will be excluded from all subsequent models, and in the forward selection once a marker is added, it will remain in all further models. On the other hand, in the stepwise selection, a marker may enter or leave the model in different steps. Therefore, the number of models visited during the search may be higher in stepwise selection, which increases the chances of selecting more good sets of cofactor markers for the CIM analysis.

10. *Graph window tools*—In the menu of the graph window, there are many functions that enable the user to customize the display of QTL mapping. For instance, (1) to display QTL summary information, click on `Tools`, then on `Show QTL information`, check `Automatic locating QTLs` and click `OK`; (2) to create a summary of QTL mapping in excel file (*.*xls*), go to `File` in the graph window menu and click on `Save as Excel File`.

11. *A general recommendation on CIM model tuning*—`Model 6` is good for starting an analysis. Start with the default values of 5 for control markers and 10 for `window size`. Fine tuning the number of control markers and `window size` will allow for better resolution of QTL mapping.

12. *Setting CIM threshold for graphic display*—The threshold shown in the `Threshold (LR)` box is the default value that will appear in the graph window. Therefore, it is important to understand how to modify the threshold displayed in the graph window when either permutation method is chosen or when more than one trait is being analyzed together. To set the appropriate value for display in the graph window, click on `Setting` in the menu of the graph window and choose `Set Display Parameters` in the drop-down list, then enter the correct threshold value for each trait in the text box on the bottom-left corner of the opened window (the default value for all traits is 2.5 in LOD units or 11.5 in LRT units). Click `OK` to save the parameters entered and to return to the graph window.

    Alternatively, the threshold values can be updated directly in the *qrt* file by editing this file with standard text editors, such as, *Notepad* or *WordPad*.

13. *LOD d support interval*—The LOD-d support interval of a QTL is a continuous genomic region that includes the position of the QTL and all positions on its left and right sides with LOD values larger than or equal to the LOD value at the position of the QTL after subtraction of a positive constant *d*. The LOD-1 support interval is generally used and has a confidence interval usually less than 95% confidence (5). We recommend using LOD-1.5 support interval which has a confidence level close to 95%.

14. *MIM model selection criteria*—The standard permutation test (14), conditional empirical threshold, and residual empirical threshold (15) seem not to be very well suitable for computing adequate thresholds in multiple-QTL models. An alternative model-based method, attractive in terms of both computational burden and statistical properties, has been proposed by

Zou et al. (17): the score-based threshold. Under some regular conditions, the score and LRT statistics are asymptotically equivalent in a large sample (19). But an interesting characteristic of the score statistic is that it can be approximated by a sum of independent parts. Motivated by this characteristic, and based on the decomposition of the score function in Cox and Hinkley (20), Zou et al. (17) derived the large-sample distribution of the score statistic for genome-wide QTL mapping, and Laurie, Wang, Carlini-Garcia, and Zeng (unpublished data) extended the score statistic for testing hypothesis in the MIM method. A detailed description of the score-based threshold algorithm can be found in E Silva and Zeng (21).

The AIC (22) and the BIC (23) select models that minimize a criterion of the form $C(\kappa) = -2\ \log(\hat{L}_\kappa) + D(n, P)$, where P is the total of parameters in model κ, n is the sample size, $\hat{L}_\kappa$ is the estimated likelihood function of model κ, and $D(n, P)$ is equal to $2P$ in the AIC and $P\log(n)$ in the BIC.

15. *MIM QTL position optimization*—In turns, positions of all QTL in the MIM model are updated by picking a QTL in the model, and holding the other QTL fixed at their current positions. The effects of the picked QTL are then removed from the model, and a new search for a QTL is done within the region delimited by the two neighboring QTL of the picked QTL, avoiding 5 cM from the neighboring QTL (the search is performed until the end of the chromosome if no neighbor QTL is found on either side of the picked QTL). The new position of the picked QTL is set to the position of the maximum LRT within the searched region, and all parameters in the model are updated. The effect of the picked QTL can then be excluded from the model if it is no longer significant. This procedure is repeated until all positions of QTL in the model are updated.

16. *MIM window size*—The neighboring regions on the left and right sides of an estimated QTL location are defined as `window size`. Therefore, an estimated QTL has two `window sizes`, unless it is located on either end of a chromosome, in which cases the estimated QTL has one `window size` only. All positions within the `window size` (left or right) of an estimated QTL are disregarded when searching for other putative QTL, because such positions are considered to be too tightly linked to the estimated QTL and could decrease the power of the test statistic due to strong correlation (collinearity). A rule of thumb is to set `window size` wider to start with and gradually reduce it if there is evidence of linked QTL.

References

1. Sax K (1923) Association of size differences with seed-coat pattern and pigmentation in *Phaseolus vulgaris*. Genetics 8:552–560
2. Soller M, Brody T (1976) On the power of experimental designs for the detection of linkage between marker loci and quantitative loci in crosses between inbred lines. Theor Appl Genet 47:35–39
3. Rebai A, Goffinet B, Mangin B (1995) Comparing power of different methods for QTL detection. Biometrics 51:87–99
4. Wu R, Ma C, Casella G (2007) Statistical genomics of quantitative traits: linkage, maps, and QTL. Springer, New York
5. Lander ES, Botstein D (1989) Mapping mendelian factors underlying quantitative traits using RFLP linkage maps. Genetics 121:185–199
6. Zeng Z-B (1993) Theoretical basis for separation of multiple linked gene effects in mapping quantitative trait loci. Proc Natl Acad Sci U S A 90:10972–10976
7. Zeng Z-B (1994) Precision mapping of quantitative trait loci. Genetics 136:1457–1468
8. Kao CH, Zeng Z-B (1997) General formulas for obtaining the MLEs and the asymptotic variance-covariance matrix in mapping quantitative trait loci when using the EM algorithm. Biometrics 53:653–665
9. Kao CH, Zeng Z-B, Teasdale RD (1999) Multiple interval mapping for quantitative trait loci. Genetics 152:1203–1216
10. Zeng ZB, Kao CH, Basten CJ (1999) Estimating the genetic architecture of quantitative traits. Genet Res 74:279–289
11. Wang S, Basten CJ, Zeng Z-B (2010) Windows QTL Cartographer 2.51. Department of Statistics, North Carolina State University, Raleigh
12. Weber K, Eisman R, Higgins S, Morey L, Patty A, Tausek M, Zeng Z-B (2001) An analysis of polygenes affecting wing shape on chromosome 2 in *Drosophila melanogaster*. Genetics 159:1045–1057
13. Zeng Z-B, Wang T, Zou W (2005) Modeling quantitative trait loci and interpretation of models. Genetics 169:1711–1725
14. Churchill GA, Doerge RW (1994) Empirical threshold values for quantitative trait mapping. Genetics 138:963–971
15. Doerge RW, Churchill GA (1996) Permutation tests for multiple loci affecting a quantitative character. Genetics 142:285–294
16. Kao C, Zeng Z-B (2002) Modeling epistasis of quantitative trait loci using Cockerham's model. Genetics 160:1243–1261
17. Zou F, Fine JP, Hu J, Lin DY (2004) An efficient resampling method for assessing genome-wide statistical significance in mapping quantitative trait loci. Genetics 168: 2307–2316
18. E Silva LDC (2010) Multiple trait multiple interval mapping of quantitative trait loci from inbred line crosses. Department of Statistics, North Carolina State University, Raleigh
19. Chang MN, Wu R, Wu SS, Casella G (2009) Score statistics for mapping quantitative trait loci. Stat Appl Genet Mol Biol 8:1–35
20. Cox DR, Hinkley DV (1974) Theoretical statistics. Chapman and Hall, London
21. E Silva LDC, Zeng Z-B (2010) Current progress on statistical methods for mapping quantitative trait loci from inbred line crosses. J Biopharm Stat 20:454–481
22. Akaike H (1969) A method of statistical identification of discrete time parameter linear systems. Ann Inst Statist Math 21:243–247
23. Schwarz G (1978) Estimating the dimension of a model. Ann Statist 6:461–464
24. Wang S, Basten CJ, Zeng Z-B (2007) Windows QTL Cartographer 2.0 user manual. Department of Statistics, North Carolina State University, Raleigh

Chapter 7

Design Database for Quantitative Trait Loci (QTL) Data Warehouse, Data Mining, and Meta-Analysis

Zhi-Liang Hu, James M. Reecy, and Xiao-Lin Wu

Abstract

A database can be used to warehouse quantitative trait loci (QTL) data from multiple sources for comparison, genomic data mining, and meta-analysis. A robust database design involves sound data structure logistics, meaningful data transformations, normalization, and proper user interface designs. This chapter starts with a brief review of relational database basics and concentrates on issues associated with curation of QTL data into a relational database, with emphasis on the principles of data normalization and structure optimization. In addition, some simple examples of QTL data mining and meta-analysis are included. These examples are provided to help readers better understand the potential and importance of sound database design.

Key words: Quantitative trait loci, Data modeling, Database design, Meta-analysis

1. Introduction: QTL Studies and QTL Databases

A quantitative trait locus (QTL) is a statistically identified genomic region hypothetically responsible for genetic variation in a trait. This specific region in a genome is thought to harbor genetic variants that make a significant contribution to the expression of a complex trait. Experimentally, QTL estimation is usually carried out within a given resource population with a specific mating scheme designed for detecting genetic segregations useful for the test. Thus, any established QTL is based on a specific population. Multiple such experiments with different resource populations can provide additional evidence of QTLs for the given species. However, results from different experiments may or may not agree with each other. To date, large numbers of QTLs have been reported in human, mouse, rat, cattle, chicken, pigs, sheep, among many other vertebrate species as well as in plants, invertebrates, and fungi (1).

Several factors limit our ability to accurately use information from the myriad of reported QTL. First, QTL information within

Scott A. Rifkin (ed.), *Quantitative Trait Loci (QTL): Methods and Protocols*, Methods in Molecular Biology, vol. 871,
DOI 10.1007/978-1-61779-785-9_7,

the public domain are scattered in many publications, each of which is the result of independent studies with similar or different statistical analysis methods. Second, QTL represent statistical evidence for cosegregation of traits and markers within a particular experimental population. Thus, each reported QTL may be biased, but when all QTL for a trait are collectively analyzed, they provide evidence of a true QTL. Third, traits are defined and measured in many different ways in different laboratories and/or countries, and there is a lack of standardized nomenclature to define similar traits for meaningful comparisons. Each alias trait name is known to different individuals and may be used under slightly different context. For example, the longissimus dorsi muscle area is referred as loin eye area (LEA), loin muscle area (LMA), meat area (MLD), ribeye area (REA), etc. This presents a challenge in terms of unambiguous identification and effective computer management of trait terms for comparisons. While the accuracy of QTL locations depends on a number of factors, such as marker density of the linkage map, the design of the experiment, the size and structure of the resource population, the method to establish significance threshold, etc., the precise location of a true QTL may be approximated by results from multiple studies.

Rapid progress has been made in the last 2 decades in the progression from marker mapping to trait/QTL mapping, to the eventual discovery of the causal variant. A vast amount of QTL data have been accumulated, which presents a challenge for human comprehension. Since the ultimate goal of QTL studies is the identification of the actual variant(s) (i.e., gene) responsible for phenotypic variation, it would be useful if: (a) QTL data can be stored in a database for archive and easy retrieval; (b) tools could be built to facilitate data translation and comparison. Since many QTL for a given trait can map to the same or similar genomic region, it is possible to combine results from different QTL studies, which will help for better estimates on the genome region to focus, thus to improve the effectiveness of identifying positional candidate genes or marker discovery.

A relational database can be employed for QTL data collection and management. To date, there have been a number of QTL databases, e.g., rat (2), mouse (3), cattle, chicken, pigs, sheep (4), and Gramene (5) among others. The backend of these databases are all based on a relational database management system (RDBMS), such as MySQL, Oracle, Sybase, PostgreSQL, etc. It is worthwhile to note that a number of factors are important for a robust database structure to warehouse QTL data, such as how QTL data may be represented in a database, how to model the related data to effectively describe a QTL, how can QTL data be managed in order for meta comparisons and analysis, etc. In this chapter, we will summarize the principles and methods in the design, implementation, and use of a QTL database. Animal QTLdb is one of the most advanced such databases in terms of the built-in functionalities, user tools, and scalability for function extension. Thus, we will reference it for most of the examples that we provide throughout the chapter.

We will focus on key issues and principles for QTL modeling and QTL database construction in this chapter, and readers are advised to refer to more specialized books and related resources on relational database design, operation, and programming, for more in-depth knowledge in order to fully comprehend the material covered. All italicized words are intended as concepts, which are essential to better understand the issues that we discuss. All fixed-width letters/words are used to show program codes.

2. QTL Database Design

There are a number of design issues that must be addressed when building a relational database for QTL data warehousing and meta-analysis. First, a good database model is needed to fit the QTL data. Second, QTL data need to be transformed and structured in the database model. Third, an effective implementation method is needed to build the database in order to facilitate data input and output. Most biological data can be entered into a relational database structure that holds a collection of data that is organized in a set of formally described tables from which data can be accessed or reassembled in many different ways without having to reorganize them. We will start by introducing some basic concepts of relational database (See Note 1).

2.1. Basic Concepts Needed to Build a Relational Database

The idea of a relational database is derived from the principles of relational algebra that were proposed by Codd (6). Briefly, the first level of a "relational" structure is as simple as a two-dimensional table with "rows" and "columns", which form the primary unit of storage in a relational database. One or more such tables, with each containing a unique set of data, can be linked together by a second level of "relation" between tables using "*keys*". A set of such related tables can form the basic structure of a so-called "relational database". However, it is not that any arbitrary relation between data can be used to build a good relational database. The "relationship" has to be well defined and structured. One must follow a number of rules in order to build a robust database. As we only discuss some basic rules as an introduction, readers are highly encouraged to refer to specialized books on how to build relational databases, should they want additional information on relational database design.

A *table* is made up of columns and rows and contains one or more data categories stored in columns. A *column* contains a set of values for the same kind of data in the same *data type* (for example,

Table 1
Basic data types defined by MySQL

Data type	Description
`CHAR(size)`	Holds a fixed length string (can contain letters, numbers, and special characters). The fixed size is specified in parenthesis. Can store up to 255 characters
`VARCHAR (size)`	Holds a variable length string (can contain letters, numbers, and special characters). The maximum size is specified in parenthesis. Can store up to 255 characters (NEW: If you put a greater value than 255, it will be converted to a TEXT type)
`TEXT`	Holds a string with a maximum length of 65,535 characters
`INT(size)`	−2147483648 to 2147483647 normal. 0 to 4294967295 UNSIGNED*. The maximum number of digits may be specified in parenthesis
`DECIMAL (size,d)`	A number stored as a string, allowing for a fixed decimal point. The maximum number of digits may be specified in the "size" parameter. The maximum number of digits to the right of the decimal point is specified in the "d" parameter
`DATE()`	A date. Format: YYYY-MM-DD (year-month-day in numbers)
`DATETIME()`	A date and time combination. Format: YYYY-MM-DD HH:MM:SS

character strings, integers, etc. See Table 1 (see Note 1) for a simple reference), and a *row* contains a sequence of related values such that a value in the nth row, column m corresponds to another piece of data in a different column, say *r*, but in the same row of the table. A RDBMS table row should hold data that have only one relationship between data stored in different columns. Each such row is called a "*record*".

A *record* is typically identified by a unique value called a *primary key*. It is possible, although not generally very useful, to create a table without a primary key. A *key* is an entity in a table that distinguishes one row of data from another. For example, an animal's identification number can be a key to uniquely identify data from different animals. Multiple data tables can be related to each other in a variety of ways, usually with keys. The simplest relationship is the *one-to-one* relationship, in which one record in a table is related to another record in a separate table. This is tricky because in theory such tables should be merged into one under the principle of data normalization (see below). However, in reality such a data structure merge reduces the efficiency for data management. For example, animal farm data and animal laboratory records are better recorded separately but with reference to each other. A *one-to-many* relationship is one in which one record in a table is related to multiple records in another table. For example, an animal may have multiple trait measurements which are attributed by dates of the measurement, method and instrument used, environmental conditions during data collection, etc., that are stored in a separate table.

A *many-to-one* relationship defines the reverse situation where more than one record in a single table relates to only one record in another table. For example, a group of animals may receive the same treatment or be sampled under one condition. A *many-to-many* relationship is where more than one record in a table relates to more than one record in another table (usually a "relationship" table is useful to link such two tables). For example, multiple markers may be associated with multiple QTL detected, and the links between them can usually be made via the animals, the experiments, etc.

In an RDBMS model, the data stored in tables are organized logically for a particular purpose. The logical organization of data helps to minimize data duplication, reduce data anomalies, and reinforce data integrity. This process is called *normalization*. Data normalization simplifies the way the data structure is defined, how data can be separated into different tables, and how these tables can be related to one another without ambiguity so that data stored in different tables can be associated in logical yet simple ways.

A *relational database* contains a set of such related tables that contain data fitted into predefined categories and relationships. The construction of a relational database should result in a set of tables with metadata and formal descriptions of the tables, columns, domains, and constraints ("relationship" in strict terms). In addition, we need to mention that the data stored within a RDBMS are manipulated with a programming language called Structured Query Language, or *SQL* (7). SQL is designed to follow English grammar. Originally, it was called a Structured English Query Language and abbreviated as SEQUEL. Even today "SQL" is still pronounced as "sequel". See following sections for actual SQL examples.

2.2. QTL Data Modeling, Transformation, and Representations

A QTL is a genome location associated with a trait, and this hypothetical association is tested and supported by statistical evidence. As such, several pieces of information are necessary in order to describe a QTL: (a) the trait name it represents and how that trait is defined and measured; (b) the genome map used and the location of the QTL on the map, e.g., the peak location and flanking boundaries; (c) the population used for the QTL test and the mating scheme in which genetic segregation was observed; (d) the statistical method(s) used and evidence that support it; and (e) other experiment details. In order for a QTL database to objectively store QTL information for analysis, all this information needs to be captured. A formal data modeling procedure for building a database involves conceptual data modeling (CDM), logical data modeling (LDM), and physical data modeling (PDM). Instead of going through each method, we will use a tutorial procedure to emphasize how to fit different QTL data types to construct a relational data structure.

2.2.1. Trait Data

Biological traits are ubiquitously used in all biological research papers. A challenge when one tries to computationally model trait data is the lack of a standard that defines how trait terms should be named, defined, measured (or observed), and recorded. Hu et al. (8) proposed the use of trait ontology to manage trait data and implemented a trait hierarchy within the Pig QTLdb, which facilitated easy organization and comparison of trait information. This hierarchy utilized two concepts, "trait class" and "trait type (super trait)", to organize trait data (Table 2).

A long trait hierarchy list as shown in Table 2 can be awkward to read and difficult for computer programs to manage. Instead of using a *hierarchy data model* (see Note 2), Hu et al. employed a simple table structure to manage the ontology relationships by partitioning the information into two tables (Tables 3 and 4) under the *relational data model*. Under this model, the two tables are linked together with "`Trait_ID`" as keys. More specifically, the column "`Trait_ID`" is used as a *primary key* in the "Traits" table, and as a *foreign key* in the "`Trait_ontology`" table. The main advantage of this simplified structure (Tables 3 and 4) is to enable the use of controlled vocabularies to easily locate a defined item with a relational database. A couple points need to be pointed out here. One, although the relationship type "`is_a`" in Table 4 may be coded in a separate table to comply with data normalization rules, for two reasons this is not done here: (a) "`is_a`" is already used by the database as a code internally; (b) therefore it is not subject to human manipulations. This is an example to show how deep one wants his/her data normalization to go (e.g., *1NF*, *2NF*, *3NF*, and so on; see Subheading 2.2.4) for optimal balances between the theoretical completeness of it and the efficiency to get things done at minimum complexities and costs. Two, by

Table 2
Example trait hierarchy with the use of "trait class" and "trait type (super trait)". The purpose of the structure is to group the traits in order for cross experiments comparisons of QTL results in which traits are defined, named, and measured differently.

Trait class	Trait type (super trait)	Traits
Meat/carcass quality	Back fat	Average backfat
		Backfat at last lumbar
		Backfat depth at maximum muscle depth
		Backfat thickness by ruler
		Backfat thickness by ultrasound
		First rib backfat
		Last rib backfat

Table 3
Trait definition information is abstracted from Table 2, with each trait name assigned to a unique identifier ("`Trait_ID`", serving as the *primary key* of the table)

***Table name*: Traits**

Trait_ID	Trait_Name
1	Meat quality
2	Back fat
3	Average backfat
4	Backfat at last lumbar
5	Backfat depth at max. mus. depth
6	Backfat thickness by ruler
7	Backfat thickness by ultrasound
8	First rib backfat
9	Last rib backfat

Table 4
Trait hierarchy relationships are abstracted from Table 2 where "`Trait_A`" and "`Trait_B`" are foreign keys to `Trait_ID` in Table 3

***Table name*: Trait_ontology**

Trait_A	Relation	Trait_B
1	is_a	0
2	is_a	1
3	is_a	2
4	is_a	2
5	is_a	2
6	is_a	2
7	is_a	2
8	is_a	2
9	is_a	2

using this structure, not only one but multiple levels of "trait-types" and "sub-trait-types" can be accommodated, allowing more complex hierarchy information to be stored (think of `Trait_A` as "children" and `Trait_B` as "parents", a child can be a parent of other children and so on, which can simply be added as more rows in Table 4).

Some users may ask why, in the "`Trait_ontology`" table, traits are represented by codes rather than by their names for easy reading. The reasons behind this are twofold. On one hand, it is easier for computers to manipulate data with codes for better accuracy and fewer errors. On the other hand, one principle of designing a relational database is that *a piece of data appears in a database only once*. This is important because, when a user looks up a piece of information, getting multiple results from multiple places in a database can be very confusing even though they may be identical. For a simple example, to correct a spelling error, one would not have to make multiple corrections in tens or hundreds of places in the database, but only at a single place. Thus, the correction process occurs only once and not multiple times, which minimizes the chance of introducing more errors. In a more complex table structure, the advantage of using *keys* is more evident. Some others may ask that, does it make it complicated by putting data into two tables, where information retrieval doesn't seem to be straightforward. The answer is no, because the SQL is designed to handle tasks like this easily. For example, the parent/child relationships of the trait terms can be retrieved with a simple SQL query:

```
SELECT parent.trait_name as parent_term,
       child.trait_name as child_term
FROM traits AS parent,
     trait_ontology,
     traits AS child
WHERE parent.trait_id = trait_ontology.trait_b AND
      child.trait_id = trait_ontology.trait_a
ORDER BY 2;
```

With a little loop through the multiple levels of the ontology relationships, the entire trait hierarchy structure shown in Table 2 can be reconstituted with information retrieved from Tables 3 and 4 (codes are not shown; Readers of this chapter should be able to compose one when done with this chapter).

Many different data display formats can be implemented as a *view* using SQL. A *view* is a virtual table. The physical form of a *view* is only a stored SQL code or function. Once an SQL query is built, it can be conveniently reused, for direct query, or for building into another SQL query. This is a good example of making complex things "simple" by using relational data model.

2.2.2. Mapping Data

QTL data are normally published in two forms: tables and/or graphs. A tabulated data sheet usually contains the QTL location, significance level supported by the test statistics, and perhaps the additive and/or dominance phenotypic effects of this QTL.

Tabulated data are generally easy to transform into a relational database table format. QTL graphs data are more complicated. While it is possible to store all data points to redraw the QTL curve, it might not worth the effort to do so because the shape of a QTL curve may not be a major focus of a QTL meta-analysis. In addition, it is difficult to obtain such data from literature, or by contacting the authors. In fact, a QTL curve is a plot of statistical estimates using segregation information from limited number of markers, thus the shape of a QTL may vary depending on the method used. What really matters are the start, the end, and the peak locations of a QTL, which are essential to describe a QTL (Fig. 1a).

Since QTL are mapping features recorded as linkage distances, we can transform the key information from a QTL curve into one-dimensional, linear coordinates (Fig. 1b). This way the key information of a QTL is preserved and the storage of data is simplified. We can record a QTL in a relational database table using 2 or 3 data

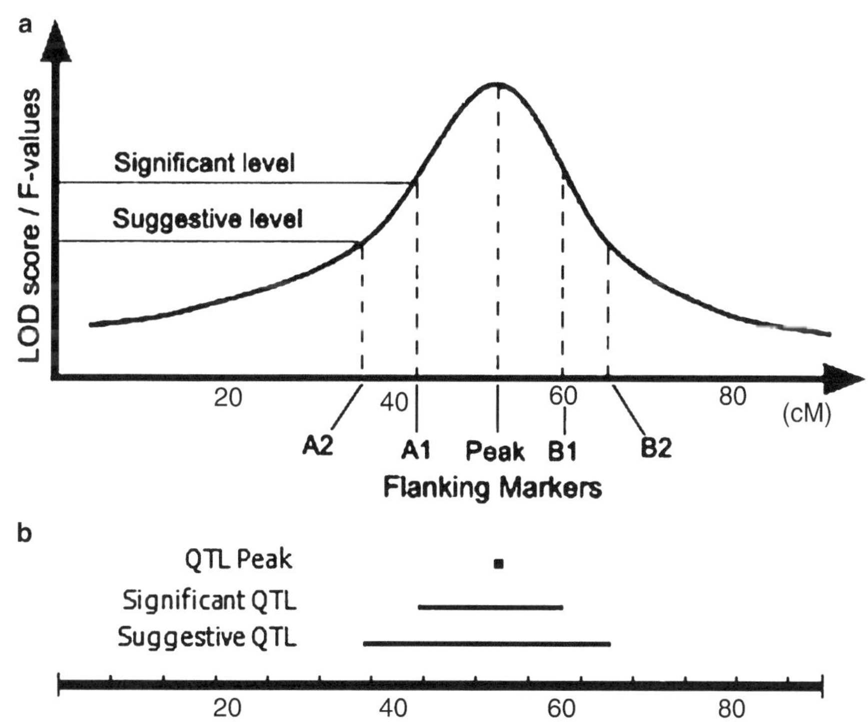

Fig. 1. A schematic QTL representation that shows how flanking marker locations are named and the QTL significance levels are defined (**a**), and how this data can be rendered into one-dimensional coordinates (**b**) for curation into a database table. Note how the QTL line coordinates on the linkage map in (**b**) correspond to the boundaries on the *x*-axis in (**a**).

points for its location (peak and boundaries), along with the test statistics and QTL effect values to describe a QTL.

2.2.3. Statistics

There are various ways to identify a QTL. These include different experimental designs and statistical analysis methods, such as analysis of variance (ANOVA) and interval mapping, among others. Depending on the statistical methods used, results from testing a number of statistical parameters may be reported, for example, LOD scores, LS means, *P*-values, *F*-values, variances, Bayes values, likelihood ratios, and so on. An incomplete form to collect these data can be in a format shown in Table 5.

When this structure is used to collect data, obviously not all cells in every row and column of Table 5 will be filled, leaving many unused. Such use of database space is not only inefficient, but also makes it cumbersome to recapture the data for representations and analysis. Table 6 demonstrates one option used in the Animal QTLdb to effectively collect such data in a simple and efficient way. One advantage of using this structure is to efficiently make use of *indices* for columns to be searched. An *index* in a relational database can be thought of a list of pre-sorted key values, each corresponding to a value in the indexed column. There are a variety of data structures and

Table 5
An initial form for collecting statistical parameters data

	Statistical parameters							
	LOD scores	LS means	*P*-value	*F*-values	Variances	Bayes values	Likelihood ratios	...
QTL 1				3.932				
QTL 2				12.877				
QTL 3			0.034					
...								

Table 6
A simplified table structure from Table 4 to hold all QTL statistics

QTL	Stat_parameter	Stat_value
1	*F*-value	3.932
2	*F*-value	12.877
3	*P*-value	0.034
...	...	...

search algorithms by which indexes are implemented, such as B-tree or R-tree. The use of an *index* can exponentially improve the speed by which data can be searched and retrieved (by default, all *keys* in a RDBMS are automatically subject to index).

2.2.4. Experiment Data

Experimental data are important to QTL results because it is the basis by which a QTL is identified and interpreted (9). However, it could be a challenge to have a uniform structure to capture all experimental data, since data to describe an experiment can vary greatly between experiments. While there are on-going efforts to develop specialized laboratory information management systems (LIMS) for complete experimental data collection and management, we can focus on data essential for QTL interpretation. These data may include a description of the population used, pedigree structure (mating types), trait definition and measurements, marker description, genotyping methods, statistical methods and software, etc. Currently, Animal QTLdb along with other QTL databases uses several free text spaces for paragraphs curated to describe an experiment (Fig. 2).

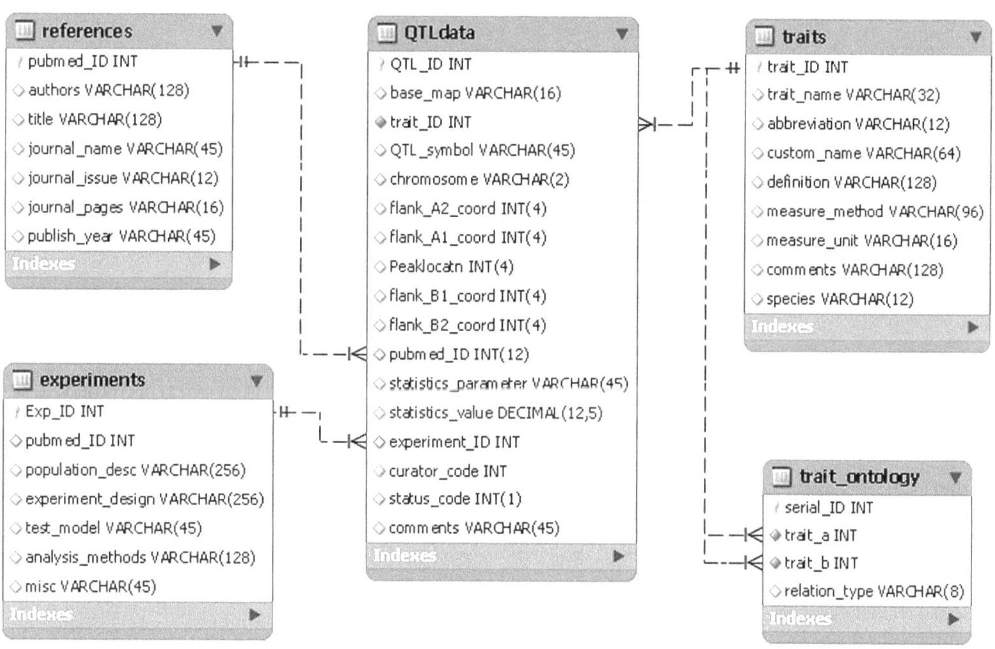

Relationship keys: references.pubmed_ID = experiment.pubmed_ID
references.pubmed_ID = QTLdata.pubmed_ID
experiment.Exp_ID = QTLdata.experiment_ID
traits.trait_ID = QTLdata.trait_ID
traits.trait_ID = trait_ontology.trait_a
traits.trait_ID = trait_ontology.trait_b

Legend: Primary key
Foreign key
Not null
One-to-many relationship
One and only one match

Fig. 2. A simplified ER diagram of Animal QTLdb that shows several of the basic concepts discussed in the text. The diagram was produced with MySQL Workbench 5.2 (8).

To summarize, Fig. 2 shows a snapshot of a simplified *entity-relationship* diagram (ERD) of the Animal QTLdb, which demonstrates the initial outcomes that we have just discussed.

An *ERD* is a form of visual representation of data objects from a database modeling process (*entity-relationship modeling*, ERM), to show an abstract and conceptual representation of data. An ERD may not be the final outcome after an initial data modeling. In fact, a good database structure is often the result of several rounds of data modeling in which a researcher is faced with a series of choices: How many tables are needed and what will they each represent? Which columns will best fit in which tables? What will be the relationships between the tables? The answers to each of these questions lies in something called *normalization*. *Normalization* is the process of simplifying the design of a database so that it achieves the optimum structure where all principles of database design apply. Normalization theory gives us the concept of normal forms to assist in achieving the optimum structure. The normal forms are a linear progression of rules that are applied to a database design, with each higher normal form achieving a better, more efficient design. A data normalization procedure may include the *first normal form* (*1NF*; *Minimal Form*), the *second normal form* (*2NF*), and the *third normal form* (*3NF*). Details of normalization procedures are beyond the scope of this chapter; users are encouraged to consult the literature for details as how each normal form is derived at each step (see "Further Reading" list).

ERD is one way to describe a database *schema*, which is the formal representation of a database model where the database tables, fields, relationships, views, indexes, functions, queues, and other elements are defined. Other ways of schema description include the use of data description language (DDL), SQL-Schema Statements, XML schema mapping, etc. An SQL-Schema Statement can not only define the data types and relationships, but it can also be used to create the database in an RDBMS environment. To move from a *conceptual design* to physical implementation is relatively straightforward with an SQL "`create`" statement, as illustrated in the following MySQL example (with comments (see Note 3) after the "#" sign on each line):

```
CREATE DATABASE QTLdb;                           # Create a database space (instance)
CREATE TABLE trait_ontology (                    # Create a table under the "QTLdb" space.
  Serial_ID INT(12) PRIMARY KEY,                 # Define the column attributes
  Trait_a   INT(12) NOT NULL,                    # Define the column attributes
  Trait_b   INT(12) NOT NULL,                    # Define the column attributes
  Relationship_type VARCHAR(8) NOT NULL,         # Define the column attributes
  INDEX indexx (Trait_a),                        # Define an index for column "trait_a"
  INDEX indexy (Trait_a)                         # Define an index for column "trait_b"
);
```

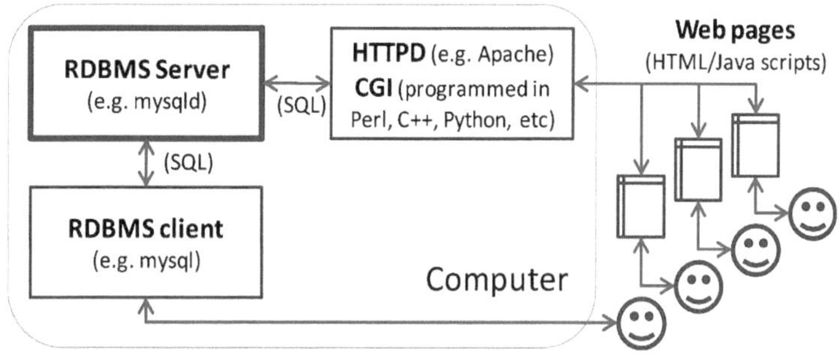

Fig. 3. A conceptual representation of the components needed to interact with the database and build more versatile user interfaces using the web technology.

In practice, the *primary key* often uses the `INT` data type and is set to `AUTO_INCREMENT`. All other tables defined in the schema may be created in the same way. This SQL statement can be executed in an SQL client environment to create the electronic table structure. Note that the relationships between tables defined by *keys* can be implemented in the SQL query statements by the "`where`" clause as in the trait ontology query example shown in Subheading 2.2.1.

2.2.5. What Are Needed to Implement a Database

If one wishes to implement a database design, a few more components are needed not only to have a virtual database structure, but also to build useful user interfaces for it to be practically useful. To do this, you will either need a local computer system administrator and a database administrator to help setting up a RDBMS environment, or you will need to do it yourself. For example, there are books that describe step-by-step procedures where to download, unpack, and install a MySQL database server and client (see "Further Reading" list at the end of this chapter).

Generally, one needs to know SQL, plus at least one of the following programming languages—Perl, Python, PHP, C++, Java, or visual basic (VB). A running SQL server/client is essential to interact with a database. A web server such as Apache would be useful to build online web tools to interact with a database. To formulate web interface for database reports, an HTML format language will be a must. The relationships between these parts are illustrated in Fig. 3. All of these components working together form a popular way to make an underlining database useable to users (similar systems include LAMP—Linux/Apache/MySQL/PHP—among others). We will give a brief introduction on each of these in the next section.

2.3. RDBMS, World-Wide Web, and QTL Database User Interfaces

There are many commercial and open source RDBMS software for use. Well-known such software packages include Ingres, Oracle, Sybase, MySQL, PostgreSQL, etc. For example, the Animal QTLdb uses MySQL as its backend RDBMS (10). The use of these databases requires the knowledge of SQL programming

Table 7
Basic SQL-schema constraints

Constraints	Specifications
PRIMARY KEY	Only one primary key column per table; the UNIQUE constraint and index automatically applies
FOREIGN KEY	The set of data in this column are foreign keys. Referential Integrity applies
NOT NULL	The column can't be set to null, or the row cannot be inserted
UNIQUE	This column has a unique value or null for all rows of the table
INDEX	This column is always automatically indexed

language. Here we introduce users to the most basic SQL statements as a start. We encourage users to explore more advanced SQL techniques as needed either online or in the "Further Reading" at the end of the chapter.

2.3.1. SQL-Schema Statements

Readers are perhaps already familiar with the `CREATE TABLE` statement from the example in the previous section. This statement uses table constraint specifications to add additional restrictions on the contents of the table. Once specified, these constraints are automatically enforced by the DBMS. The most common table/column constraints are shown in Table 7.

For a routine complex data query viewed as a simple table, a permanent SQL query can be implemented to generate a virtual table — *view* — by a statement similar to `create table`:

```
CRETAE VIEW name as (select .. from .. where .. AND ..);
```

Tables and Views can be deleted when no longer needed using `DROP` statement:

```
DROP TABLE table_name;
DROP VIEW view_name;
```

2.3.2. SQL-Data Statements

There are four basic SQL-data statements for data manipulations. The examples below show the backbone of each statement type. The text in square brackets would be replaced with actual content. Query tables and views in the database:

```
SELECT [column] FROM [tables] WHERE [table relation
constraints and search constraints] ORDER BY [column]
```

Add rows to tables:

```
INSERT INTO [table] (list of fields) VALUES (list of
values);
```

Modify data in columns by table rows:

```
UPDATE [table] SET column=value WHERE [table relation
constraints and search constraints];
```

Remove rows from tables:

```
DELETE FROM [table] WHERE [table relation constraints
and search constraints];
```

2.3.3. World-Wide Web and an HTML Form Starter

Traditional RDBMS used to be operated on a computer console, which is limited to only one local user, or multiple users whose computers may be physically networked with the server computer where the RDBMS is setup in server-client mode, and the local computer has a RDBMS client installed. The world-wide web (WWW) has provided the opportunity for traditional RDBMS to greatly increase its user scope by allowing remote users to access the database using the internet through a programmable common gateway interface (CGI; may be programmed in Perl, C++, and other languages) or through server-enabled PHP scripts working with a web server. Depending on how these interface layers are programmed, the ability of users to access databases can range from browsing through the contents to managing day-to-day operations of a database. The CGI programs can add additional capabilities to web interfaces because they allow more handles to be built in order to implement customizable constraints, logistics, and features during the data input/output process.

To accept user data for input, a web form can be made to take data, as in this HTML FORM example which uses defined internal names for each data field (e.g., `name="symbol"`, etc.) so that a CGI program can handle them. The "`action`" line specifies to which CGI program the form data shall be sent.

```
<FORM method=post action="/cgi-bin/yourCGIprogram">
QTL_symbol:                 <INPUT type="text" name="symbol">
QTL peak position (cM):     <INPUT type="text" name="Positn">
QTL span interval (cM):     <INPUT type="text" name="interv">
Flank Marker A2:            <INPUT type="text" name="fMarkA2">
Flank Marker A1:            <INPUT type="text" name="fMarkA1">
......
LOD score:                  <INPUT type="text" name="LODscore">
Likelihood Ratio:           <INPUT type="text" name="likeratio">
<INPUT type="submit" name="submit" value="Submit">
</FORM>
```

In this example, the dotted lines represent omitted similar constructs, possibly with the use of "`INPUT`", "`SELECT`", "`RADIO`", etc. Refer to an HTML resource book for form elements to use. Figure 4 shows a sample QTL input data form produced this way.

For database query input, a similar form can be built to send one or more query strings:

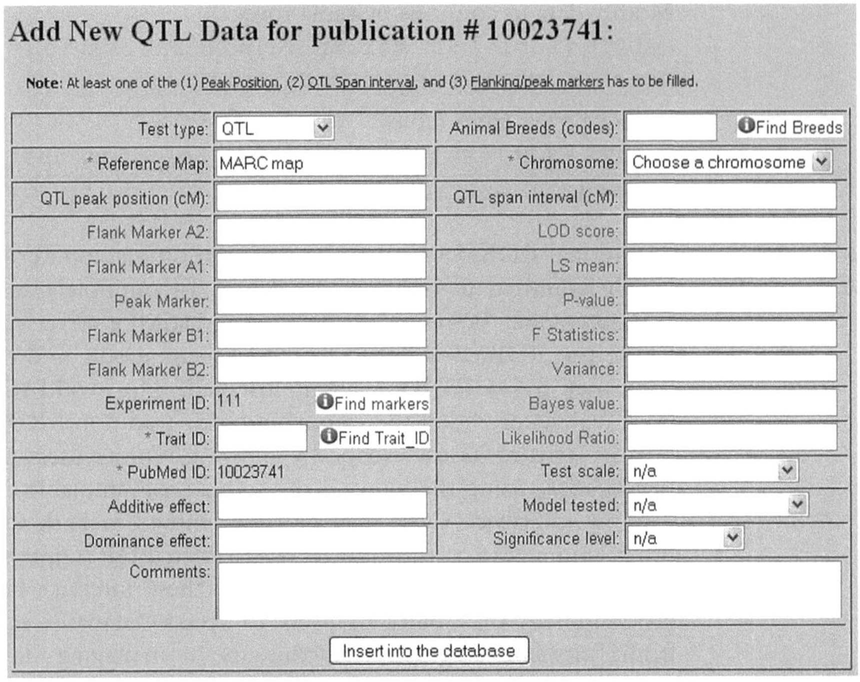
Add New QTL Data for publication # 10023741:

Note: At least one of the (1) Peak Position, (2) QTL Span interval, and (3) Flanking/peak markers has to be filled.

Test type:	QTL	Animal Breeds (codes):	Find Breeds
* Reference Map:	MARC map	* Chromosome:	Choose a chromosome
QTL peak position (cM):		QTL span interval (cM):	
Flank Marker A2:		LOD score:	
Flank Marker A1:		LS mean:	
Peak Marker:		P-value:	
Flank Marker B1:		F Statistics:	
Flank Marker B2:		Variance:	
Experiment ID:	111 Find markers	Bayes value:	
* Trait ID:	Find Trait_ID	Likelihood Ratio:	
* PubMed ID:	10023741	Test scale:	n/a
Additive effect:		Model tested:	n/a
Dominance effect:		Significance level:	n/a
Comments:			

Insert into the database

Fig. 4. A sample QTL data curation web form created with standard HTML FORM syntax. Note that you can optionally use "TABLE" tags in HTML to format the page so that the columns can be aligned for a better visual effect.

```
Search: <INPUT type="text"name="qTrait" value="" size="30">
        <INPUT type="submit" name="submit" value="Search">
```

2.3.4. CGI: A Data Bridge

When an HTML form is ready to submit data, a CGI program handles the data submission and passes it on to the database. Here is a simple Perl script to handle the submitted data:

```
#!/usr/bin/perl
require "cgi-lib.pl";
&ReadParse(*FORM); # To get the form data into a Perl hash structure "%FORM"
use DBI;
$dbh = DBI->connect("dbi:mysql:QTLdb","$dbuser","$dbpass");
$sql = "INSERT INTO QTLdata (QTL_symbol, chromosome,
       flank_A2_coord, flank_A1_coord, .., ..) VALUES
      ($FORM{symbol}, $FORM{Positn}, $FORM{interv},
       $FORM{FMarkA2}, $FORM{FMarkA1}, .., ..);
$dosql = $dbh -> prepare ("$sql");
$dosql -> execute;
$dosql -> finish;
print "Content-type: text/html\n\n";
print "<HTML><HEAD><TITLE>test</TITLE></HEAD>\n";
print "<BODY>\n";
print "<H2>QTL Data Submission results</H2>\n";
print "Your data is submitted.\n";
print "</BODY></HTML\n";
```

There are a few tricks that need to be explained in this example. First, the perl DBI/DBD library is employed for it to talk to the backend MySQL database. It uses object-oriented constructs for you to program the parts needed to interact with the database. Second, the perl library "`cgi-lib.pl`" is used to parse out the submitted data from the web form into Perl internal variable holders for further processing. This CGI program is triggered by web submission actions and can take the data from the web form and insert them into the database.

For making database queries, one would only need to change the SQL (what *scalar* variable "`$sql`" holds) to a `SELECT` statement in the CGI example and modify the related lines as in:

```
$sql = "SELECT * from QTLdata where QTL_symbol like % grow% ;
$dosql = $dbh -> prepare ("$sql");
$dosql -> execute;
@values = $ dosql -> fetchrow_array;
```

The data retrieved from the database and held in the *array* `@values` can be parsed out and displayed with a `foreach` loop:

```
foreach $value(@values) {
  print "$value";
}
```

This can be inserted somewhere in the CGI example between the lines printing the HTML `BODY` codes (between the starting `<BODY>` and ending `</BODY>` tags). In a similar way, by using a Perl::GD library, Hu et al. (4) was able to implement CGI code to graphically display QTL maps on a web browser (Fig. 8a) so that users can visually compare results across studies. Customized QTL data reports may be built, either in a tabular form or in some sort of graph. The "combined dairy cattle QTL traits" (http://www.vetsci.usyd.edu.au/reprogen/QTL_Map/) web site demonstrates an alternative way to display QTL data.

2.4. Literature Curation, Data Flow, and Quality Controls

The quality of a database relies not only on a robust design aimed at logistically holding QTL data for search and retrieval, but also on how the database is designed to curate, enter, and check data for integrity, reuse, and so on.

A number of constraints and checkpoints can be enforced on data entry at the HTML FORM (using Javascripts), CGI, or SQL level. For example, one can check for the correct data type, remind the curator if a required field is unintentionally left empty, etc. During and after data entry, codes can be implemented to verify data integrity, consistency, and check for possible errors.

Under a simple scenario, by assuming that most errors can be caught by going through three proof readings by different eyes, Hu et al. (4) implemented a three-tier data curation structure in the

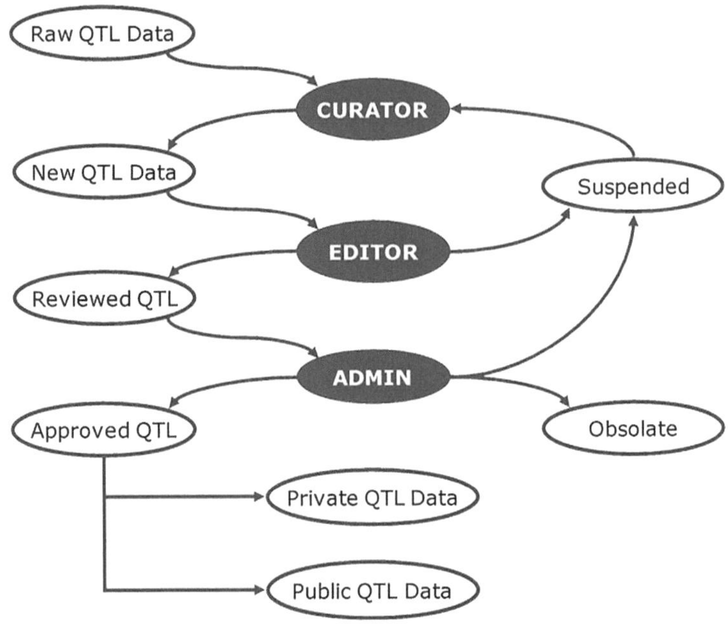

Fig. 5. Data flow during the data curation: considerations for data quality control.

Animal QTLdb to move the QTL data flow from curators to editor, and finally to the database administrator for final passage (Fig. 5). To implement this, we need to record which curator is responsible for the data input on which record (see Fig. 2 for details). The newly entered data goes through the pipeline to be checked by the editor (the data "`status`" will change), and so on. Under this structure, the curator, editor, and database administrator have to work together and share responsibilities in a workflow to ensure data quality and smooth process control. Such a process helps to minimize the errors, being it grammar, wording, or data format issue.

The data flow process described in Fig. 5 can be implemented with a "status code" on each QTL record (Fig. 2). A list of sample status codes is listed in Table 8. This way, the location of a record in the curator/editor pipeline at a given time can be determined by the status code. The change of the code number represents the movements and locations of the record in the pipeline.

What we have discussed in this chapter are only some basic principles on a QTL database design and ways to implement them. The examples given are not exhaustive as to what is actually needed to deploy a QTL database. The topics not covered include version tracking, historical data keeping, backup, and recovery. Readers should explore further for technical feasibilities to implement database designs.

Table 8
Examples of QTL data flags used to code for the status of a record

Code	Meaning
0	New data
1	Reviewed by editor
2	Approved by admin (public data)
3	Approved by admin (private data)
4	Suspended
5	Obsoleted
6	Sent for reprocessing

Refer to Fig. 2 for how it is implemented

3. Design QTL Database as a Research Tool

In this chapter, we started with the term "warehouse" to address the role a database can bring to QTL research. In fact, the function of a database is far beyond a "warehouse". In order to design a useful QTL database, two aspects of the problems should be well reviewed. First, it is essential to decide what parameters to include. The Animal QTLdb developmental works by Hu et al. have led to a proposed set of minimal information standards when reporting a QTL (http://miqas.sourceforge.net/), which provides a general guide for items to include. Second, it is always useful to keep in mind the utility you wish the database to bring to the end users. In this section, we will demonstrate some examples of how the Animal QTLdb was designed and can be used as a research tool to open up new research possibilities.

3.1. Structural Genomics and QTL Data Mining

QTL is a mapping feature. One potential goal of a QTL database would be to directly align genes, transcripts, SNPs, and other mapping features to QTL to assist researchers in identifying candidate genes or markers. However, in order to do so, QTL map locations measured by linkage distances in centiMorgans (cM) must be converted to their physical distances in base pairs (Mbp). Figure 6 illustrates a situation where a QTL defined by its linkage map locations cannot be precisely linked to the physical (sequence) map for lack of needed anchor marker information. There are two ways to transfer the QTL information over to the physical map:

1. To display both maps independently and draw links between the two as shown in Fig. 6. In this way, users can visualize the

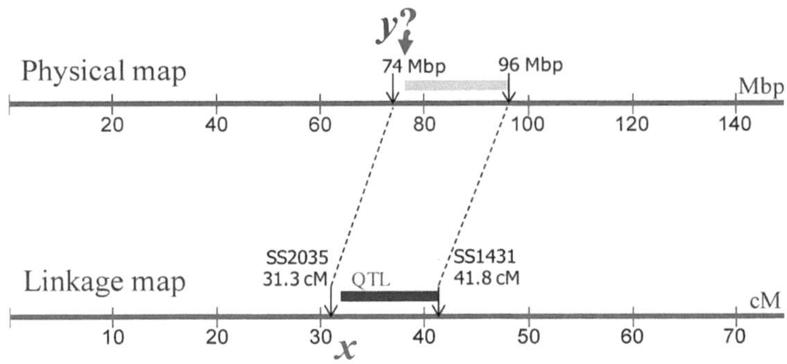

Fig. 6. Diagram to illustrate how a QTL location on linkage map may be interpolated to its physical map location with referencing to the closest "anchoring" marker locations.

linkage between the two maps to locate regions on the physical map for identification of underlining genes. Although this method is not precisely accurate, it is good enough to serve the purpose since a QTL span is normally in terms of ±1 cM (≈1 Mb) and a gene is usually much smaller.

2. A simple mathematical formula can be used to estimate the QTL size by interpolation using information from the nearest anchor markers (let L be linkage locations; P be physical locations; x be known QTL location on linkage map, and y be unknown location on physical map; refer to Fig. 6 for the variable foot-notations):

$$P_y = P_{SS1431} - \frac{(L_{SS1431} - L_x)(P_{SS1431} - P_{SS2035})}{L_{SS1431} - L_{SS2035}}$$

Alternatively, one can use the empirical 1 cM ≈ 1 Mbp units, or use actual chromosomal lengths to derive the cM/Mbp conversion ratio. This can be built into a CGI program to "translate" the locations on the fly.

3.2. Comparative Genomics and QTL Data Mining

Structural genomics information can be brought across species for the purposes of comparative studies by the methods we discussed in Subheading 3.1. This can be accomplished by using *comparative anchor markers* or functional mapping of genes across species. For example, corresponding links between human and mouse chromosomes can be established using markers mapped in both genomes. The more such anchor markers are placed in both genomes, the more precise the QTL location can be estimated. A comprehensive example of such comparative alignment is shown in Fig. 7, where pig chromosome 6 with an interesting QTL is aligned with human chromosomes 1, 18 and 19 via RH comparative mapping. A gene expression profile can also be also linked, which adds more strength for QTL data mining.

3.3. QTL Metadata and Simple Meta-analysis

We already know that QTL data from multiple experiments can be aligned (Fig. 8a). Subsequently, multiple QTL results on the same

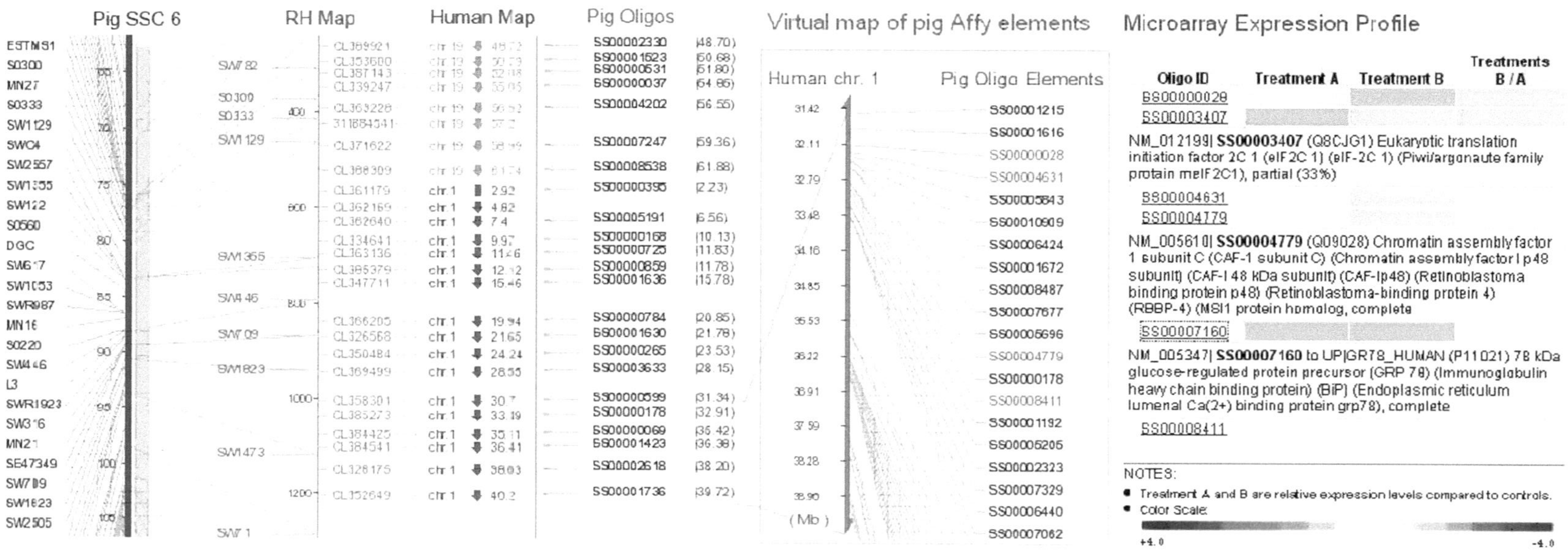

Fig. 7. A snapshot of pig chromosome 6 showing an interesting QTL region (gray bar along Pig SSC6 chromosome line). The pig map is aligned with human chromosomes 1, 18, and 19 via RH comparative mapping. To the *right* are a gene expression profiles-linked human genome locations by BLAST of oligo sequences used in the experiment (The color coded expression patterns are converted to gray scales in this print (11))

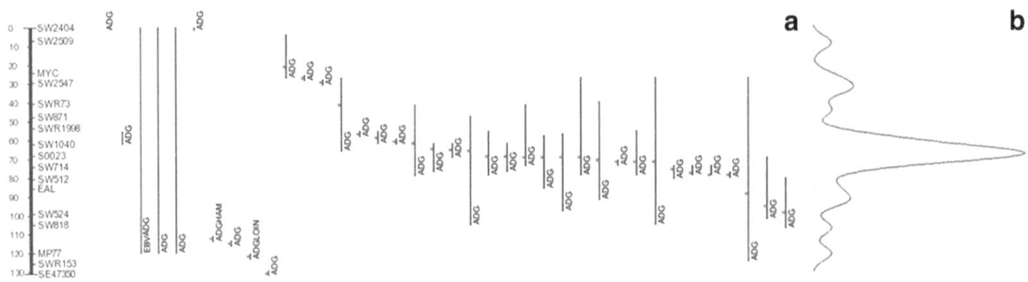

Fig. 8. A sample graphical display of QTL found on porcine chromosome 4, showing how do they align and support a generalized meta count (*source*: Animal QTLdb).

trait can be combined to describe a generalized "QTL" using the original QTL as metadata. Figure 8b shows a curve whose elevations (note the curve in Fig. 8b has been turned 90° clockwise) from the base line are simple counts of the presence of QTL at small intervals (e.g., 1 cM).

Although this can be done all in one program, for demonstration purposes we show it as a two-step procedure. First, all QTL spans (left and right boundary coordinates) for trait "ADG" on chromosome 4 are queried with a simple SQL statement:

```
SELECT A1_coord, B1_coord
FROM QTLdata a, traits b
WHERE a.trait_ID=b.trait_ID AND
        a.chromosome=4 AND
        b.trait_name='ADG';
```

and the results are saved into a file called "`Chr4.ADG.txt`". Next, a simple Perl script can loop through the entire length of the chromosome 4 (131 cM), count for the presence of a QTL, and add up the counts for every cM:

```
#!/usr/bin/perl
open(IN,"Chr4.ADG.txt");
while (<IN>) {
      chomp;
      ($lowcm,$hicm) = split(/\t/,"$_");
      for($i=0;$i<=131;$i++) {
            if (($i >= $lowcm) && ($i <= $hicm)) {
                  $qhash{$i}++;
            }
      }
}
close(IN);
foreach $key(sort {$a <=> $b} keys %qhash) {
     print "$key\t$qhash{$key}\n";
}
```

Please note that in this example we assumed that these meta ADG QTL were produced from identical experimental designs, i.e., assuming the testing statistics thresholds, confidence intervals, and degree of freedoms are all equal between each original experiment. In fact, this cannot be possibly true in the real world. This is a simplified scenario to count the raw QTL stored in a QTL database for a gross estimate of roughly where the most likely causal variant is located based on the meta-QTL reports. A formal meta-QTL analysis method would be more robust and statistically sound, and we refer the reader to Chapter 8 by Xiaolin WU in this book for more details.

4. Summary

This chapter focused on key issues and techniques necessary for QTL data modeling, conceptual design of a relational database, and its physical implementation. The introduction to several entry level programming techniques is meant to serve as a starter and was therefore brief. While there are multiple ways to accomplish a task, we tried to give clues rather than to imply that there is only one approach to accomplish something. We strongly encourage readers to explore further in "Further Reading".

5. Notes

1. The examples used in this chapter will be mainly based on MySQL unless otherwise indicated.
2. Hierarchy model, relational model, network model, Object-Oriented Model, Object-relational Model, etc. are among many data models that can be used to build a database. In this chapter, we only use relational model. Users can explore more on other data models.
3. "Comments" are constructs in program source codes where arbitrary notes can be inserted. "#" is a character to start a comment in most programming language, and anything after it will not be read by a compiler.

References

1. Korstanje R, Paigen B (2002) From QTL to gene: the harvest begins. Nat Genet 31:235–236
2. Rat Genome Database, QTL. HU http://rgd.mcw.edu/objectSearch/qtlQuery.jsp UH. Accessed 21 Feb 2012
3. The Jackson Laboratory QTL Resources. HUhttp://pga.jax.org/qtl/ UH. Accessed 21 Feb 2012
4. Hu Z-L, Fritz ER, Reecy JM (2007) AnimalQTLdb: a livestock QTL database tool set for positional QTL information mining and

beyond. Nucleic Acids Res 35(database issue): D604–D609

5. Gramene QTL Database. HUhttp://gramene.agrinome.org/qtl/UH. Accessed 21 Feb 2012
6. Codd EF (1970) A relational model of data for large shared data banks. Commun ACM 13:377–387
7. MySQL Workbench 5.2. http://wb.mysql.com/. Accessed 12 May 2010
8. Hu Z-L, Dracheva S, Jang W-H, Maglott D, Bastiaansen J, Rothschild MF, Reecy JM (2005) A QTL resource and comparison tool for pigs: PigQTLDB. Mamm Genome 16:792–800
9. Aerts J, Burt D, Carre W, DeKoning DJ, Haley C, Hu Z-L, Law A, Reecy J et al. MIQAS—minimum information for QTLs and association studies. http://miqas.sourceforge.net/. Accessed 21 Feb 2012
10. MySQL. http://www.mysql.com/. Last updated 1 Sep 2010. Accessed 21 Feb 2012
11. Hu Z-L, Park CA, Fritz ER, Reecy JM (2010) QTLdb: a comprehensive database tool building bridges between genotypes and phenotypes. In: Invited lecture with full paper published electronically on The 9th World Congress on Genetics Applied to Livestock Production (WCGALP), Leipzig, Germany, 1–6 Aug 2010

Further Reading

Hernandez MJ (2003) Database design for mere mortals: a hands-on guide to relational database design. Addison-Wesley, Reading, MA, USA

Widenius M, Axmark D, Arno K (2002) MySQL reference manual—documentation from the source. O'Reilly Media, O'Reilly Media, Sebastopol, CA, USA

Chang E (2003) Practical perl with CGI applications. Addison Wesley, Reading, MA, USA

Chapter 8

Meta-analysis of QTL Mapping Experiments

Xiao-Lin Wu and Zhi-Liang Hu

Abstract

Meta-analysis is an important tool for integrating information from multiple quantitative trait loci (QTLs) studies. Pooling of results from several studies allows greater statistical power for QTL detection and more precise estimation of their genetic effects. Hence, a meta-analysis can yield conclusions that are stronger than those of individual studies and can give greater insight into the genetic architecture of complex traits. In this chapter, we present basic theories and methods for meta-analysis of QTL mapping experiments. The meta-analytic procedures are described in a general context. The statistical methods cover both parametric and nonparametric statistical models. Finally, we illustrate the features of these statistical methods using simulated and real datasets.

Key words: Likelihood, Literature review, Markov chain Monte Carlo, Meta-analysis, Nonparametric models, Quantitative trait loci

1. Introduction

Meta-analysis is emerging as an essential tool for quantitative aggregation and synthesis of knowledge from independent studies on the same or a similar subject. In the past decade, there has been an explosion of QTL mapping experiments in animals and plants. These QTL studies, however, were conducted using various reference populations and experimental designs, and reported QTL may not be directly comparable between each other. As always, there have been questions regarding whether QTL locations identified for a given trait in one population correspond to those detected in other populations, or whether QTL locations identified in one species correspond to QTL or other types of loci detected in corresponding regions of other species. Meta-analysis can help answer such questions (1–3). A well-conducted meta-analysis allows a more objective appraisal of the evidence, resolving uncertainty and disagreement among studies. The availability of public QTL databases, such as Animal QTLdb (4, 5), GRAMENE (6), and QTL MatchMaker (7),

Scott A. Rifkin (ed.), *Quantitative Trait Loci (QTL): Methods and Protocols*, Methods in Molecular Biology, vol. 871, DOI 10.1007/978-1-61779-785-9_8,

encourages systematic description of QTL studies and facilitates comparing and combining of available QTL data.

The term, meta-analysis, was coined by G. V. Glass in 1976 when he proposed that distinct methods are needed to integrate the findings from a body of research (8). Since then, meta-analysis has become a widely accepted research tool in a variety of disciplines such as medical, social, and behavioral sciences (9). Broadly speaking, a meta-analysis can be defined as the quantitative review and synthesis of the results of related and independent studies using appropriate statistical methods (10). The objectives of a meta-analysis of QTL data can be several-fold. First of all, a meta-analysis can increase QTL detection power. In practical situations, QTL studies with small sample sizes are common and they often fail to find QTL with small effects even when they exist (11). Putting results together can increase the effective sample size and therefore allows more precise effect estimation of QTLs leading to increased power. In addition, a meta-analysis can assess the amount of variability between studies, identify study characteristics associated with particular QTLs, and it can also help gain insight into the genetic architecture of complex traits (12). Methodologically, a meta-analysis involves the application of standard statistical principles (i.e., hypothesis testing and statistical inference) to situations where only summary information (published and unpublished reports) is available and not the original data (e.g., phenotypes and genotypes of individuals, and pedigree when applicable). Analogously, combining information by pooling original data into a single dataset is called "mega-analysis" (13).

However, combining results of QTL mapping across several studies is a challenge because many aspects of these studies may differ, such as marker density, linkage, sample size, population type, experimental design, and statistical methods. In order to study QTL congruency, Goffinet and Gerber (1) proposed a meta-analysis strategy to resolve the number of QTL and their locations based on model selection. Etzel and Guerra (14) developed a meta-analytic approach to overcome the between-study heterogeneity and to refine both QTL location and the magnitude of the genetic effects. Veyrieras et al. (15) proposed a two-stage meta-analysis to integrate multiple independent QTL mapping experiments, implemented using the MetaQTL package. These methodological developments have stimulated dozens of QTL meta-analysis studies in the past 10 years (e.g., refs. (16–19)).

In what follows, we will present basic theories and general frameworks for meta-analysis of QTL mapping experiments. The general procedures typically include the following: (Subheading 2.1) defining objectives (formulating a specific purpose); (Subheadings 2.2 and 2.3) literature search (identifying relevant primary studies); (Subheadings 3.1 and 3.2) data abstraction and acquisition (coding data and defining the study outcome measures); (Subheading 3.3) combining results (aggregating and synthesizing results using appropriate statistical methods); and (Subheading 3.4) reporting results (interpreting and reporting the results and deciding follow-up steps).

2. Planning for a Meta-analysis

2.1. Defining Objectives and Meta-analysis Designs

Good planning is half the battle. A meta-analysis begins with a well-formulated design and questions. First of all, the study objectives need to be defined. For example, is the purpose of the study to validate QTL results in a broader population or to guide new studies? The design of the meta-analysis may differ with the answer to this question. Next, what are the operational definitions of the research outcome? As far as QTL effect is concerned, is it measured as the difference between QTL genotypic means (e.g., additive and dominance effects) or as QTL variance? This difference is related to experimental designs and reference populations used in the primary studies. The former is a typical measure of QTL effect in inbred crosses, whereas the latter is used for outbreed populations. Also relevant is the question of what contribute to the variation across individual studies. The answer to this question has an impact on choice of statistical models for inference, and on the interpretation of the results.

2.2. Literature Search

Search methods and strategies. Sources to be searched include public literature databases, technical reports, research manuscripts, and even work in progress if available. Reliance on only published reports leads to so-called publication bias, because most journals tend to selectively publish results that are statistically significant. This is sometimes called the "file drawer problem" because studies not reaching significance effect sizes are hard to publish and are relegated to file drawers. In general, bias is due to that studies selected in a meta-analysis are insufficiently representative of the totality of research being carried out. A practical way to minimize publication bias is to include information from unpublished QTL data. Egger et al. (20) and Sterne et al. (21) present some intuitive discussion on detecting and correcting bias in the context of meta-analysis.

We usually start a literature search with popular bibliographic reports, such as the Science Citation Index (e.g., http://apps.isiknowledge.com.ezproxy.library.wisc.edu/) and PubMed (http://www.ncbi.nlm.nih.gov/pubmed). A manual search of these databases requires specification of a search statement and a method of searching. Most research libraries add controlled vocabulary terms to bibliographic records. For example, classification codes and subject headings for books and descriptors for articles comprise controlled vocabulary. In contrast, natural language terms are those that appear in titles or abstracts and are not assigned by the research library.

A search statement typically combines the two sets of terms. In PubMed, for example, a search for body weight QTL published in Genetics would be specific as follows: `((QTL) ANDbodyweight) AND "Genetics"[Journal]`. As of 7 Sep 2010, this search extracted a total of 22 reports. Here, both "QTL (quantitative trait loci)" and "body weight" are Mesh headings used in PubMed (Mesh is the acronym for "Medical Subject Headings," which is the authority list of vocabulary terms used for subject analysis of biological literature at the US National Library of Medicine), and "`[Journal]`" is a search field tag for the name of journal. Com monly used search filed tags in PubMed are listed in Table 1.

Table 1
List of search filed tags in PubMed

Fields	Tag names
Affiliation	[AD]
Article identifier	[AID]
All fields	[ALL]
Author	[AU]
Book	[book]
Editor	[ED]
First author name	[1AU]
Full author name	[FAU]
Grant number	[GR]
Investigator	[IR]
ISBN	[ISBN]
Issue	[IP]
Journal title	[TA]
Language	[LA]
Mesh major topic	[MAJR]
Mesh subheadings	[SH]
NLM unique ID	[JID]
Publication date	[DP]
Publication type	[PT]
Text words	[TW]
Title	[TI]
Title/abstract	[TIAB]
UID	[PMID]
Volume	[VI]

There are two basic methods of literature searching. A backward search involves identifying a publication and then moving to earlier items in the citation, whereas a forward search identifies a publication and then searches all items that later cite the publication. The search loop is repeated until it exhausts. Using either method, the selection principles of the search need to be documented, such as the scope (including the subject headings, language constraints) and the domain (including sources that failed to yield studies) throughout the search and data synthesis.

As unpublished literature databases, dissertations and master's theses at various universities can be searched. At the UW-Madison libraries, for example, the Dissertations & Theses databases include doctoral dissertations in all subject areas completed at US accredited institutions. Some master's theses and foreign language dissertations are also included. Citations for dissertations dated back to 1980 and citations for master's theses started from 1988. Some public bibliographic databases can also be considered. For example, the NTIS (National Technical Information Service) summarizes completed researches sponsored by more than 600 US Federal agencies (http://www.ntis.gov/).

2.3. Evaluation of Retrieved Literature and Search Success

Evaluating quality and relevance of retrieved literature. The type of items to be collected in a meta-analysis typically include the characteristics of the report (author, year, source of publication), the study (scope of the sample, types of populations), species and breeds (including demographic features), and QTL location and effect size (sample size, outcome statistics, estimate, and standard error). Then, we need to determine the quality of the coding process and to decide some criteria for either accepting or rejecting a study to be meta-analyzed (22). However, the rules for assessing the quality of the studies and determining their relevance to the objectives of the meta-analysis are not clear, but they depend on the current state-of-art. Cook and Campbell (23) provided a framework describing several features of a study, which, if violated, impact the interpretation and quality of primary studies. In a QTL study, for example, if there is randomization bias with regarding to factors other than the QTL affecting the trait, we would expect either a larger or smaller difference in estimated QTL effect. Such bias would impact the internal validity of the study. Likewise, if the power to detect a QTL is low, it would threaten the statistical validation of the study. Limitations to the extent to which studies can be generalized to populations or breeds compromise the external validity of a study. Chalmers et al. (24) proposed a scoring method for inclusion and exclusion of studies. Their framework assesses three areas: study design, implementation, and analysis. For example, two readers, who are blinded to the authors, source, results, and discussion of the primary study, make ratings regarding the quality of studies, resulting in a percentage score that may be incorporated into a sensitivity analysis at the analytic stage.

This allows one to examine how overall inference changes if the analysis is restricted to high quality studies. As a formal approach, the ultimate inclusion status of a study may be decided by a panel of judges or experts.

Measuring the success of the search process. Given the unprecedented volume of information available nowadays, it is not practically feasible for us to obtain every piece of literature that is related to a search topic. Two concepts in information retrieval, *recall* and *precision*, can be used to describe the success of the search process. Recall measures the success of the retrieval process, computed as:

$$\text{Recall} = \frac{\text{number of relevant documents retrieved}}{\text{total number that should be retrieved}} \times 100$$

A higher percent recall corresponds to a more successful search. The second concept, precision, relates to the false rate and is calculated as:

$$\text{Precision} = \frac{\text{number retrieved and relevant}}{\text{total number retrieved}}$$

The goal is to have high recall and high precision literature retrievals. In practice, this goal can be accomplished by using a combination of search strategies.

In reality, however, the total number of documents that should be retrieved (TND) is unknown, because we have no way of knowing whether the set of located studies is representative of the full set of existing studies. Instead, more elaborate methods, such as estimation of population size using capture-recapture models (25), can be employed. Let N be TND, which is the number we wish to estimate, and M be the number of documents that were obtained ("captured"), marked (or tagged), and "released." After some time of literature search, there should be sufficient documents to mix: n documents were "captured," and m of them were recognized to be "marked" documents. Under the assumption that the proportion of "recaptured" documents is equal to the proportion of "marked" documents, that is, $m/n = M/N$, TND can be estimated as: $N = nM/m$.

3. Meta-analysis

3.1. Building a Consensus Map

Combining multiple QTL mapping experiments by alignment to a common reference or consensus map offers a more complete picture of the genetic control of a trait than can be obtained in any one study. This can be done using one of several software packages such as the *MetaQTL* package (15). Prior to building the consensus map, one needs to determine the overlap between marker names in different individual maps. Markers whose orders are not consistent across different individual maps ought to be removed from subsequent analysis.

In a meta-analysis, a consensus map is typically constructed based on a weighted least squares method, which takes into account the distances between markers in each individual map, and rescaled if necessary in Haldane units, with their accuracy determined by the population size and type. This method assesses the goodness-of-fit parameter λ of the consensus model, computed for each chromosome:

$$\lambda = \sum_{i=1}^{n} \sum_{jk} \frac{\left[d_{ijk} - (\gamma_k - \gamma_j)\right]^2}{\gamma_{ijk}^2}$$

where n is the number of QTL mapping experiments, d_{ijk} is the estimate in the ith map of the distance between adjacent markers j and k in cM, γ_{ijk}^2 is the corresponding expected variance of the distance estimate based on the population type and its size, γ_k and γ_j are the positions (in cM) of markers j and k on the consensus map, respectively. Here, a high value of λ corresponds to a low level of consistency between the marker distances in the different individual maps. Under the null hypothesis (assuming the same actual maps for all experiments), the goodness-of-fit value of the consensus map for each linkage group is affected only by sampling errors in individual maps and follows a χ^2 distribution: $\lambda \sim \chi^2_{q-m+1}$ where q is the total number of marker intervals over n individual maps, and m is the total number of markers for the chromosome. Thus, it is possible to build a statistic test, for example, using a 5% type I risk level. Finally, an estimation of QTL positions and their confidence intervals (CI) can be projected onto the consensus map based on a scaling rule between the positions of flanking markers of these QTL on the original map and the positions of markers on the consensus map.

3.2. Defining the Study Outcome

After the primary studies have been collected and coded, one needs to identify a summary (outcome) measure common to all studies and then combine results from these studies. In the context of QTL studies, a summary measure can be QTL location, effect size, any statistic (such as LOD score), or even significance level computed in the primary studies. Often, there is little control over the choice of the summary measure because most of the decision is dictated by what is available in the primary studies.

QTL number and position. As far as QTL number is relevant, QTL locations are typically grouped based on this number in a parametric meta-analysis. Assume that there are a total of n studies, each reporting a QTL on a particular chromosome. The first question would be how many consensus QTLs (also referred to as meta-QTL hereafter) they represent. Potentially, there can be a single meta-QTL, two meta-QTLs, and so on, up to n distinct meta-QTL. Assessment of the number of QTLs can be made by selecting from amongst the best-fitting models with $1, 2, \ldots, n$ QTL on the basis of a likelihood ratio test (LRT), Akaike Information Content (AIC), or adjusted AIC (AIC*) (1). Briefly, the method considers QTL positions and corresponding CI in individual experiments, after projection on the consensus map. For a given number of hypothetical (meta-) QTLs, a Gaussian mixture model can be used to perform a quantitative clustering of the individual QTL to different meta-QTL. Models with different numbers of meta-QTLs are treated as different models, and the number of meta-QTLs is determined by choosing the most probable model based on some criterion.

With QTL locations reported in primary studies, their standard errors may not be available but can be estimated. Thus, for a report to be included in the meta-analysis, it ideally provides the interval map (test statistic profile). In addition to providing estimates of QTL location ($\hat{d}_j$), the interval map enables estimation of the standard error for the QTL location, $\sigma_j = se(\hat{d}_j)$, if not directly reported, after conversion of the test statistic approximately to a log-likelihood (ln L) scale. The standard error can be estimated from the curvature (Fisher information) of the log-likelihood profile at the estimated map position:

$$\sigma_j = [-\partial^2 \ln L/\partial d^2|_{d=\hat{d}_j}]^{-1/2}$$

The curvature can be estimated by fitting a local quadratic near the maximum of ln L and determining the coefficient of the quadratic term.

Conveniently, the variance associated with the position of a given QTL (say σ_j^2) can be determined from the 95% CI of QTL position, by noting:

$$\mathrm{CI} = 2 \times 1.96 \times \sigma_j$$

Here, the CI is either the value reported directly in the studies when available or the value derived the percentage of the variance explained by the QTL (R^2) using the following empirical formula (26):

$$\mathrm{CI} = \frac{530}{N \times R^2}$$

where N is the population size. In practice, this formula tends to give larger CI (more conservative) than those reported in the primary studies.

QTL effects. Here, we focus on effect size of single meta-QTL, one at a time, instead of QTL effect sizes projected on to a grid of locations on each chromosome (13). For a report to be included in this part of meta-analysis, it has summary data about effect size and its standard error of the QTL (or the data information that is sufficient to derive these quantities). In inbred crosses, for example, QTL additive effect (or allele substitution effect) may be the most relevant study measure. Let $\mu_{QQ(i)}$, $\mu_{Qq(i)}$, and $\mu_{qq(i)}$ represent the means of genotypes QQ, Qq, and qq, respectively, in the *i*th study. The additive effect of the QTL is computed as:

$$a_{(i)} = \frac{1}{2}(\mu_{QQ(i)} - \mu_{qq(i)})$$

Assuming homogeneous variance for the three genotypes, the variance of QTL additive effect in the *i*th study is estimated by:

$$\hat{\sigma}^2_{(i)} = \frac{(n_{qq(i)} - 1)s^2_{qq(i)} + (n_{Qq(i)} - 1)s^2_{Qq(i)} + (n_{QQ(i)} - 1)s^2_{QQ(i)}}{(n_{qq(i)} + n_{Qq(i)} + n_{QQ(i)} - 3)}$$

where, for example, $n_{aa(i)}$ and $s^2_{aa(i)}$ are the number of individuals and the sample variance of genotype aa. The standard error of the additive effects is calculated as:

$$\mathrm{se}(a_{(i)}) = \sqrt{\frac{\hat{\sigma}^2_{(i)}}{4}\left(\frac{1}{n_{QQ(i)}} + \frac{1}{n_{qq(i)}}\right)}$$

The dominance effect (and its standard error) of a QTL can be computed similarly.

For outbreed populations, QTL variance is a relevant study measure. Suppose that we have a collection of $i = 1, 2, \ldots, k$ primary sib-pair studies that tested for linkage to the same QTL by using $j = 1, 2, \ldots, m$ markers within the same chromosome segment *L* cM long. QTL variance (σ^2_g) can be estimated by observing (14):

$$E(\hat{\beta}_{ij}) = -2(1 - 2\theta_{ij})^2\sigma^2_g$$

where $\hat{\beta}$ represents the Haseman–Edston regression (27) coefficient for marker *j* of study *i*, and θ_{ij} is the recombination fraction between the QTL and marker M_{ij}.

Other measures. When the summary data from the primary studies consist of test statistics, we can recover the estimated effect size if the appropriate information is reported (26). Sometimes, the study summaries are significance levels (*p*-values). The *p*-values may also be combined in the meta-analysis (9), but this type of literature review adds little insight into size and direction of QTL effect.

3.3. Choosing Statistical Models

A variety of statistical methods can be used for meta-analysis of QTL mapping experiments. Here, we describe a fixed-effects model, a random-effects model, a two-point mixture model, and a Bayesian nonparametric model using a Dirichlet process prior (DPP). The choice of an appropriate model depends on the assumption about the variation between studies and on study objectives as well.

Meta-analytic fixed-effects model. Assume that we plan to combine results from a total of *n* primary studies. For each primary study, say *i*, let γ_i be a point estimate of the true parameter θ_i, such that

$$\gamma_i = \theta_i + e_i$$

where e_i is a residual term. If the study sizes are moderate or large, each γ_i is asymptotically normally distributed (by the central limit theorem) and approximately unbiased. That is,

$$\gamma_i \sim N(\theta_i, s_i^2), \quad \text{for } i = 1, \ldots, k$$

where s_i^2 is the variance of γ_i and this quantity is typically assumed to be known in a meta-analysis.

As the simplest case, the analysis under homogeneity assumes that the unknown parameter is identical in all independent studies, that is $\theta_1 = \theta_2 = \cdots = \theta_n = \theta$, and the only source of uncertainty comes from the sampling of individuals into studies. In practice, however, a bias correction, normalization, and/or variance stabilizing transformation may be needed to ensure that the homogeneity assumption is valid or approximately so. Then, the maximum likelihood (ML) estimation of θ is given by

$$\hat{\theta}_{\text{ML}} = \frac{1}{\sum_i w_i} \sum_i w_i \gamma_i \quad \text{with standard error se}(\hat{\theta}_{\text{ML}}) = \frac{1}{\sqrt{\sum_i w_i}}$$

where $w_i = 1/s_i^2$. The ML estimate of θ is the weighted average of true effects in the set of n studies, with weights equal to $w_i = 1/s_i^2$. This provides the basis for the traditional meta-analysis. Use of inverse variance weights minimizes the variance of the common effect size parameter θ. If all the weights are equal (i.e., $s_1 = \cdots = s_k = s$), then $\hat{\theta}_{\text{ML}}$becomes

$$\hat{\theta} = \frac{1}{k} \sum_i \gamma_i \quad \text{with standard error se}(\hat{\theta}) = \frac{s}{\sqrt{k}}$$

The meta-analytic fixed-effects model provides a conditional inference about the set of n studies included in the meta-analysis. It addresses the question of how large the average true QTL effect is in the set of n studies included in the meta-analysis. As such, a fixed-effects model also provides valid inference (e.g., conclusion about the average effect) under heterogeneity, as long as the inference is restricted to the set of studies included in the meta-analysis. If the true effects are actually identical in all individual studies (i.e., $\theta_1 = \theta_2 = \cdots = \theta_n = \theta$), the distinction between the various models disappears.

A statistical test for the homogeneity of study means can be done by testing the null hypothesis of no effect ($H_0 : \theta_1 = \theta_2 = \cdots = \theta_n = \theta$) vs. the alternative ($H_1$: At least one θ_i is different). Under H_0, for large sample sizes, we have

$$Q = \sum_i w_i (\gamma_i - \hat{\theta}_{\text{ML}})^2 \sim \chi_{k-1}^2$$

where χ_{k-1}^2 represents a χ^2 distribution with $k - 1$ degrees of freedom. If the null hypothesis is not rejected (i.e., when $Q$is no greater than the $100(1-\alpha)$ percentile of the χ^2_{k-1} distribution), we would conclude that the n studies share a common mean θ (which is estimated by $\hat{\theta}_{\mathrm{ML}}$). Otherwise, the alternative hypothesis would be accepted. Then, we would proceed either by attempting to identifying covariates that stratify studies into the homogeneous population or by estimating a meta-analytic random-effects model instead.

Meta-analytic random-effects model. In real situations, heterogeneity can be present, and should be part of the analysis. In a meta-analysis of QTL mapping experiments, two types of heterogeneity are of primary interest (28): locus and size heterogeneity. Under the scenario of locus heterogeneity, study populations may differ in their genetic backgrounds, so that a locus affecting the trait of interest in one population might have no effect in another one. Likewise, the same locus may influence the trait in all populations, but its effect size may vary with these populations. This is called size heterogeneity, which happens, for example, when the frequency of the causal allele is much smaller in some populations or interacts with other loci or with the environment or other risk factors. In the presence of heterogeneity, differences among studies arise from both between-study variation of true effect size and chance variation due to sampling of individuals into studies. Thus, a fixed-effects model tends to underestimate the true degree of variability of θ and generate p-values which are artificially low. If between-study variation is not accounted for properly, meta-analytic results will appear to be more significant than they actually are.

The analysis under heterogeneity assumes that the true study-specific effect θ_i, for $i = 1, \ldots, k$, is different and arises from some distribution, say a norm distribution with mean θ, such that

$$\theta_i = \theta + u_i$$

where $u_i \sim N(0, \tau^2)$ and τ^2 is the between-study variance of effect size. Then, y_i can be expressed linearly as

$$\begin{aligned} y_i &= \theta_i + e_i \\ &= \theta + (\theta_i - \theta) + e_i \\ &= \theta + u_i + e_i \end{aligned}$$

This is a random-effects model. Marginally, the distribution of y_i is

$$y_i \sim N(\theta, \tau^2 + s_i^2)$$

If $\tau^2 = 0$, the above model becomes identical to the fixed-effects model.

Thus, assuming τ^2 is known, the ML estimate for θ is obtained similarly as

$$\hat{\theta}(\tau)_{\mathrm{ML}} = \frac{1}{\sum_i w(\tau)_i} \sum_i w(\tau)_i y_i$$

where $w(\tau)_i = 1/(\tau^2 + s_i^2)$. Thus, in a random-effects model, the estimated θ is also considered as a weighted average, but the weight is adjusted to take into account the additional variability between studies (τ^2). The above formula also works if τ^2 is estimated and the estimated value is plugged in. The restricted maximum likelihood (REML) approach can be used to estimate the variance component in the model. Iteratively, the REML estimate of τ^2 is the solution to

$$\hat{\tau}^2_{\text{REML}} = \frac{1}{\sum_i w(\tau)_i} \sum_i w(\tau)_i^2 \left(\frac{k}{k+1} (\gamma_i - \hat{\theta}_{\text{REML}})^2 - s_i^2 \right)$$

and $\hat{\theta}_{\text{REML}}$ is calculated using the same formula as that of $\hat{\theta}(\tau)_{\text{ML}}$ but replacing $w(\tau)_i$ with $w(\hat{\tau}_{\text{REML}})_i = 1/(\hat{\tau}_{\text{REML}} + s_i^2)$.

Meta-analytic models with moderates. It is possible to include study-level covariates, also called moderators, in meta-analysis models. With one or more moderators added to a fixed-effects model, it yields a fixed-effects-with-moderators model:

$$\gamma_i = \theta + \mathbf{x}'_i\beta + e_i$$

where β is a vector containing all study-level covariates, and $\mathbf{x}'_i$ is a row incidence vector (which takes values of 0 and 1, respectively). If one or more moderator variables are included in the random-effects model, it produces a so-called meta-analytic mixed-effects model:

$$\gamma_i = \theta + \mathbf{x}'_i\beta + u_i + e_i$$

where $u_i \sim N(0, \tau^2)$. In the above model, the value of τ^2 represents the "amount of residual heterogeneity" in the true effects or outcome, that is, the amount of variability among the true effects or outcome that is not accounted for by the moderators included in the model.

Bayesian implementation. Within the Bayesian framework, all variables and data are treated as random. For a meta-analytic fixed-effects model, a normal prior distribution, $\theta \sim N(\theta_0, \sigma_0^2)$, is typically assumed, where θ_0 and σ_0^2 are known hyperparameters (representing are mean and variance, respectively, of the normal prior distribution). Then, the Bayesian analysis incorporates information from both the prior and the data to obtain so-called posterior inference of unknown parameters. By the properties of conjugacy, the posterior distribution of θ is also normal.

$$\theta|\text{else} \sim N\left(\left(\sigma_0^{-2} + \sum_i w_i \right)^{-1} \left(\sigma_0^{-2}\theta_0 + \sum_i w_i\gamma_i \right), \left(\sigma_0^{-2} + \sum_i w_i \right)^{-1} \right)$$

where "else" is used to represent the data, all parameters excluding θ, and all known hyperparameters. From the above, the posterior mean of θ is given as:

$$E(\theta|\text{else}) = \left(\sigma_0^{-2} + \sum_i w_i \right)^{-1} \left(\sigma_0^{-2}\theta_0 + \sum_i w_i\gamma_i \right)$$

If $w_1 = w_2 = \cdots = w_k = s^{-2}$, then we have

$$E(\theta|\text{else}) = \frac{\sigma_0^{-2}}{\sigma_0^{-2} + ks^{-2}}\theta_0 + \frac{ks^{-2}}{\sigma_0^{-2} + ks^{-2}} \frac{\sum_i \gamma_i}{k}$$

The posterior mean of θ can be interpreted as the weighted average of the prior mean (θ_0) and the data mean ($(\sum_i \gamma_i)/k$), and the weights are $\sigma_0^{-2}/(\sigma_0^{-2} + ks^{-2})$ and $ks^{-2}/(\sigma_0^{-2} + ks^{-2})$, respectively. If σ_0^2 is very large (e.g., assuming a flat prior distribution for θ), then $\sigma_0^{-2} + \sum_i w_i \to \sum_i w_i$ and the poster mean of θ coincides with its maximum likelihood estimate because

$$E(\hat{\theta}|\text{else}) \to \frac{1}{\sum_i w_i} \sum_i w_i \gamma_i \quad \text{with se}(\hat{\theta}) = \frac{1}{\sqrt{\sum_i w_i}}$$

For the random-effects model, if τ^2 were known and if the same normal prior distribution were assumed for θ, the posterior mean of θ would take a similar form:

$$E(\hat{\theta}|\text{else}) = \frac{1}{(\sigma_0^{-2} + \sum_i w(\tau)_i)} \left(\sigma_0^{-2}\theta_0 + \sum_i w(\tau)_i \gamma_i \right)$$

However, τ^2 is unknown. In the Bayesian model, a scaled inverse χ^2 prior distribution is typically assumed to τ^2: $p(\tau^2) \sim \chi^{-2}(\upsilon_\tau, S_\tau^2)$, where υ_τ and s_τ^2 are the known degrees of freedom parameter and scaling parameter, respectively. Then, θ and τ^2 can be simulated using a Gibbs sampler, by iteratively generating values from their fully conditional distributions:

$$\tau^2|\text{else} \propto \chi^{-2}\left(\upsilon_\tau + k, \upsilon_\tau S_\tau^2 + \sum_i u_i^2 \right)$$

$$\theta|\text{else} \sim N\left(\left[\sum_i s_i^{-2} + \sigma_0^{-2} \right]^{-1} \left(\sigma_0^{-2}\theta_0 + \sum_i s_i^{-2}(\gamma_i - u_i) \right), \left[\sum_i s_i^{-2} + \sigma_0^{-2} \right]^{-1} \right)$$

$$u_i|\text{else} \sim N((s_i^{-2} + \tau^{-2})^{-1}(s_i^{-2}(\gamma_i - \theta)), (s_i^{-2} + \tau^{-2})^{-1}), \quad \text{for } i = 1, \ldots, k$$

Again, the posterior mean of θ can be interpreted as the weighted average of the prior mean and the data mean. A similar interpretation can be made on the posterior means of u_i as well.

A two-point mixture model for locus heterogeneity. If there is evidence that the QTL influences the trait in some populations under investigation and not at all in others, this type of heterogeneity can be modeled using a two-point mixture model at the study level:

$$\gamma_i \sim N(\theta_i, s_i^2)$$

and

$$\theta_i = \begin{cases} \theta & \text{with probability } \alpha \\ 0 & \text{with probability } (1 - \alpha) \end{cases}$$

Intuitively, the two-point mixture model can be interpreted as follows. The QTL affects the quantitative trait in a portion, say α, of the populations and θ is the common effect size of the QTL in these populations, but it has not material effects in the remaining populations (say $1 - \alpha$). The marginal distribution of γ_i is:

$$\gamma_i \sim \alpha N(\theta, s^2) + (1 - \alpha) N(0, s_i^2)$$

The EM algorithm can be used to estimate this mixture of normal distributions. Let $\phi(x; \mu, \sigma^2)$ denote the normal density function with mean μ and variance σ^2. The *E* (expectation) step at stage $m + 1$ of the iterative procedure computes the posterior probability $p_i^{(m+1)}$ that γ_i have arisen from a normal distribution with mean $\theta^{(m)}$ given the prior mixing proportion $\alpha^{(m)}$:

$$p_i^{(m+1)} = \frac{\alpha^{(m)} \phi(\gamma_i; \theta^{(m)}, s_i^2)}{\alpha^{(m)} \phi(\gamma_i; \theta^{(m)}, s_i^2) + (1 - \alpha^{(m)}) \phi(\gamma_i; 0, s_i^2)}$$

In the *M* (maximization) step, parameters $\alpha^{(m+1)}$ and $\theta^{(m+1)}$ are updated as:

$$\alpha^{(m+1)} = \frac{1}{n} \sum_i p_i^{(m+1)}$$

$$\theta^{(m+1)} = \frac{\sum_i p_i^{(m+1)} \gamma_i / s_i^2}{\sum_i p_i^{(m+1)} / s_i^2}$$

The model parameters α and θ are constrained to lie in [0,1] and $[0, +\infty)$, respectively. Notice that the two-point mixture model can be extended to account for both size heterogeneity and locus heterogeneity.

Nonparametric model using a DPP. A Bayesian nonparametric model using a Dirichlet process prior (referred to as the DPP model) can be used, which can be interpreted as extending the mixture model to the infinite case. The normality assumption, $u_i \sim N(0, \sigma_b^2)$, is typically made in a parametric model, but it has neither theoretical justification nor any empirical data support. In reality, population stratification and admixture is common, leading to multimodal distributions of the data. In contrast, the DPP model makes a weaker assumption about study-specific effect size or outcome measure.

To relax the normality assumption about study-specific outcome measure, we replace $u_i \sim N(0, \tau^2)$ with $u_i \overset{\text{iid}}{\sim} G, \forall i$, where G is some general distribution, $G \sim \pi$, and π is a "nonparametric prior." A choice for π is the Dirichlet process (29, 30), i.e.,

$$G \sim \mathrm{DP}(\alpha G_0)$$

Here, G_0 is a "baseline" distribution function, which is also referred to as the "center" of the DP prior, in the sense that

$E(G(.)) = G_0(.)$, and α is interpreted as a precision parameter indicating the degree of concentration of the prior on G around some parametric family. In particular, we assume that $G_0 \equiv N(u_i|u_0, \tau^2)$, where u_0 can take a fixed value (e.g., $u_0 = 0$) or it can be treated as an unknown quantity in the model. In the latter case, a prior distribution about u_0 is also assumed in the Bayesian hierarchical model specifications.

Inference about θ and τ^2 in the DPP model can be made similarly as they are in a parametric model (30). However, inference about u_i's in the DPP model is different than in the parametric model. For simplicity, assume that $u_0 = 0$. It can be shown that the posterior distribution of u_i takes the following form:

$$p(u_i|\text{else}) \propto q_0 G_0(.) + \sum_{i' \neq i}^{N} q_i \delta(u_{i'})$$

where $q_{i'} \propto N(\gamma_{i'}|\theta + u_{i'}, s_{i'}^2)$, and $q_0 \propto \alpha \int N(\gamma_i|\theta + u_i, s_i^2) N(u_i|0, \sigma_u^2)\, \mathrm{d}u_i = \alpha N(\theta, s_i^2 + \sigma_u^2)$. Thus, the fully conditional posterior distribution of u_i is a mixture of $N - 1$ degenerate distributions, $\delta(u_{i'})$, with point mass at $u_{i'}$ $(i' \neq i)$, and of the parametric conditional distribution $G_0(.)$ under the assumption of a baseline distribution. The u_i's can be simulated as follows: (1) $u_i = u_{i'}$ with probability $q_{i'}$, for $i' = 1, \ldots, i-1,\ i+1, \ldots, N$, or, (2) u_i is drawn from $G_0(.)$ with probability q_0.

A notable feature of the DPP model is that the posterior distribution of g is discrete, because the distribution of u_i has point masses located at previous draws $u_{i'}$ $(i' \neq i)$. This implies a clustering property: the values of u_i's for the primary studies are clustered by the DPP model. For example, if u_i represent a QTL location, the clusters of u_i's on a specific chromosome can have meaningful implication for the number of putative QTL and their locations. Let $g_1, \ldots, g_q$ be q distinct values among n estimates of QTL locations $u_1, \ldots, u_n$, where $1 \leq q \leq n$ at each iteration of Markov chain Monte Carlo sampling. Then, the unique values of $u_1, \ldots, u_n$ induce a partitioning into m clusters. For each cluster, say j, all the u's belonging to this cluster take on the same value g_j. Biologically, each cluster can represent a hypothetic (meta-)QTL. Given that $u_1, \ldots, u_n$ are random; this induces a random portion as well. In the Bayesian context, the marginal posterior distribution of the number of clusters (i.e., number of QTL) can be constructed conveniently by directly counting the number of distinct values of u_i's at each iteration of the sampler. Following Bush and MacEachern (31), g's can be simulated from their fully conditional distributions. The precision parameter α can be treated either as known or as unknown and estimated in the analysis (32).

3.4. Reporting Meta-analysis Results

Meta-analysis reports may vary with the purposes of studies. At a minimum, a report consists of an abstract and a main body of the report. The abstract typically summarizes study objectives, operational definitions of outcome measures, populations, meta-analysis design, search strategies, results, and conclusions and implications. In the body of the report, data collection procedures, as well as potential biases in the retrieved literature, should be described in detail. The estimated size of all possible studies to be collected and recall and precision of the retrieved literature are also relevant. The key elements of each primary study are typically listed in a table and the overall effect size is compared to those reported in primary studies. Often, plots and graphs are useful to show the contrast of the primary data and the estimated effect size by the meta-analysis, for publication bias and for sensitivity analysis. The conclusions of the meta-analysis need to be made as appropriate as possible and the significance (or lack thereof) of the statistical results should be clearly stated. With Bayesian statistical methods, posterior distributions of parameters of interest should be summarized in either tables or graphs. Implications of the results for future research and possibly follow-up studies need to be stated as well. Finally, limitations associated with the methods and results ought to be mentioned.

4. Illustrative Examples

4.1. Meta-analysis Using Simulated Data

In this section, features of the statistical methods are illustrated using a simulated dataset. For the sake of simplicity in the illustration, we skip all "upstream" steps, and focus on combing parameter estimates using three different statistic methods. We consider only a single meta-QTL evaluated by 30 primary studies. In the simulation, most QTL variance for the first ten populations are immaterial, as they are generated from gamma distribution with a mean close to zero (i.e., shape = 0.1 and scale = 1, leading to a mean of 0.1). The QTL variance in the remaining 20 primary studies is generated from gamma (shape = 8, scale = 0.5), and the mean is equal to 4.0 (=8 × 0.5). For each primary study population, the sample variance s_i^2 of QTL is assumed to be known and generated from gamma (shape = 1, scale = 0.25).

The simulated summary data for the 30 studies are as follows:

```
> simuqtl<-read.table(simudat_adgq1.csv,head=T,
sep=,)
> simuqtl
     qtlID     yi     vi
1        1 0.0000 0.1993
2        2 0.0000 0.2826
3        3 1.2129 0.1377
```

```
4        4 0.1165 0.1945
5        5 0.0000 0.2176
......
21      21 5.0183 0.2496
22      22 5.8010 0.5916
23      23 4.2098 0.0016
24      24 2.2349 0.5278
25      25 4.4397 0.6851
......
30      30 4.6959 0.5314
```

Fitting parametric models using the metaphor package. An R package called metaphor (33), is used to implement the meta-analysis. Installation instructions can be found in the CRAN Web page (http://cran.r-project.org/). After the metaphor library has been loaded, various meta-analytic models can be fitted using the `rma.uni()` function (with alias name `rma()`). A fixed-effects model is fitted using the rma() function with `method=FE`. Under the assumption of homogeneous means among studies, a common effect size (QTL variance) across the 30 populations is estimated to be 2.178, with its standard error being 0.026. The χ^2 test, however, rejects the null hypothesis for homogeneous QTL variance among studies ($p < 0.001$).

```
>library(metafor)
>fixmod<-rma(yi,vi,data=simuqtl,method="FE")
>fixmod
Fixed-Effects Model (k = 30)
Test for Heterogeneity:
Q(df = 29) = 6709.6942, p-val < .0001
Model Results:
estimate se zval pval ci.lb ci.ub
2.1783 0.0261 83.4549 <.0001 2.1271 2.2295 ***
Signif. codes: 0 *** 0.001 ** 0.01 * 0.05 . 0.1  1
```

Then, a random-effects model assuming heterogeneous mean among the studies could be more appropriate. This is done by calling the rma() function without defining a specific method, because it fits a random-effects model by default. In this example, the common effect size estimated by the random-effects model is closer to the weighted mean of simulated QTL variances than that estimated by the fixed-effects model. The between-study variance of the effect size (QTL variance) is estimated to be 5.180 with a standard error of 1.427. The 95% CI of between-study variance is between 3.178 and 9.439.

```
>ranmod<-rma(yi,vi,data=simuqtl)
>ranmod
Random-Effects Model (k = 30; tau^2 estimator: REML)
```

```
tau^2 (estimate of total amount of heterogeneity):
5.1800 (SE = 1.4273)
tau (sqrt of the estimate of total heterogeneity):
2.2760
I^2 (% of total variability due to heterogeneity):
99.44%
H^2 (total variability / within-study variance):
179.92
Test for Heterogeneity:
Q(df = 29) = 6709.6942, p-val < .0001
Model Results:
estimate se zval pval ci.lb ci.ub
2.9711 0.4258 6.9779 <.0001 2.1366 3.8056 ***
Signif. codes: 0 *** 0.001 ** 0.01 * 0.05 . 0.1  1
```

In a meta-analysis, forest plots can be used to show the relative strength of effect size in multiple primary studies (34). A forest plot consists of at least two columns. The left-hand column lists the names of the studies, and on the right-hand side is a plot of the measure of effect size for each of these studies (often represented by a rectangle) and their CIs represented by horizontal lines. The area of each rectangle is proportional to the study's weight in the meta-analysis. The common effect size estimated by the meta-analysis is usually plotted as a diamond. A vertical line representing no effect is also plotted. If the CI for an individual study overlaps with this line, the effect size for the individual study is not significant. The same interpretation applies to the common effect size estimated by the meta-analysis. In this example, the effect size estimated by the meta-analysis is significant because its 95% CI does not overlap with the vertical line representing no effect (Fig. 1).

```
> forest(ranmod, slab=simuqtl$qtlID, cex=1.0)
> op<-par(cex=1.0,font=2)
> text(-3,34,"Primary studies",pos=2)
> text(15,34,"QTL variance",pos=2)
> par(op)
```

Then, we make a scatterplot of QTL effect size against a measure of study size (which is the standard error of QTL variance in this example), as shown in Fig. 2. This is known as a funnel plot (35, 36). A symmetric inverted funnel shape arises from a "well-behaved" dataset, indicating that publication bias is unlikely. In contrast, an asymmetric funnel suggests a relationship between effect size and study size, which is possibly due to publication bias or a systematic difference between smaller and larger studies ("small study effects").

```
> funnel (ranmod, main="Fixed-effects model")
```

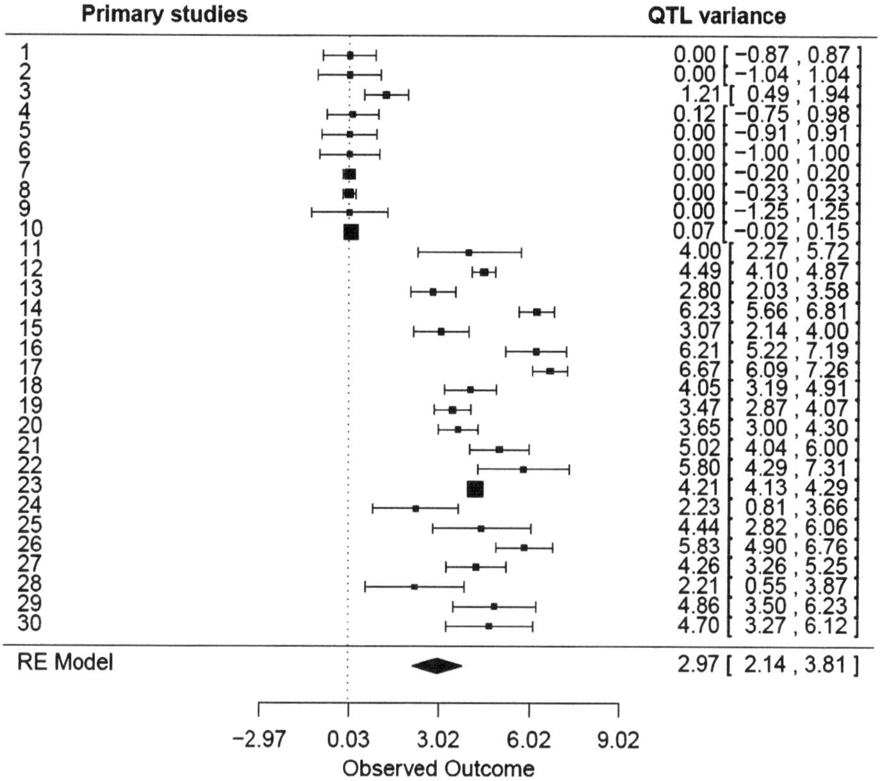

Fig. 1. Forest plot showing QTL variance obtained from 30 primary studies (*rectangles*) and a common estimate from the meta-analysis (*diamond*).

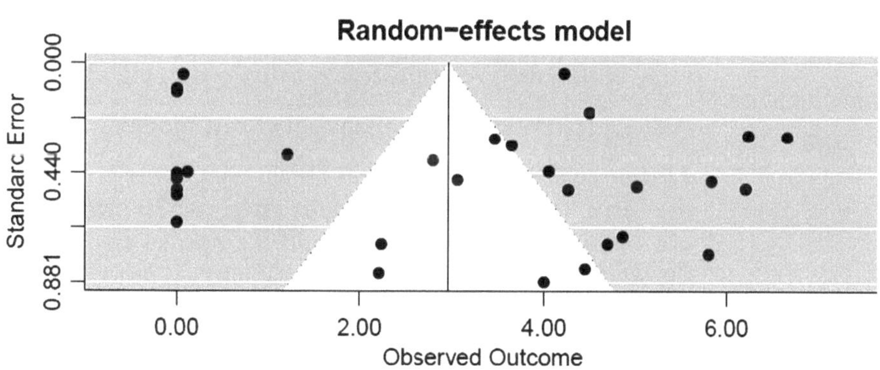

Fig. 2. Funnel plot for the meta-analytic random-effects model of QTL variance obtained from 30 primary simulation studies.

Radial (or Galbraith) plots provide a way to assess the consistency of observed outcomes that have differing precisions (e.g., due to heteroscedastic sampling variances). For a fixed-effects model, the plot shows the inverse of the standard errors on the horizontal axis (i.e., $1/\sqrt{s_i^2}$) against the individual observed outcomes

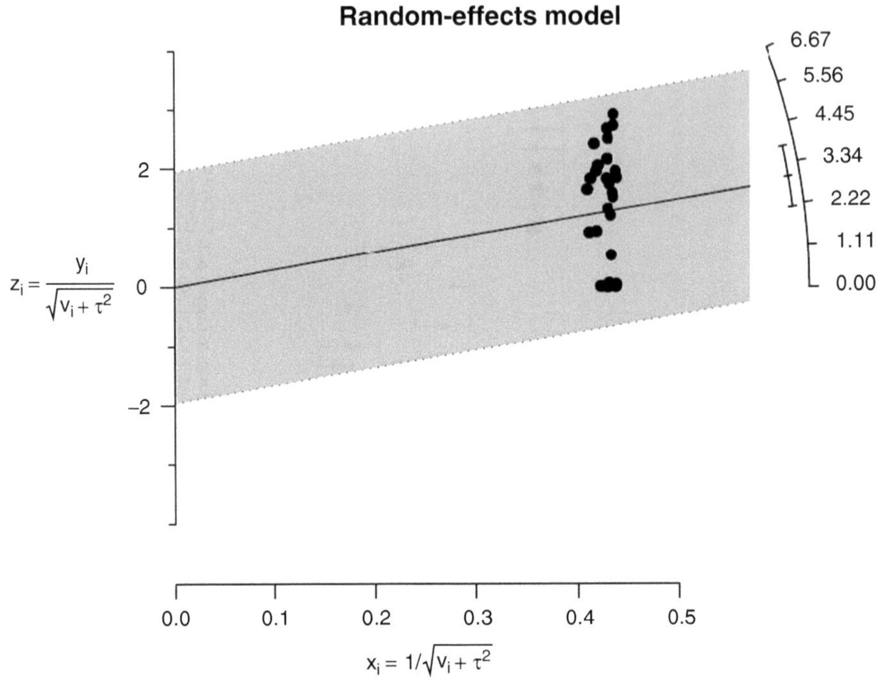

Fig. 3. Radial plot for the meta-analytic random-effects model of QTL variance obtained from 30 primary simulation studies.

standardized by their corresponding standard errors on the vertical axis (i.e., $y_i/\sqrt{s_i^2}$). For a random-effects model, it uses $1/\sqrt{\sigma_b^2 + s_i^2}$ for the horizontal and $y_i/\sqrt{\sigma_b^2 + s_i^2}$ for the vertical axis. On the right size of the plot, an arc is drawn. A line projected from (0,0) through a particular point within the plot onto this arc indicates the value of the observed outcome for that point (Fig. 3).

```
> radial (ranmod, main="Random-effects model")
```

Fitting the DPP model using the DPpackage. In the present example, the kernel density of QTL variance from the 30 primary studies is obviously multimodal (Fig. 4), and the normal assumption about the study-specific effect size (QTL variance) is not valid. A mixture model would be appropriate in this case. Because the exact number of components is unknown, we fit a Bayesian nonparametric model with a DPP. As mentioned before, this can be viewed as an infinite mixture model.

We assume that the DPpackage has been downloaded and installed ((37); http://cran.r-project.org/). In R, we first load the DPpackage library and then proceed to the meta-analysis. In the Bayesian analysis, the Markov chain Monte Carlo sampling consists of 20,000 saved iterations, with a burn-in period of 10,000 iterations. The saved samples are used for posterior inference. The number of clusters is estimated to be 4.16, with a 95% highest posterior density (HPD) interval between 4 and 5 clusters.

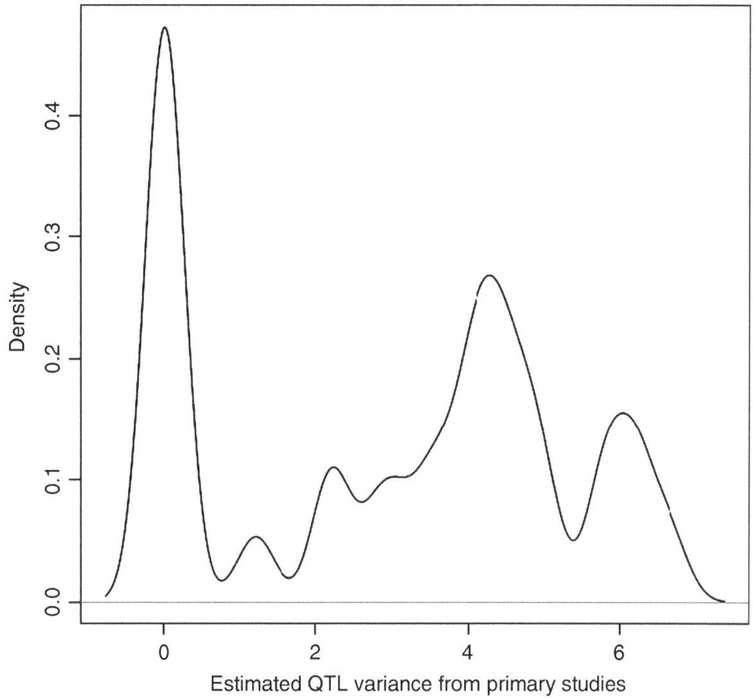

Fig. 4. Kernel density plot of QTL variance obtained from 30 primary simulation studies.

For the baseline distribution, the mean and variance are estimated to be 3.518 and 1.429, respectively.

```
> library(Dppackage)
> yi<-simuqtl$yi; vi<-simuqtl$vi
> y <- cbind(yi,vi)
> prior<-list(alpha=0.05,tau1=20,tau2=10,mub=0,
Sb=100) # Prior information
> state < NULL # Initial state
> nburn<-10000; nsave<-20000; nskip<-20; ndisplay <-
100 # MCMC parameters
> mcmc <- list(nburn=nburn,nsave=nsave,nskip=nskip,
ndisplay=ndisplay)
> fit1<-DPmeta(formula=y~1,prior=prior,mcmc=mcmc,
state=state,status=TRUE) # fit the model
> summary(fit1) # Summary with HPD and Credibility
intervalsBayesian semiparametric linear mixed
effects meta-analysis
......Regression coefficients:
Mean Median Std. Dev. Naive Std.Error 95%HPD-Low 95%
HPD-Upp
yi 2.973784 2.974683 0.410719 0.004107 2.124092
3.739124
```

```
Baseline distribution:
Mean Median Std. Dev. Naive Std.Error 95%HPD-Low 95%
HPD-Upp
mu 3.518220 3.525928 0.617367 0.006174 2.282208
4.710285
sigma2 1.429125 1.346000 0.462647 0.004626 0.709066
2.354514
Precision parameter:
Mean Median Std. Dev. Naive Std.Error 95%HPD-Low 95%
HPD-Upp
ncluster 4.166000 4.000000 0.443468 0.004435 4.000000
5.000000
>plot(fit1,ask=FALSE) # Plot model parameters
```

4.2. Meta-analysis of ADG QTL Locations in Swine Chromosome 1

As an application, we conduct a meta-analysis of average daily gain (ADG) QTL locations on swine chromosome 1 (SSC1). The summary data include mean and 95% CI of QTL position, extracted from the Animal QTLdb database (http://www.animalgenome.org/cgi-bin/QTLdb/index). The example data represent 21 ADG QTL reported by 13 independent studies (Table 2). Estimated QTL position (POS) are obtained from the original studies and the corresponding standard errors (SE) are computed based on the 95% CI of QTL positions (26). For the QTL locations without reported CI (whose QTLID are marked by "*"), we assign the average SE to each of them, for the sake of simplicity.

```
> adgqtl<-read.table("PigADGqtl.csv",head=T,
sep=",")
> adgqtl$VI<-adgqtl$SE^2
> summary(fit1)Bayesian semiparametric linear mixed
effects meta-analysis
......Regression coefficients:
Mean Median Std. Dev. Naive Std.Error 95%HPD-Low 95%
HPD-Upp
yi 104.61564 104.99803 7.78270 0.07783 89.39264
119.35588
Baseline distribution:
Mean Median Std. Dev. Naive Std.Error 95%HPD-Low 95%
HPD-Upp
mu 76.98523 76.98686 8.88818 0.08888 60.12954
95.21049
sigma2 460.87975 434.86365 146.37506 1.46375
231.18716 752.22395
Precision parameter: Mean Median Std. Dev. Naive Std.
Error 95%HPD-Low 95%HPD-Upp
ncluster 6.732200 7.000000 0.720233 0.007202 6.000000
8.000000
alpha 0.334775 0.318720 0.127279 0.001273 0.122692
0.595187
```

Table 2
Estimated positions and standard errors for average daily gain (ADG) QTL on swine chromosome 1 (data extracted from animal QTLdb)[a]

REFID	QTLID	CHR	POS	SE	Trait	SIGLEV
ISU0007	841	1	43.73	1.51	ADG	++
16978171	2,846	1	101	4.52	ADG	++
16978171	2,847	1	115	4.52	ADG	++
16415521	*2,885	1	119.5	5.52	ADG	NA
16415521	*2,886	1	67.6	5.52	ADG	NA
16478944	3,133	1	143	6.51	ADG	++
12807782	3,665	1	133.8	3.42	ADG	++
12807782	3,673	1	60	3.91	ADG	++
17121599	3,914	1	86.1	17.22	ADG	++
17121599	3,917	1	105.8	17.22	ADG	++
9922390	448	1	139	5.36	ADG	++
9922390	447	1	139	5.36	ADG	++
10656927	139	1	79	0.18	ADG	++
10656927	140	1	79	0.19	ADG	++
11403749	170	1	140.5	2.42	ADG	++
12081807	659	1	140.5	8.80	ADG	++
ISU0002	319	1	12	1.86	ADG	+
ISU0002	*320	1	121.3	5.52	ADG	NA
9922390	446	1	139	5.36	ADG	+
9263050	*495	1	102.9	5.52	ADG	NA
11048919	*549	1	134	5.52	ADG	NA

[a] *REFID* reference ID; *QTLID* QTL ID; *CHR* chromosome where the QTL is localized; *POS* reported map position of the QTL; *SE* standard error of reported map position of the QTL

Plots of the 21 reported ADG QTL locations clearly show a wide range of QTL locations on SSC1 among the studies (Fig. 5), possibly representing several ADG QTL on SSC1. In the presence of such heterogeneity, a common (central) estimate of QTL location has no biological meaning. So a fixed-effects model is not a valid solution to this problem. A random-effects model is also not desirable in this case because the kernel density of the reported ADG QTL locations is multimodal (Fig. 6—left), which by no means looks like a normal

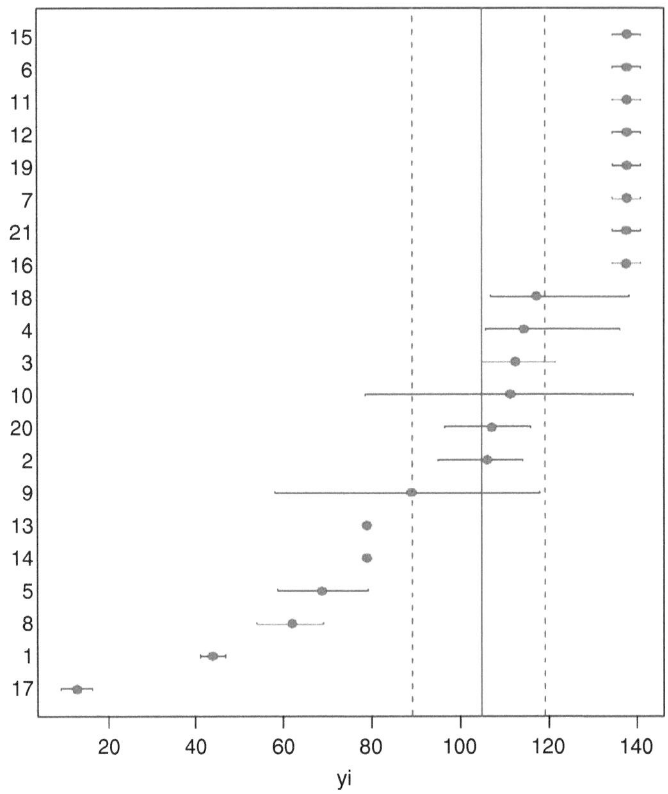

Fig. 5. Plots of average daily gain (ADG) QTL locations on swine chromosome 1, obtained from 21 primary studies.

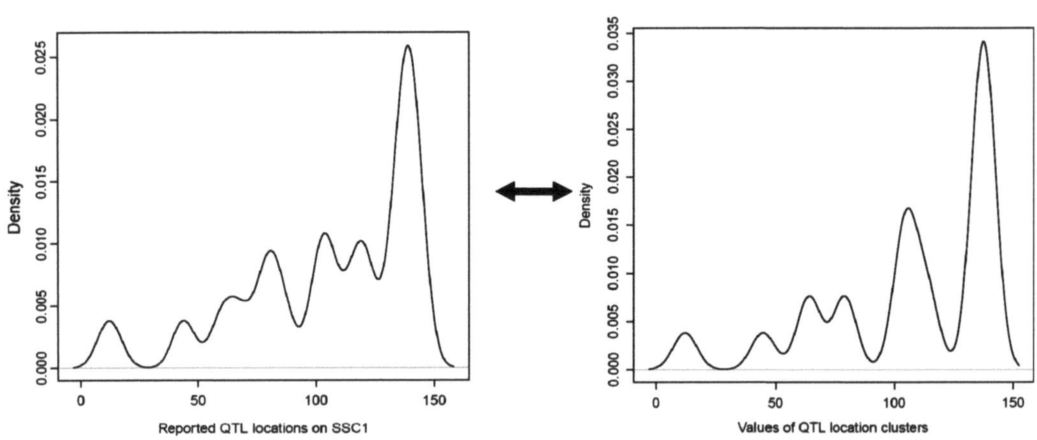

Fig. 6. Comparison of the kernel density plot of average daily QTL locations reported by 21 primary studies (*left*) and the posterior distribution of clusters values of QTL locations inferred using the nonparametric model with a Dirichlet process prior (*right*).

distribution. Hence, a Bayesian nonparametric model with a DPP is used.

The DPP model makes a weaker assumption about the study-specific QTL locations. Noticeably, the DPP model introduces a clustering property, and each cluster could represent a distinct QTL. The posterior distribution of the cluster values (Fig. 6—right) is in good agreement with the kernel density plot of the 21 reported ADG QTL locations (Fig. 6—left). This coincidence demonstrates that the DPP model could fit the data well when the distribution of QTL location (or any effect size or outcome measure) deviates from a normal distribution.

The distribution of the number of clusters in the DPP model depends on the parameter α. This parameter is given a fixed value ($\alpha = 0.05$) in the DPP model for the simulated data. In reality, however, the value of this parameter is not known. So this parameter is treated as unknown in the DPP model for the ADG QTL data (30). In the Bayesian context, a prior distribution needs to be assumed to the parameter α, for example, $\alpha \sim \beta$ (2, 20), and the value of α is estimated from its fully conditional distribution. In this example, the posterior mean (standard error) of α is 0.335 (0.319). The number of clusters for the ADG QTL locations is estimated to be 6.73 with 95% HPD interval being between 6 and 8, indicating that the 21 reported ADG QTL could present from 6 to 8 ADG QTL on SSC1. The mean and variance for the baseline distribution are 76.99 and 460.8, respectively. The posterior distributions of the mean and variance of the baseline distribution and of the cluster number are shown in Fig. 7.

Finally, it is worth commenting on the role of the parameter α in the DPP model. The parameter α measures the degree of belief in G_0 (which is typically assumed to be normal). So, α is interpretable as a measure of how close G_0 is to the true but unknown distribution G. As $\alpha \to \infty$, the prior for G "concentrates" on G_0. Simply put, a small value of α indicates that the data is diffuse, and that the nonparametric model using the DPP would fit the data better than the parametric methods assuming a normal distribution of u_i's. This was exactly the case with our examples. As α becomes large, the prior distribution of u_i's in the meta-DPP model would approach a normal distribution, and their estimates from the parametric and nonparametric models would become comparable to each other.

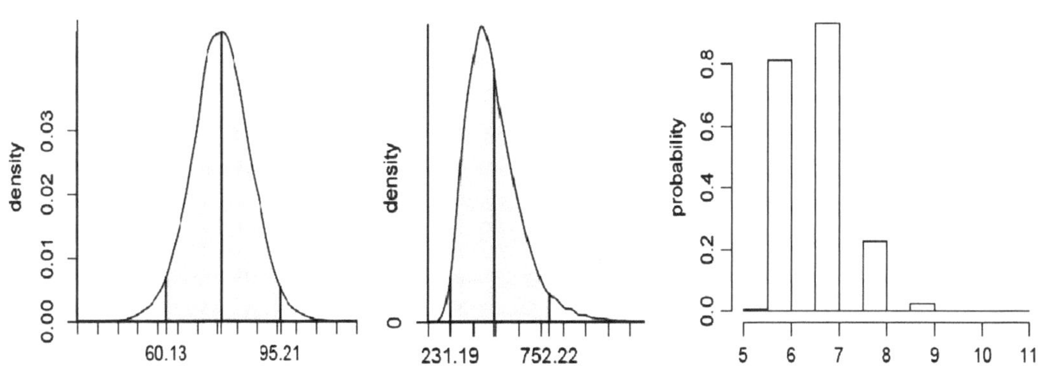

Fig. 7. Posterior distributions of the mean and variance of the baseline distribution and of the number of clusters, all pertaining to ADG QTL on swine chromosome 1.

References

1. Goffinet B, Gerber S (2000) Quantitative trait loci: a meta-analysis. Genetics 155:463–473
2. Hayes B, Goddard ME (2001) The distribution of the effects of genes affecting quantitative traits in livestock. Genet Sel Evol 33:209–229
3. Khatkar MS, Thomson PC, Tammen I, Raadsma HW (2004) Quantitative trait loci mapping in dairy cattle: review and meta-analysis. Genet Sel Evol 36:163–190
4. Hu ZL, Dracheva S, Jang W, Maglott D, Bastiaansen J, Rothschild MF, Reecy JM (2005) A QTL resource and comparison tool for pigs: PigQTLDB. Mamm Genome 16:792–800
5. Hu ZL, Fritz ER, Reecy JM (2007) AnimalQTLdb: a livestock QTL database tool set for positional QTL information mining and beyond. Nucleic Acids Res 35:D604–D609
6. Ni J, Pujar A, Youens-Clark K, Yap I, Jaiswal P, Tecle I, Tung CW, Ren L, Spooner W, Wei X, Avraham S, Ware D, Stein L, McCouch S (2009) Gramene QTL database: development, content and applications. Database (Oxford) 2009:bap005
7. Star KV, Song Q, Zhu A, Böttinger EP (2006) QTL MatchMaker: a multi-species quantitative trait loci (QTL) database and query system for annotation of genes and QTL. Nucleic Acids Res 34(Database issue):D586–D589
8. Glass GV (1976) Primary, secondary and meta-analysis of research. Educ Res 5:3–8
9. Hedges LV, Olkin I (1985) Statistical methods for meta-analysis. Academic, New York
10. Normand ST (1999) Meta-analysis: formulating, evaluating, combining, and reporting. Stat Med 18:321–359
11. Ball RD (2005) Experimental designs for reliable detection of linkage disequilibrium in unstructured random population association studies. Genetics 170:859–873
12. Salih H, Adelson DL (2009) QTL global meta-analysis: are trait determining genes clustered? BMC Genomics 10:184
13. Goldstein DR, Guerra R (2010) A brief introduction to meta-analysis, genetics and genomics. In: Guerra R, Goldstein DR (eds) Meta-analysis and combining information in genetics and genomics. Chapman & Hall/CRC, Boca Raton
14. Etzel CJ, Guerra R (2002) Meta-analysis of genetic-linkage analysis of quantitative-trait loci. Am J Hum Genet 71:56–65
15. Veyrieras J-B, Goffinet B, Charcosset A (2007) MetaQTL: a package of new computational methods for the meta-analysis of QTL mapping experiments. BMC Bioinformatics 8:49
16. Ioannidis JP, Ntzani EE, Trikalinos TA, Contopoulos-Ioannidis DG (2001) Replication validity of genetic association studies. Nat Genet 29:306–309
17. Hanocq E, Laperche A, Jaminon O, Laine A-L, Le Guis J (2007) Most significant genome regions involved in the control of earliness traits in bread wheat, as revealed by QTL meta-analysis. Theor Appl Genet 114:569–584
18. Rong J, Feltus FA, Waghmare VN, Pierce GJ, Chee PW, Draye X, Saranga Y, Wright RJ, Wilkins TA, May OL, Smith CW, Gannaway JR, Wendel JF, Paterson AH (2007) Meta-analysis of polyploid cotton QTL shows unequal contributions of subgenomes to a complex network of genes and gene clusters implicated in lint fiber development. Genetics 176:2577–2588
19. Truntzler M, Barriere Y, Sawkins MC, Lespinase D, Betran J, Charcosset A, Moreau L (2010) Meta-analysis of QTL involved in silage quality of maize and comparison with the position of candidate genes. Theor Appl Genet 121:1468–1482
20. Egger M, Smith GD, Schneider M, Minder C (1997) Bias in meta-analysis detected by a simple, graphical test. BMJ 315:629–634
21. Sterne JA, Egger M, Smith GD (2001) Investigating and dealing with publication and other biases in meta-analysis. BMJ 323:101–105
22. Sands ML, Murphy JR (1996) Use of kappa statistic in determining validity of quality filtering for meta-analysis: a case study of the health effects of electromagnetic radiation. J Clin Epidemiol 49:1045–1051
23. Cook TD, Campbell DT (1979) Quasi-experimentation: design & analysis issues for field settings. Houghton Mifflin, Boston
24. Chalmers TC, Smith H Jr, Blackburn B, Silverman B, Schroeder B, Reitman D, Ambroz A (1981) A method for assessing the quality of a randomized control trial. Control Clin Trials 2:31–49
25. Seber GAF (2002) The estimation of animal abundance and related parameters. Blackburn Press, Caldwell
26. Darvasi A, Soller M (1997) A simple method to calculate resolving power and confidence interval of QTL map location. Behav Genet 27:125–132
27. Haseman JK, Elston RC (1972) The investigation of linkage between a quantitative trait and a marker locus. Behav Genet 2:3–19

28. van Houwelingen HC, Lebrec JJP (2010) Heterogeneity in meta-analysis of quantitative trait linkage studies. In: Guerra R, Goldstein DR (eds) Meta-analysis and combining information in genetics and genomics. Chapman & Hall/CRC, Boca Raton
29. Ferguson TS (1973) A Bayesian analysis of some non-parametric problems. Ann Statist 1:209–230
30. Ferguson TS (1974) Prior distribution on spaces of probability measure. Ann Statist 2:615–629
31. Bush CA, MacEachern SN (1996) A semi-parametric Bayesian model for randomized block designs. Biometrika 83:275–285
32. Gianola D, Wu XL, Manfredi E, Simianer H (2010) A non-parametric mixture model for genome-enabled prediction of genetic value for a quantitative trait. Genetica 138:959–977
33. Viechtbauer W (2010) Conducting meta-analysis in R with the metaphor package. J Stat Softw 36:1–48
34. Lewis S, Clarke M (2001) Forest plots: trying to see the wood and the trees. BMJ 322:1479–1480
35. Light RJ, Pillemer DB (1984) Summing up: the science of reviewing research. Harvard University Press, Cambridge
36. Sterne JA, Egger M (2001) Funnel plots for detecting bias in meta-analysis: guidelines on choice of axis. J Clin Epidemiol 54:1046–1055
37. Jara A (2007) Applied Bayesian non- and semiparametric inference using DPpackage. R News 7:17–26

Further Reading

Normand ST (1999) Meta-analysis: formulating, evaluating, combing, and reporting. Stat Med 18:321–359

van Houwelingen HC, Lebrec JJP (2010) Heterogeneity in meta-analysis of quantitative trait linkage studies. In: Guerra R, Goldstein DR (eds) Meta-analysis and combining information in genetics and genomics. Chapman & Hall/CRC, Boca Raton

Part III

Extending the Power of Quantitative Trait Locus Analysis

Chapter 9

Using eQTLs to Reconstruct Gene Regulatory Networks

Lin S. Chen

Abstract

In recent years, a new type of experiment has emerged. It involves genetic crosses and simultaneous measurements of the genome-wide gene expression and genotype information of the offspring. In this chapter, I discuss how to reconstruct gene regulatory networks from this type of data. Subheading 1 provides an overview of the topic. In Subheading 2, I review previous methods of constructing gene networks from expression data alone and point out the difficulties of inferring causal relationships from observational studies. I also introduce the concept of Mendelian randomization of genotypes during a genetic cross. Based on this concept, several methods have been proposed that utilize the genetically randomized genotype information (expression quantitative trait loci information) to infer gene regulatory relationships. Subheading 3 describes the development and details of these methods. I also discuss the pros and cons of each. Subheading 4 addresses a major challenge of inferring gene regulation: how to adequately consider the existence of hidden variables, and points out that further research is still needed.

Key words: eQTL, Gene regulatory network, Causation, Mendelian randomization, Hidden causal variable

1. Introduction

The advance of high-throughput technology opens a new gateway for modern molecular biology. Nowadays various kinds of genomic information can be readily measured. For example, microarray technology can simultaneously measure thousands of mRNA expression levels (1). Genome-wide expression profiling allows us to peek into a living biological system and provides us the opportunity to understand the structure and dynamic rules of gene regulation and to reconstruct gene regulatory networks (2).

This is a daunting task because biological systems are notoriously complex, and the quality of microarray gene expression data is largely limited by many experimental factors. More importantly, expression profiles are often measured at a static time, while gene

Scott A. Rifkin (ed.), *Quantitative Trait Loci (QTL): Methods and Protocols*, Methods in Molecular Biology, vol. 871,
DOI 10.1007/978-1-61779-785-9_9,

regulation is a dynamic process that involves many factors other than expression (3, 4). Without dynamic information or information on all the unmeasured potential causal factors, correlations between genes can be due to real regulation, coregulation of unmeasured factors, or coexpression under certain conditions, and these relationships are often indistinguishable based on statistical criteria. It can be misleading to conclude causation (here meaning one gene regulating the other) based on data from gene expression profiling alone.

In the post-genome era, new technology enables us to measure genome-wide genetic information in addition to expression on the same samples. This was proposed and first demonstrated with yeast. Brem et al. (5) genetically crossed two strains of yeast, a lab strain and a wild type strain, and produced 112 segregants. They measured the expression of ~6,000 genes and genotypes of ~3,000 genetic markers on these segregants. By treating each gene's expression as a quantitative trait and identifying the expression quantitative trait loci (eQTLs) that each was linked to, they revealed the genetic architecture of transcriptional variation in yeast. Similar experiments were subsequently conducted on mice, plants, and other organisms (6–9). In addition to genome-wide eQTL analysis, integrating expression data with genome-wide genotype information also provides a nice experimental setting for reverse engineering gene networks.

2. Why Do We Need eQTLs?

2.1. Reconstructing Gene Networks from Expression Data

A gene network is conceptually different from a gene regulatory network. A gene network represents the relationships among a set of genes, often through undirected edges. An edge between two genes indicates that these two genes tend to have correlated expression. However, that does not necessarily mean that one gene transcript is regulating or is causal for the transcriptional expression of the other. Gene regulatory networks or, more precisely, transcriptional regulatory networks portray the regulatory relationships among a set of genes through directed edges. A directed edge from gene G_1 to G_2 indicates that transcriptional variation of G_1 is directly or indirectly causing the variation in expression of G_2, i.e., G_1 is regulating G_2.

In an observational study, correlation does not imply causation. Figure 1 displays a simple example in which the expression levels of two genes are correlated, and their correlation can be due to at least three possible scenarios: both are regulated by a common locus L; G_1 is causal for G_2; or G_2 is causal for G_1. When the causal factor L is unobserved, for example in a gene expression microarray experiment, the three possible scenarios are indistinguishable and all will

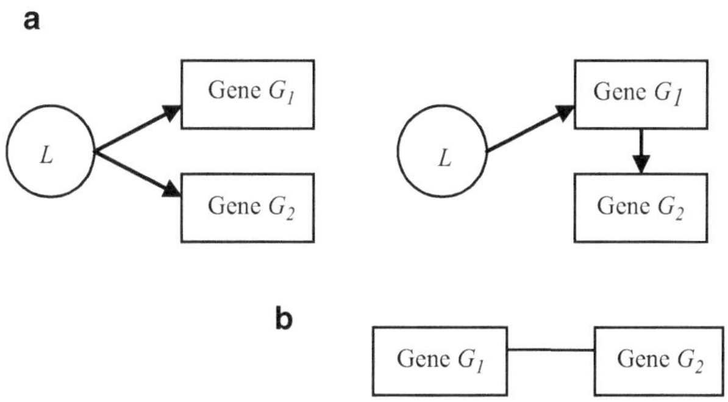

Fig. 1. A simple example: gene G_1 is correlated with G_2. This correlation can be entailed by at least three types of relationships. Let L denote a genetic locus. When L is causal for both G_1 and G_2, G_1 is causal for G_2, or G_2 is causal for G_1, the two genes will be correlated. (**a**) Directed graphs, (**b**) an undirected graph.

be represented by a same undirected edge between the two genes in a gene network. Because a biological system is complex with many genomic features causally interacting, an expression network inferred from correlations is often not informative.

2.2. Natural Randomization in Genotypes

Randomization is a gold standard to infer causation (10). For example, in a simple and ideal setting where all other factors are controlled, if a drug has been properly randomized across subjects, and, following the randomization, the outcome variable changes, a causal relationship from the drug to disease outcome can be inferred.

More recently, in the literature of genetic epidemiology, a similar concept has been proposed called Mendelian randomization of genotypes (11, 12). Genotype, the DNA constitution of an individual at a particular locus, is formed and fixed during meiosis. Based on Mendel's law of inheritance, the parental alleles of a particular locus are independently segregated to different offsprings in a genetic cross (13). This independent segregation of DNA imitates a naturally occurring randomization process, where the "treatment (or control)" here can be seen as the allele from (or not from) one parent (e.g., Parent P_1 in Fig. 2). At a particular locus, offspring randomly inherit the allele from this parent with a certain probability. Across the entire genome, numerous natural genotype randomization processes occur at different loci in a genetic cross, resulting in the genome of any offspring being a random recombinant version of the original parental genomes. Note that genotype randomization processes at two nearby loci can be highly dependent. For example, loci L_1 and L_2 in Fig. 2 are dependent and always segregate together. However, the genotype at a particular locus, e.g., L_1 is genetically randomized to offspring. In other words, when there is no segregation distortion, a haploid offspring O_1 has 50/50 chance of inheriting the piece of DNA at locus L_1 from parent P_1 or P_2. For a different offspring O_2, the inheritance is also 50/50 and is independent of what any other offspring inherit.

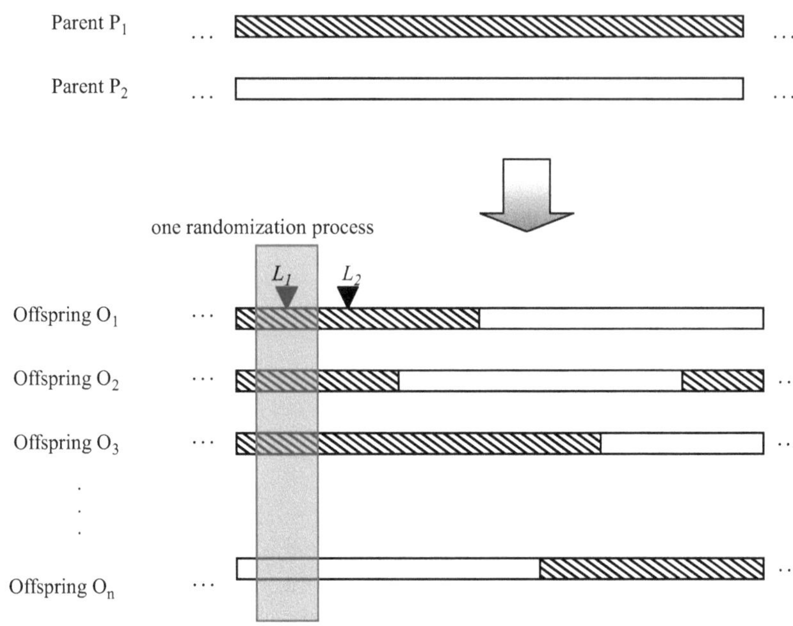

Fig. 2. A graphical illustration of Mendelian randomized genotypes from a haploid cross. Due to independent inheritance of different offsprings from a randomized genetic cross of two or more backgrounds, the genotype at any particular locus in the genome, for example locus L_1, can be seen as a random variable with P(Genotype at L_1 is inherited from P_1) = 0.5 if there is no segregation distortion. The genotype inheritance occurred in the whole genome consists of many Mendelian randomization processes. Though these natural randomizations might be related, for example the randomization occurred at locus L_1 is highly correlated with its nearby locus L_2, it does not invalidate our model or arguments in this chapter, most of which only consider one randomization process at one locus, e.g., L_1, at a time.

The naturally occurring Mendelian randomization of genotypes is analogous to a randomized experimental design. It provides us an opportunity to unambiguously infer causation among gene transcripts or from gene transcripts to a complex trait. If the transcriptional variation in two genes, G_1 and G_2, are both statistically linked to a same locus L in a segregating population (note that G_1 and G_2 are not necessarily physically linked), since L has been naturally randomized to offsprings, it indicates that $L \rightarrow G_1$ and $L \rightarrow G_2$. Here $\rightarrow$ means causation. The genetic variation near the locus affects the transcriptional variation in both G_1 and G_2, directly or indirectly. Several methods have been proposed to further elucidate the relationship between G_1 and G_2 for each pair of potential genes and to reconstruct gene regulatory networks.

3. Methods

The reconstruction of gene regulatory networks involves using a probabilistic graphical model to represent the conditional dependence and conditional independence for a set of random variables. Consider a finite set of n genes $\{G_1, G_2, \ldots, G_n\}$. The relationships among these genes are depicted by a directed acyclic graph (DAG) (14). Given the network topology of these genes in the DAG, it is often assumed that each gene is independent of its nondescendants, given its parents in the network, where descendants are defined as the immediate reactive genes, and parents are defined as the immediate causal genes. The joint probability density function of these genes can be written as the product of the density functions of individual genes, conditional on their parent variables in the DAG:

$$P(G_1, \ldots, G_n) = \prod_{i=1}^{n} P(G_i | Parents(G_i)).$$

A Bayesian network is a probabilistic graphical model that represents a set of random variables and their conditional dependencies via a DAG. For example, given the Bayesian network $G_1 \to G_2 \to G_3$, the joint probability density function of (G_1, G_2, G_3) can be written as $P(G_1, G_2, G_3) = P(G_3|G_2)P(G_2|G_1)P(G_1)$. In this section, we introduce several methods for reconstructing gene networks.

3.1. Optimization-Based Search

Friedman et al. (2) adapts Bayesian networks to reconstructing gene networks from expression data. For a set of n genes, Friedman et al. proposed a scoring method that evaluates each possible network with respect to the data to search for the optimal network according to this score. One method for deriving a score is to evaluate the posterior probability of a network given the data. The score of a network is also decomposable and can be rewritten as the sum

$$S(Network : Data) = \sum_i Score\ Contribution(G_i, Parents(G_i) \colon Data).$$

Since the number of potential candidate networks increases super exponentially with the number of genes, even the highest posterior probability is very small and is often not much different from that of the second best network. The best network for one dataset is rarely reproducible for another dataset of similar type. Some later work uses a similar idea and incorporates eQTL information in the graph (15). In general, scoring methods have the advantage of being able to operate even with small samples. However, they focus on discovering Bayesian networks but not on causally interpreting them. They do not consider the potential effects of unknown or unmeasured factors and largely disregard stochastic variation between datasets.

3.2. A Likelihood-Based Model Selection Approach

Compared with finding a best fit network for each dataset, a more robust way to build networks is to build a Bayesian network from bottom up, i.e., focusing on one pair of genes (or a gene and a complex trait) at a time and connecting the causal pieces into a regulatory network.

Schadt et al. (7) proposed an integrative genomics approach, which is a multistep procedure to identify the potential causal genes for complex traits. For any gene and a complex trait of interest, they first test if both are linked to a same genetic locus. If so, they argue that there are only a limited number of relationships are possible. Figure 1a shows three possible relationships between the locus L, a gene G_1, and a complex trait G_2. Other more complicated relationships involve the combination of two or more of these three relationships. In a subsequent step, they propose a likelihood-based causality model selection test. It calculates the likelihoods associated with each of the potential models and chooses the one with the smallest Akaike Information Criterion (AIC) value as the best model supported by the data. The selected model predicts the causal relationship between the gene and the complex trait.

Specifically, the algorithm works in the following steps:

1. For a complex trait (or a particular gene) of interest, G_2, identify the quantitative trait loci that are significantly linked to G_2. For example, a locus L with logarithm of odds (LOD) score >3.
2. Identify the genes with significant correlations to G_2. Compute the p-values corresponding to Pearson correlation coefficients for all genes to G_2. Keep the ones with significant correlations (e.g., p-value < 0.001) as potential causal genes for G_2.
3. For each QTL, L, identified in Step 1, further filter out the genes that are not significantly linked to L. The remaining genes after this step (G_1s) are those jointly linked to L with G_2 and are significantly correlated with G_2.
4. For each trio (L, G_1, G_2), fit the three models in Fig. 1a. Compute the AIC value for each model. The model with lowest AIC is chosen as the model entailed the relationship among (L, G_1, G_2). Note that here Ls are identified in Step 1, G_1s are identified in Steps 2 and 3, and G_2 is a fixed trait or gene of interest.

Using the above algorithm, for each fixed trait or gene, G_2, one can identify the genes with the relationship $L \rightarrow G_1 \rightarrow G_2$. The G_1s are the causal genes for G_2. Generalized to a set of G_2s or even the entire genome, one can reconstruct a gene regulatory network based on the detected causal relationships by connecting them together.

This likelihood-based model selection approach incorporates eQTL information and is a pioneering work that moves beyond correlation-based reconstruction of gene networks. However, it has several limitations. First, it is difficult to jointly control the significance level in a multistep procedure. For example, the false discovery rates (FDRs) incurred in the first, second, third, and fourth steps are 4, 5, 3, and 8%, respectively. It is not clear how many false discoveries are incurred in all four steps together. Among the gene pairs that have been identified with a regulatory relationship, it is difficult to quantify and compare the confidences of them. Second, the effects of unmeasured causal variables in the genome are inadequately considered, while those effects often cannot be ignored. For example, there may exist a major transcription factor or some unmeasured environmental effects that influence the variation of multiple genes. Third, model selection procedures can be used to select a model that best fits the data, but they are not appropriate to determine causal relationships. Even without the consideration of hidden variables, the model that depicts the real causal relationship of two genes does not always have the lowest AIC. For example, G_1 affects the expression of G_2 and meanwhile G_2 is coregulated with G_1, and these two relationships can have same or opposite directions. In this situation, the model gives lowest AIC can depend on the effect sizes of different relationships. AIC (similarly, Bayesian Information Criterion) assumes that the true underlying model is among the set of models being considered. In reality, many genes are involved in a more complicated setting than being considered. When the true underlying model is not considered, model-selection based on AIC criterion might arbitrarily force one model to be selected and lead to many falsely predicted relationships. In the work by Schadt et al. (7), ~100 genes are predicted to be causal for abdominal obesity in the mouse but only a few have been experimentally validated.

3.3. Structural Equation Modeling

Li et al. (9) proposed to use structural equation modeling (SEM) to model the causal relationships among multiple genes. SEM is a hierarchical system of regressions that is an extension of standard multiple linear regression. The model structure of a directed graph can be decomposed into several causal relationships and each is represented by a linear model. In each model, the causes are put in the right-hand side and the responses are put in the left-hand side. For example, a simple gene regulatory network $L \rightarrow G_1 \rightarrow G_2$ corresponds to the SEM,

$$\begin{cases} G_1 = \alpha L + \varepsilon, \\ G_2 = \beta G_1 + \delta, \end{cases} \tag{1}$$

where the parameters α and β are called path coefficients, ε and δ are independently distributed and here the "=" sign implies causal relationship. It means " $\leftarrow$," i.e., "is determined by."

Li et al. (9) point out that in a genetic inbred cross, the genotypes have been properly randomized to offspring and thus causal relationships can be inferred in the context of eQTL mapping. Since the genotype L is genetically randomized, causal effects from L to a gene have a defined direction, i.e., if a gene is linked to L, then L is causal for the expression of the gene. Based on eQTLs, they develop the following SEM approach to analyze complex genetic systems:

1. For a gene of interest, G_2, perform a genome scan and identify the eQTLs linked to it.

$$G_2 = \beta_0 + \beta_1 L + \varepsilon. \tag{2}$$

2. Identify pleiotropic eQTLs. Perform conditional genome scans using one gene as a covariate in the analysis of another gene.

$$G_2 = \beta_0 + \beta_1 L + \beta_2 G_1 + \varepsilon. \tag{3}$$

3. Define an initial path model. For example, comparing the LOD scores of L in (2) and (3), if there is a substantial change in the LOD scores after conditioning on G_1, this suggests that G_1 is causally connected to L and to G_2. Edges should be drawn from the eQTL to both genes and an edge from G_1 to G_2 should also be drawn.
4. Assess the model using the goodness-of-fit test. The test statistic is defined as $(N-1)F(\Theta)$, where $F(\Theta)$ is the maximized log likelihood function given the SEM (for example, a SEM entailed in (1)). The test statistic follows a χ^2 distribution with $p(p+1)/2 - q$ degrees of freedom, where p is the number of variables (genes and loci) included in the model, $p(p+1)/2$ is the number of unique elements in the covariance matrix and q is the number of model parameters (path coefficients). If the p-value of the goodness-of-fit test is less than 0.05, it suggests that the model does not provide a good fit to the data and the model needs to be reassessed.
5. Refine the model. If a model does not provide a good fit to the data, refine the model by adding a new path to the initial model, removing a path, or reversing the causal direction of a path. The addition is supposed to improve the goodness of fit. The removal should not dramatically reduce the goodness of fit.
6. Iterate between Steps 4 and 5 until the final model provides a good fit to the data, is parsimonious, and each path coefficient is significant and nontrivial.

This approach shares intrinsic similarity with the approach proposed in Schadt et al. (7). They both utilize the randomized genotype information to narrow the search spaces of potential models. In contrast to the model-selection approach based on AIC criterion, this approach provides a more refined procedure that iteratively assesses and modifies the model until a final model is reached. However, the approach also suffers from similar caveats to the model-selection approach: the control of false discoveries in this multistep procedure is not addressed, the consideration of hidden variables is inadequate, and the causal interpretation of the model is still difficult. According to the founder of SEM (16) (p. 240), "prior knowledge of the causal relations is assumed as prerequisite." SEM was developed to quantitatively assess the cause–effect relationships among a set of variables by combining the qualitative cause–effect information with statistical data. SEM was intended to be used to estimate the path coefficients, e.g., the parameters α and β in (1), when the causal relations among a set of variables are already known. SEM should be used with caution in causal exploration to identify the causal relationships among variables of interest.

3.4. Constructing Gene Regulatory Network Based on Natural Randomization of Genotypes

Chen et al. (17) directly utilized the natural randomization of genotypes, and derived a *Causality Equivalence Theorem* that establishes the equivalence between three statistically testable conditions and a type of causal relationship that is not affected by any hidden variables. Specifically, when considering a locus L, and two genes (or a gene and a trait) G_1 and G_2, a causal relationship $L \rightarrow G_1 \rightarrow G_2$ not affected by any hidden variable can be established if

1. $L \rightarrow G_1$, i.e., G_1 is linked to L
2. $L \rightarrow G_2$, i.e., G_2 is linked to L
3. $L \perp G_2 | G_1$, i.e., conditional on G_1, L is independent of G_2

Here "not affected by any hidden variable" is not an assumption. Rather, it is a property that will be met when conditions (1)–(3) are all true. The intuition behind this idea is if both G_1 and G_2 are linked to L, while L is properly randomized, then L is directly or indirectly causal for G_1 and G_2. Furthermore, if L is independent of G_2 given the variation of G_1, it indicates that the causal effect from L to G_2 can be fully captured by G_1, and thus G_1 is an intermediate cause for G_2 in the relationship, implying $L \rightarrow G_1 \rightarrow G_2$. Chen et al. (17) further proposed an empirical Bayesian approach to quantify the probability of each testable condition. The joint probability of $L \rightarrow G_1 \rightarrow G_2$ can be quantified as the products of the three probabilities.

$$\begin{aligned}
&\Pr(\mathrm{L} \rightarrow \mathrm{G}_1 \rightarrow \mathrm{G}_2) \\
&\quad = \Pr(L \rightarrow G_1 \text{ and } L \rightarrow G_2 \textit{ and } L \perp G_2 | G_1) \\
&\quad = \Pr(L \rightarrow G_1) \times \Pr(L \rightarrow G_2 | L \rightarrow G_1) \\
&\qquad \times \Pr(L \perp G_2 | G_1 | L \rightarrow G_1 \text{ and } L \rightarrow G_2).
\end{aligned}$$

To compute the joint posterior probability, the basic algorithm works as follows:

1. Transform the expression data for each gene to follow a standard normal distribution. This step not only removes potential outliers in expression data, but also facilitates the estimation of conditional independence probability in Step 4.

2. For each gene transcript of interest, G_1, test the null hypothesis of no *cis* linkage to a nearby locus L, $H_0 : L \perp G_1$, vs. the alternative hypothesis of *cis* linkage, $H_A : L \rightarrow G_1$. In a haploid example, a locus L consists of two genotypes. If G_1 is linked to L, the genotypic variation at L affects the expression of G_1, i.e., the mean expression of G_1 with one genotype would be different from the mean expression of G_1 with the other genotype. Therefore, testing linkage is equivalent to testing different mean expression of G_1 among two genotype groups. The likelihood ratio statistic, S_1, can be calculated as

$$S_1 = -2\ln\left(\frac{\text{likelihood under } H_0}{\text{likelihood under } H_A}\right) = N \ln \frac{\hat{\sigma}_0^2}{\hat{\sigma}_A^2},$$

where N is the sample size, $\hat{\sigma}_0^2$ and $\hat{\sigma}_A^2$ are the estimated variance of G_1 under the null and the alternative, respectively.

To obtain the null statistics, permute the expression of G_1 across offspring B times and for each permuted G_1^0, calculate the likelihood ratio statistics $\{S_1^{0b}, b = 1, 2, \ldots, B\}$. Compare the observed statistic with null statistics and estimate the empirical Bayesian posterior probability of $\Pr(L \rightarrow G_1)$ (18).

3. For each of the other gene transcripts, G_2, test the null hypothesis of no linkage of L to G_2 vs. the alternative of linkage between L and G_2. Same as Step 2, calculate the likelihood ratio test statistic S_2 and permute the expression of G_2 across offspring B times to obtain the null statistics $\{S_2^{0b}, b = 1, 2, \ldots, B\}$. Compare the observed statistic with null statistics and estimate the probability $\Pr(L \rightarrow G_2)$, which is a conservative estimate of $\Pr(L \rightarrow G_2 | L \rightarrow G_1)$.

4. For each trio (L, G_1, G_2), carry out the following procedure. Given the normal distribution G_1 and G_2 (Step 1), calculate the conditional distribution of $G_2|G_1$. Test the null hypothesis of $G_2|G_1$ being uncorrelated to locus L vs. the alternative of being correlated. For normal distribution, no correlation implies independence. Similar as in Steps 2 and 3, obtain the likelihood ratio statistic S_3 and the null statistics $\{S_3^{0b}, b = 1, 2, \ldots, B\}$ by permutation across offspring, and compare the observed with null ones to estimate the probability $\Pr(L \rightarrow G_2|G_1)$. $\Pr(L \perp G_2|G_1|L \rightarrow G_1 \text{ and } L \rightarrow G_2)$ is shown to be equal to $\Pr(L \perp G_2|G_1) = 1 - \Pr(L \rightarrow G_2|G_1)$.

5. Multiplying the posterior probabilities in Steps 2–4, one can obtain an estimate of $\Pr(L \rightarrow G_1 \rightarrow G_2)$, which is a conservative estimate of the posterior probability $P_{12} = \Pr(G_1 \rightarrow G_2)$.

Applying the algorithm to all possible pairs of genes in the genome and thresholding them at a certain posterior probability, one can reconstruct a gene regulatory network that consists of the gene regulatory pairs not affected by any hidden variables. Furthermore, FDR of the network can be estimated as

$$\mathrm{FDR}(\lambda) = \frac{\sum_{i,j}(1-\hat{P}_{ij})1(\hat{P}_{ij} \geq \lambda)}{\#\{\hat{P}_{ij} \geq \lambda\}},$$

where $\hat{P}_{ij}$ is the estimated posterior probability of gene G_i regulating G_j, and i, j are any two genes in the genome; $1(\hat{P}_{ij} \geq \lambda)$ is 1 or 0 according to if $\hat{P}_{ij} \geq \lambda$ and $\#\{\hat{P}_{ij} \geq \lambda\}$ is the total number of significant gene pairs at threshold λ.

In contrast to previous methods, the approach by Chen et al. (17) directly utilizes the randomized genotype information and derives a rigorous causal framework to infer causation. Unlike other multistep procedures, this work quantifies the posterior probability of each step and calculates the joint posterior probability of regulation by multiplying the probabilities together. This provides a nice control of false discovery for a multistep procedure. Furthermore, the joint posterior probabilities of regulation for pairs of genes can be compared across the genome and can be used to calculate FDR or other confidence measures of a gene regulatory network.

Realizing the challenges of potential hidden variables, the causal framework by Chen et al. (17) only aims to identify the causal relationships that are not affected by any common hidden variables. For those gene pairs that might be affected by a common causal variable, the conditional independence condition would fail, L would not be independent of $G_2|G_1$ (17, 19, 20). Thus, based on their work, one cannot estimate the complete transcriptional regulatory network, but only part of it. On the other hand, the causal framework is derived from rigorous causal inference based on Mendelian randomization of genotypes and moves beyond correlation or model-selection based approaches for identifying causation. The key part of this idea is to test and quantify the probability of conditional independence among any pair of genes that are jointly linked to the same eQTL.

In addition to the methods discussed above, there are other novel and interesting approaches. For example, Chaibub-Neto et al. (19) proposed a QTLnet approach to jointly infer gene regulatory network and associated eQTLs. They use conditional LOD scores to measure conditional independence between genes/traits and eQTLs, and gradually modify the gene regulatory network and fit the genetic architecture conditional on the newly proposed network. In previous work, eQTLs are mostly used to facilitate the detection of causal relationships among genes and traits, and they are assumed to be either known or inferred independent of network structure. QTLnet, instead, emphasizes both the construction of gene regulatory network and the detection of genetic architecture. A major challenge, though, is that the potential network search space also grows super-exponentially with the number of genes/traits/eQTLs in the network. Exhaustive searches are impossible and heuristic searching approaches are used in QTLnet algorithm.

4. The Consideration of Hidden Variables

The reconstruction of gene regulatory networks is complicated by the possible presence of hidden variables. In a simple example, when $L \rightarrow G_1 \rightarrow G_2$ and a hidden variable, H, affects the variation of both G_1 and G_2, this is statistically and graphically equivalent to $L \rightarrow G_1 \leftrightarrow G_2$ (20). Without knowing and explicitly modeling H, it is hard to infer the causal relationship $G_1 \rightarrow G_2$ based on statistical criteria.

This example is neither unique nor rare. In fact, it is ubiquitous in a complex biological system. For example, there are many master transcription regulators in genomes, and they often affect the expression of many genes (21). However, for simplicity, a lot of the methods in the literature choose to assume that hidden variables are not present or simplify the complexity of hidden variables (for example, by assuming that H affects G_1 and G_2 with the same effect). When simplified in this way, the causal inference and the subsequently reconstructed gene regulatory networks hardly reflect the real ones.

Some other methods attempt to carefully deal with the hidden variable issue. Chen et al. (17) proposed to only identify the causal relationships that are not affected by any hidden variables. Hartemink et al. (22) incorporated external information to fully consider hidden variables within a relatively small network. When hidden variables have widespread effects on many genes in the genome, they could also be modeled (23) and be potentially included or adjusted in the causal framework.

5. Summary and Discussion

To elucidate the regulatory relationships among thousands of simultaneously measured expression variations, the most challenging question is how to distinguish genuine causation (or gene regulation) from spurious correlation.

Randomization has been used as the gold standard to infer causation in clinical trials.

More recently, "Mendelian randomization" of genotypes has been introduced in genetic epidemiology. According to Mendel's law of inheritance, meiosis in an experimental cross works as a naturally occurring randomization process, distributing parental genetic variation to offspring independently. This naturally occurring randomization of genetic variation provides a basis for the statistical analysis of gene regulation. We treat gene expression as a quantitative trait. Suppose there is a genetic locus to which the trait is linked. Given that the genetic variation at the locus has been properly randomized to offspring, and if, following the randomization, we observe offspring with one genotype at the locus have different expression level than those with other genotypes, we conclude that the genetic variation at the locus is causal for the variation in gene expression.

When considering multiple genes and loci together, it is possible to infer causal relationships among genes and reconstruct gene regulatory networks from this experimental design. In this chapter, we review several methods addressing this topic. In some earlier attempts, scoring methods of Bayesian network have been proposed and they incorporated eQTL information to narrow the search space. However, the number of potential networks increases super-exponentially with the number of genes. When the number of genes in a network is large, the score differences between the best fitted network and other ones diminish. The resulting regulatory networks are often hard to reproduce. Many other approaches build networks from bottom up: they start with a subnetwork, e.g., a locus and two genes (or a gene and a complex trait) and infer the relationships among them using eQTL information. After analyzing all potential subnetworks, they build regulatory networks by connecting all causal relationships.

Schadt et al. (7) proposed a likelihood based model-selection approach. For a gene and a complex trait, it evaluates AICs of several possible models and predicts the one with the lowest AIC to be the true underlying model for the gene and the trait. This approach tends to predict too many genes to be causal. Li et al. (9) use a SEM approach to identify gene regulations. Similarly, the fit of a model given the data cannot accurately predict causation. Chen et al. (17) proposed a causal framework that infers a type of causal relationship from randomization of genotypes. They derived a theorem showing that three statistically testable conditions are sufficient to conclude one type of causation. They further proposed to calculate the empirical Bayesian probability of each condition, and the joint product of them can serve as the estimate for probability of regulation. This approach rigorously infers causation from randomized experimental design. It only focuses on one type of causation which is not affected by any hidden variables. If there are hidden variables affecting two genes, even if one gene is causal for the other, the approach would not have the power to detect them.

The existence of unknown or unmeasured hidden causal variables complicates the reconstruction of gene regulatory networks, but hidden variables have been inadequately considered in the literature. Most works assume hidden variables do not exist for modeling and computation simplicity. In fact, hidden variables are ubiquitous in a complex biological system, for example, a master transcriptional factor or a linkage "hotspot" that cannot be measured at either genetic or expression level. It is also not satisfactory to simply assume that hidden variables affect all genes in the same direction with the same effect size (20). Further work is still needed on how to properly consider and model these effects.

After reading this chapter, it may seem complicated to infer causation or regulation and to reconstruct a gene regulatory network. In fact, it is. However, we are making good progress towards better methods. The reader needs to be aware that one should always be cautious in the causal interpretation of a statistical model. The biological system is much more complex than what we had imagined in the past, and is probably more complex than what we think now. The current literature is mostly focused on DAGs, i.e., the causation is $G_1 \rightarrow G_2$, but not directed cyclic graphs, $G_1 \leftrightarrow G_2$, while in reality, both types of relationships may be common. Clearly, more innovative methods are needed.

Given our current knowledge, it would be extremely helpful to incorporate external information to reconstruct networks, and eQTL information is one type of such information. Hartemink et al. (22, 24) incorporated location information and expert knowledge in building networks for a set of genes of interest. The integration of prior information could greatly facilitate the search for the true underlying model and provides the best interpretability of the constructed network. The discussion in this chapter does not only apply to the reconstruction of transcriptional regulatory network but also apply to protein–protein interaction network and networks of other types of genomic information.

Combining eQTL and expression profiling from randomized genetic crosses helps to reconstruct gene regulatory networks. In addition to statistical and computational predictions, follow-up experimental validations also need to be performed. The work presented in this chapter can be used to grasp a whole picture of the structure of gene regulation and sort out the potential genes that are likely to have an impact on a complex trait or are involved in a disease pathway. Further experimental validations are useful to rule out false positives and validate the predictions. The ultimate goal is to contribute to the understanding of the biological systems in organisms and to develop new drug targets or treatments for complex diseases.

References

1. Eisen MB, Spellman PT, Brown PO, Botstein D (1998) Cluster analysis and display of genome-wide expression patterns. Proc Natl Acad Sci USA 95:14863–14868
2. Friedman N, Linial M, Nachman I, Pe'er D (2000) Using Bayesian networks to analyze expression data. J Comput Biol 7(3–4): 601–620
3. Spirtes P, Glymour C, Scheines R (2000) Constructing Bayesian network models of gene expression networks from microarray data. In: Proceedings of the Atlantic symposium on computational biology, genome information systems and technology. Durham, North Carolina
4. Pearl J (2000) Causality: models, reasoning, and inference. Cambridge University Press, Cambridge
5. Brem RB, Yvert G, Clinton R, Kruglyak L (2002) Genetic dissection of transcriptional regulation in budding yeast. Science 296:752–755

6. Schadt EE, Monks SA, Drake TA, Lusis AJ, Che N et al (2003) Genetics of gene expression surveyed in maize, mouse, and man. Nature 422:297–302
7. Schadt EE, Lamb J, Yang X, Zhu J, Edwards S et al (2005) An integrative genomics approach to infer causal associations between gene expression and disease. Nat Genet 37:710–717
8. Bing N, Hoeschele I (2005) Genetical genomics analysis of a yeast segregant population for transcription network inference. Genetics 170:533–542
9. Li R, Tsaih S-W, Shockley K, Stylianou IM, Wergedal J et al (2006) Structural model analysis of multiple quantitative traits. PLoS Genet 2:1046–1057
10. Greenland S (1990) Randomization, statistics, and causal inference. Epidemiology 1:421–429
11. Gray R, Wheatley K (1991) How to avoid bias when comparing bone marrow transplantation with chemotherapy. Bone Marrow Transplant 7(suppl 3):9–12
12. Smith GD, Ebrahim S (2003) Mendelian randomization: can genetic epidemiology contribute to understanding environmental determinants of disease? Int J Epidemiol 32:1–22
13. Mendel GJ (1950) Gregor mendel's letters to Carl Nageli. Genetics 35:1–29
14. Pearl J (1985) Bayesian networks: a model of self-activated memory for evidential reasoning. In: Proceedings of the 7th conference of the cognitive science society. Irvine, California, pp 329–334
15. Kulp D, Jagular M (2006) Causal inference of regulator-target pairs by gene mapping of expression phenotypes. BMC Genomics 7:125
16. Wright S (1923) The theory of path coefficients: a reply to Niles's criticism. Genetics 8:239–255
17. Chen LS, Emmert-Streib F, Storey JD (2007) Harnessing naturally randomized transcription to infer causal regulatory relationships among genes. Genome Biol 8:R219
18. Storey JD, Akey JM, Kruglyak L (2005) Multiple locus linkage analysis of genomewide expression in yeast. PLoS Biol 3:1380–1390
19. Chaibub-Neto E, Ferrara CT, Attie AD, Yandell BS (2008) Inferring causal phenotype networks from segregating populations. Genetics 179:1089–1100
20. Richardson T, Spirtes P (2002) Ancestral graph Markov models. Ann Stat 30:962–1030
21. Breitling R, Li Y, Tesson BM, Fu J, Wu C et al (2008) Genetical genomics: spotlight on QTL hotspots. PLoS Genet 4:e1000232
22. Hartemink A, Gifford D, Jaakkola T, Young R (2002) Combining location and expression data for principled discovery of genetic regulatory network models. In: Pacific symposium on biocomputing. Lihue, Hawaii, pp 437–449
23. Price AL, Patterson NJ, Plenge RM, Weinblatt ME, Shadick NA, Reich D (2006) Principal components analysis corrects for stratification in genome-wide association studies. Nat Genet 38:904–909
24. Hartemink A, Gifford D, Jaakkola T, Young R (2001) Using graphical models and genomic expression data to statistically validate models of genetic regulatory networks. In: Proceedings of the 6th Pacific symposium on biocomputing. Big island, Hawaii, pp 422–433

Chapter 10

Estimation and Interpretation of Genetic Effects with Epistasis Using the NOIA Model

José M. Álvarez-Castro, Örjan Carlborg, and Lars Rönnegård

Abstract

We introduce this communication with a brief outline of the historical landmarks in genetic modeling, especially concerning epistasis. Then, we present methods for the use of genetic modeling in QTL analyses. In particular, we summarize the essential expressions of the natural and orthogonal interactions (NOIA) model of genetic effects. Our motivation for reviewing that theory here is twofold. First, this review presents a digest of the expressions for the application of the NOIA model, which are often mixed with intermediate and additional formulae in the original articles. Second, we make the required theory handy for the reader to relate the genetic concepts to the particular mathematical expressions underlying them. We illustrate those relations by providing graphical interpretations and a diagram summarizing the key features for applying genetic modeling with epistasis in comprehensive QTL analyses. Finally, we briefly review some examples of the application of NOIA to real data and the way it improves the interpretability of the results.

Key words: Change of reference, Epistasis, Genetic effects, Hardy–Weinberg disequilibrium, Multiple alleles, NOIA, QTL

1. Introduction

Fisher (1) set the foundations of quantitative genetics, almost one century ago. He did so by developing models of genetic effects that provided a suitable mathematical description of the compatibility between multifactorial Mendelian inheritance and the findings biometricians had noted since the mid 1800s. Assisting genetic breeding—particularly eugenics (2, 3)—by focussing on the additive, heritable component of the genetic variance eventually became a major motivation for Fisher's work. It is thus not surprising that he (4) consigned epistasis to a nuisance term with analogous evolutionary implications to that of genetic-independent environmental variance. However, several key notions—such as the shifting balance theory (5), speciation by hybrid incompatibilities

Scott A. Rifkin (ed.), *Quantitative Trait Loci (QTL): Methods and Protocols*, Methods in Molecular Biology, vol. 871,
DOI 10.1007/978-1-61779-785-9_10, © Springer Science+Business Media New York 2012

(6, 7), and canalization (8)—soon highlighted the significance of epistasis within the synthetic theory of evolution. In time, landmark implementations of genetic modeling and decomposition of the genetic variance accounting for epistasis were simultaneously proffered by Kempthorne (9, 10) and Cockerham (11).

As QTL studies started to become more common, Cheverud and Routman (12, 13) warned against potential misinterpretations of estimates of genetic effects and suggested applying population-independent parameters when analyzing interacting loci, which they called physiological—as opposed to statistical—epistasis. This concept is indeed related to Fisher's (1) population-independent formulation, later called the F_∞ model (14). Hansen and Wagner (15) further inspected the relationship between physiological and statistical genetic effects with epistasis and introduced a key concept in genetic modeling, the change of reference. They preferred to refer to functional (rather than physiological) genetic effects, which are more recently being referred to as compositional (16).

This way, the concepts of functional (or compositional) and statistical genetic effects (with or without epistasis) got established. The first ones describe the genotype-to-phenotype map as allele substitutions made from one reference individual genotype regardless of the population where those genotypes occur, whereas the second ones describe properties of genetic systems in particular populations (15–18). In parallel, Tiwari and Elston (19) set a convenient matrix notation for statistical models and Yang (20) proffered a statistical model of genetic effects providing orthogonal estimates of QTL effects in spite of departures from the Hardy–Weinberg proportions in the experimental population under study.

In the last few years, there has been an increasing interest in mapping epistatic QTL (16, 21–25). Throughout this chapter, we assume that a QTL mapping experiment has been performed leading to QTL locations and their genotype probabilities for the individuals under study. We focus on how to apply genetic modeling to harness this information for unconventional genetic analyses (whether applied to studying evolutionary phenomena, developing breeding programs, or dissecting disease incidence), particularly in the presence of epistasis. To this end, we review the NOIA (natural and orthogonal interactions) model of genetic effects (17, 18, 26). NOIA has been (and continues to be) developed for generalizing and unifying the different approaches to genetic modeling by using convenient matrix notation—in particular, for merging all approaches mentioned above into a common framework. We also briefly comment on a regression method that enables the properties of NOIA to hold despite lack of genotype information. We diagram the use of NOIA for the interpretation of QTL analyses using graphical interpretations and review real-data applications.

2. Methods

2.1. Regression-Based Estimation of QTL Effects

The NOIA model consists of a set of expressions of the form $\mathbf{G} = \mathbf{S} \cdot \mathbf{E}$ (19), where $\mathbf{G}$ is the vector of genotypic values, $\mathbf{S}$ is the genetic-effect design matrix, gathering the genetic contrasts or scales, and $\mathbf{E}$ is the vector of genetic effects, accounting for also the reference point of the genetic system. Different mathematical formulations within the genetic-effect design matrices lead to different decompositions of the genotypic values of a trait in a population, as detailed in the following section. An example of genetic-effect design matrix of common use is the one with the scales providing the statistical decomposition of genotypic values in an ideal F_2 population (17, 27):

$$\begin{pmatrix} G_{11} \\ G_{12} \\ G_{22} \end{pmatrix} = \begin{pmatrix} 1 & -1 & -\frac{1}{2} \\ 1 & 0 & \frac{1}{2} \\ 1 & 1 & -\frac{1}{2} \end{pmatrix} \cdot \begin{pmatrix} \mu \\ \alpha \\ \delta \end{pmatrix} \tag{1}$$

In any case, the expression $\mathbf{G} = \mathbf{S} \cdot \mathbf{E}$ does not by itself allow the estimation of the genetic effects from data consisting of a set of N individuals with known marker-genotypes and phenotypes for a trait under study. When the genotypes of those individuals at one biallelic QTL are known, the connection between the vector of observed phenotypes, $\mathbf{Y}$, and the vector of genotypic values can be made through the regression $\mathbf{Y} = \mathbf{Z} \cdot \mathbf{G} + \varepsilon$, which expands to:

$$\begin{pmatrix} y_1 \\ y_2 \\ \\ \vdots \\ \\ y_N \end{pmatrix} = \begin{pmatrix} 1 & 0 & 0 \\ \vdots & & \\ 0 & 1 & 0 \\ \vdots & & \\ 0 & 0 & 1 \\ \vdots & & \end{pmatrix} \cdot \begin{pmatrix} G_{11} \\ G_{12} \\ G_{22} \end{pmatrix} + \varepsilon \tag{2}$$

where the incidence matrix, $\mathbf{Z}$, assigns each observed phenotype to its corresponding genotypic value and $\boldsymbol{\varepsilon}$ is the vector of error terms. The extension of (2) to any number of alleles and loci is straightforward.

A model of genetic effects in the form $\mathbf{G} = \mathbf{S} \cdot \mathbf{E}$ can enter expression (2) by just substituting the vector of genotypic values into it. This way, we obtain the regression:

$$\mathbf{Y} = \mathbf{X} \cdot \mathbf{E} + \varepsilon \tag{3}$$

where $\mathbf{X} = \mathbf{Z} \cdot \mathbf{S}$. This expression enables direct estimation of genetic effects from data. The specific meaning of the genetic effects is given by the particular parameterization chosen for $\mathbf{S}$ (e.g., (1)).

It is convenient to initially use parameterizations of $\mathbf{S}$ leading to orthogonal estimation of genetic effects of QTL (20, 28). Regression (3) provides orthogonal estimates when the model of genetic effects used (i.e., the scales in the genetic-effect design matrix, **S**) is orthogonal for the genotype frequencies of the experimental population under study (17). However, this property holds only when the **Z**-matrix is built with definite assignments for all individuals of the experimental population (i.e., each row consists in one unity and zeros elsewhere), as represented in (2). This requirement is very stringent—it does not apply whenever QTL are located within marker intervals or markers associated to QTL display missing data for some individuals. For those cases, it is still possible to obtain orthogonal estimates by using interval mapping by imputations (IMI) (29). This regression method consists in splitting each row (i.e., each individual) of the original **Z**-matrix into as many rows as the number of possible genotypes, n, each of these rows bearing a unity in a different column and zeros otherwise—i.e., the **Z**-matrix becomes then a column of N identity matrices of dimension n. The resulting rows of the **Z**-matrix are next weighted by multiplying the **Z**-matrix by an additional diagonal matrix containing the genotype probabilities of each possible genotype (see Note 1).

2.2. The NOIA Model

Models of genetic effects are reparameterizations of the genotypic values from which required genetic and biological implications can be drawn (26). As an example, Fisher (1) meant the additive (average) effects of allele i, α_i, to capture the contribution of individuals carrying that allele to the population mean phenotype of the next generation under random mating. Here, we describe how to construct **S**-matrices leading to $\mathbf{G} = \mathbf{S} \cdot \mathbf{E}$ formulations intended to fit any potentially desired property or meaning of the genetic effects. We start with the simplest case of a genetic architecture underlying a trait—one biallelic locus. Some extensions to multiple alleles and multiple loci follow. We close this section by linking all different formulations within a common framework.

2.2.1. One Locus and Two Alleles

Following Álvarez-Castro and Carlborg (17), the statistical formulation of NOIA for one locus and two alleles, $\mathbf{G} = \mathbf{S}_S \cdot \mathbf{E}_S$ (where the subscript S stands for statistical), can be expressed as a function of the genotypic frequencies of the population under study, p_{ij}, and the allele frequencies, $p_i = p_{ii} + \frac{1}{2}p_{ij},\ i, j = 1, 2,\ j \neq i$, as:

$$\begin{pmatrix} G_{11} \\ G_{12} \\ G_{22} \end{pmatrix} = \begin{pmatrix} 1 & -2p_2 & -\dfrac{p_{12}p_{22}}{2p_1p_2 - \frac{1}{2}p_{12}} \\ 1 & p_1 - p_2 & \dfrac{p_{11}p_{22}}{p_1p_2 - \frac{1}{4}p_{12}} \\ 1 & 2p_1 & -\dfrac{p_{11}p_{12}}{2p_1p_2 - \frac{1}{2}p_{12}} \end{pmatrix} \cdot \begin{pmatrix} \mu \\ \alpha \\ \delta \end{pmatrix} \qquad (4)$$

where α and δ are the additive and dominant statistical genetic effects, respectively. The reference point of the model is the population mean,

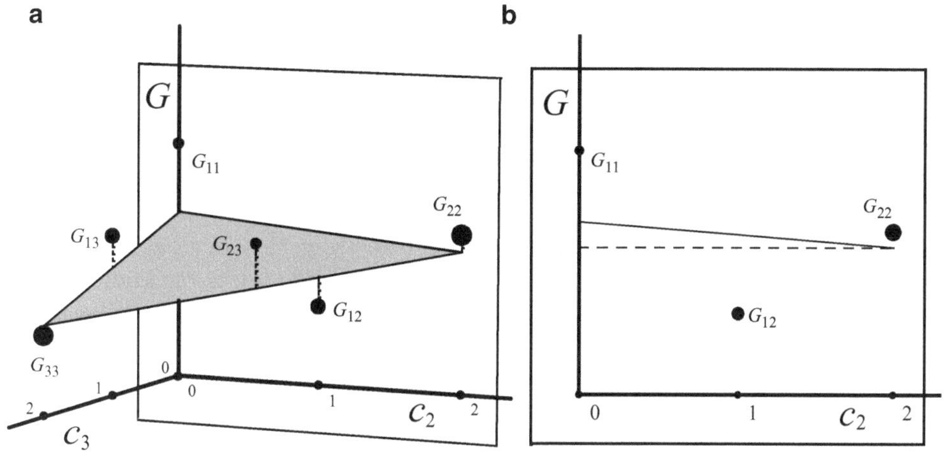

Fig. 1. (**a**) Graphical interpretation of the statistical formulation of the one-locus three-allele genetic system in Table 1. The genotypic values (G_{ij}) are spheres whose size represents the corresponding genotypic frequencies (p_{ij}). The *dark-gray plane* is the linear regression of the genotypic values on the gene content of alleles "2" and "3" (c_2 and c_3, respectively). The *dashed lines* stand for the deviations of the genotypic values and the breeding values, at the regression plane. The slice corresponding to the axes for the genotypic values and the content of allele "2" (*light-gray plane*) is detached in (**b**). (**b**) Slice corresponding to the axes *G* and c_2 (*light-gray plane* in (**a**)). The *solid line* marks the intersection with the regression plane (*dark-gray plane* in (**a**)). The *dashed line* is the corresponding linear regression in the absence of allele "3"—the remaining genotypes keeping their relative frequencies.

μ, from which the other parameters measure departures. This formulation fits Fisher's (1) linear regression of the genotypic values on their gene content—the number of copies of, for example, allele 1 in the genotypes (17) (see Fig. 1). It provides a decomposition of the genotypic values leading to an orthogonal decomposition of the genetic variance and to key biological concepts such as breeding value and heritability. Although Fisher originally introduced his decomposition for an F_2 population, note that expression (4) is parameterized, as Cockerham's (11) and Yang's (20), to account for any set of genotype frequencies.

Fisher (30) formulated the genetic effects in another way of interest for the study of selection in non-equilibrium populations (31), the average excesses. These are defined as the difference of the average individual carrying one copy of one allele and the average individual in the population. As opposed to the average effect, the average excess of one allele accounts for the correlation of that allele with other alleles in the population. Using the mathematical definitions of average excesses, it is possible to build the statistical-excess formulation of NOIA as:

$$\begin{pmatrix} \mu \\ \alpha^* \\ \delta^* \end{pmatrix} = \begin{pmatrix} p_{11} & p_{12} & p_{22} \\ -\dfrac{p_{11}}{p_1} & \frac{1}{2}\left(\dfrac{p_{12}}{p_2} - \dfrac{p_{12}}{p_1}\right) & \dfrac{p_{22}}{p_2} \\ -\frac{1}{2} & 1 & -\frac{1}{2} \end{pmatrix} \cdot \begin{pmatrix} G_{11} \\ G_{12} \\ G_{22} \end{pmatrix} \qquad (5)$$

Note that by using the definition of the average excesses for building the NOIA formulation, we get to an expression of the form $\mathbf{E} = \mathbf{S}^{-1} \cdot \mathbf{G}$, which is interchangeable with $\mathbf{G} = \mathbf{S} \cdot \mathbf{E}$ by just performing a matrix inversion. This is called the direct approach and it is convenient because inverted genetic-effect design matrices, $\mathbf{S}^{-1}$, are often simpler than their equivalent $\mathbf{S}$-matrices (17, 18, 26). We use the asterisks in (5) to differentiate these genetic effects, associated to average excesses, from the previous ones (4), associated to average effects. This formulation is parameterized in the same way as (4), thus accounting also for any possible genotype frequencies. Expressions (4) and (5) match under the Hardy–Weinberg proportions, which agrees with Fisher's observations (30).

Expressions (4) and (5) lead to dividing by zero if trying to express the genetic effects solely from the reference of an individual genotype—i.e., if setting the genotype frequencies of the two other genotypes to zero. This is not at all surprising since these expressions are associated with linear regressions (see Subheading 3.1) and there is no possible regression to one only point in a plane. However, it is possible to express the genotypic values as effects of allele substitutions from one individual genotype using a different formulation, the functional formulation of the NOIA model (17, 18). The functional formulation of NOIA for one locus and two alleles can be expressed as a function of the genotypic and allele frequencies as (17):

$$\begin{pmatrix} R \\ a \\ d \end{pmatrix} = \begin{pmatrix} p_{11} & p_{12} & p_{22} \\ -\frac{1}{2} & 0 & \frac{1}{2} \\ -\frac{1}{2} & 1 & -\frac{1}{2} \end{pmatrix} \cdot \begin{pmatrix} G_{11} \\ G_{12} \\ G_{22} \end{pmatrix} \tag{6}$$

We now use Latin instead of Greek letters to differentiate these new set of genetic effects from the previous ones ((4) and (5)). In this expression, the genotypic frequencies are assumed to be zero except for the frequency of the individual genotype chosen as reference, R, which equals one.

2.2.2. Several Alleles

We now show how to extend the biallelic NOIA functional formulation (6) to an arbitrary number of alleles, r, with $n = r(r+1)/2$ possible genotypes, using again the direct approach. For the functional formulation, (6) can be extended to three alleles rather easily as (18):

$$\begin{pmatrix} R \\ a^{12} \\ d^{12} \\ a^{13} \\ d^{13} \\ d^{23} \end{pmatrix} = \begin{pmatrix} p_{11} & p_{12} & p_{22} & p_{13} & p_{23} & p_{33} \\ -\frac{1}{2} & 0 & \frac{1}{2} & 0 & 0 & 0 \\ -\frac{1}{2} & 1 & -\frac{1}{2} & 0 & 0 & 0 \\ -\frac{1}{2} & 0 & 0 & 0 & 0 & \frac{1}{2} \\ -\frac{1}{2} & 0 & 0 & 1 & 0 & -\frac{1}{2} \\ 0 & 0 & -\frac{1}{2} & 0 & 1 & -\frac{1}{2} \end{pmatrix} \cdot \begin{pmatrix} G_{11} \\ G_{12} \\ G_{22} \\ G_{13} \\ G_{23} \\ G_{33} \end{pmatrix} \tag{7}$$

Here, superscripts are needed for differentiating genetic effects associated with all possible pairs of alleles. The missing additive effect in the new vector of genetic effects can be recovered by $a^{23} = a^{13} - a^{12}$. The upper-left quarter of the three-allele matrix in (7) coincides with the two-allele matrix in (6), which facilitates us to build (7). The extension from r to $r + 1$ alleles can be done in a completely analogous way—further technical details are provided by Yang and Álvarez-Castro (18).

The biallelic statistical-excess formulation of NOIA (5) can be extended to three and higher numbers of alleles in a similar way to the functional formulation ((5) and (6)). The average effects for multiple alleles are provided implicitly in the literature (10, 18). However, it is also possible to extend the statistical formulation of NOIA (4) to multiple alleles, thus providing explicit expressions for multiallelic average effects (26).

2.2.3. Several Loci

A major advantage of the $\mathbf{G} = \mathbf{S} \cdot \mathbf{E}$ notation in genetic modeling is to enable straightforward extensions to multiple loci. Indeed, the genetic effect design matrix for a multiple-locus genetic system can be obtained by just computing the Kronecker product of the single-locus matrices (19). This can be expressed for an arbitrary number, l, of loci as (17):

$$\bigotimes_{k=l}^{1} (\mathbf{S}_{L_k}) \tag{8}$$

with putatively different numbers of alleles at each of the l loci, L_k. The Kronecker product of two matrices consists in just multiplying the first matrix to each of the scalars of the second one (see Note 2).

Although matrix (8) includes by default all levels of gene interaction among loci, the resulting model can be easily constrained to a particular, chosen set of genetic effects—for instance to only pairwise interactions. This can be done by just setting to zeros the columns of the **S**-matrix (equivalently, the rows of the inverted **S**-matrix) associated with the discarded genetic effects. For instance, setting the last columns of the matrix in expression (4) to zeros, or equivalently the last rows in (5), leads to discarding dominance. The Kronecker product also allows the inclusion of environmental effects into the model. However, for the statistical and the statistical-excess formulations, the Kronecker product assumes random association among the effects represented by each of the matrices (see Note 3).

2.2.4. Transformations

Here, we present a last and consequential expression of the NOIA model framework. Let $\mathbf{G} = \mathbf{S}_1 \cdot \mathbf{E}_1$ and $\mathbf{G} = \mathbf{S}_2 \cdot \mathbf{E}_2$ be two different decompositions of the genotypic values for the genetic architecture underlying a trait. It is straightforward to transform the genetic effects of the first decomposition into the ones of the second decomposition as (17):

$$\mathbf{E}_2 = (\mathbf{S}_2)^{-1} \cdot \mathbf{S}_1 \cdot \mathbf{E}_1. \tag{9}$$

This is a change-of-reference tool sensu Hansen and Wagner (15). The power of this simple expression relies on the generality of the developments we have shown above, which in their turn gain significance through it. We can thus perceive (9) as the cornerstone of the NOIA model. In fact, the use of the common $\mathbf{G} = \mathbf{S} \cdot \mathbf{E}$ matrix notation connects the different kinds of decompositions of genetic effects shown above ((4)–(8)).

Van der Ween (27) provided a way to translate parameters between a few models of genetic effects of common use in the 1950s—the F_2, the F_∞ and a combination of both. Expression (9) generalizes that concept in two ways. First, it can be used to change the meaning of the genetic effects by translating them across three different formulations ((4)–(6)). Second, each of those different formulations having been parameterized by the genotypic frequencies enables expression (9) to provide parameters reflecting effects of allele substitutions measured in relation to diverse reference points, whether these are individual genotypes or population means (under linkage equilibrium). In brief, expression (9) encapsulates the motivation for NOIA as a general (within formulations) and unified (across formulations) theoretical framework for modeling genetic effects.

3. Applications

3.1. Graphical Interpretation

Figure 1 depicts the graphical interpretation of the statistical formulation of genetic effects for one locus and three alleles that is summarized in Table 1. The breeding values of the six genotypes are the predictions of the regression plane (dark-gray plane in Fig. 1a) and the dominance deviations (dashed vertical lines) are the difference between the breeding values and the genotypic values scaled by the mean phenotype. The genotype "11" has the highest breeding value. In particular, it has a higher breeding value than the other two genotypes not bearing allele "3." This can be better perceived in Fig. 1b as the negative slope of the solid line. However, when allele "3" is withdrawn from the population (the remaining genotypes keeping their relative frequencies) this is no longer true. Instead, the three remaining genotypes would actually have exactly the same breeding values (i.e., zero), as shown by the dashed horizontal line. In other words, the genetic properties of genotypes bearing a pair of alleles at one locus depend not only upon the relative frequencies of the genotypes involving those

Table 1
Genotype values, genotype frequencies, and breeding values for the six genotypes of a one-locus three-allele genetic system

	11	12	22	13	23	33
G_{ij}	1.5	0.5	1	1	1	0.5
p_{ij}	0.05	0.15	0.30	0.15	0.05	0.30
α_{ij}	0.26	0.18	0.10	0.01	0.07	0.23

alleles but also upon the presence of further genotypes for that locus in the population.

This can also be demonstrated for the other two possible pairs of alleles. Allele "2" is dominant over allele "3" (see Table 1), which implies that if withdrawing allele "1" the breeding value of "22" could not possibly be lower than its genotypic value (both being measured as departures from the population mean, in order to be compared). The mismatch between the three-allele system and the biallelic one without allele "2" is even easier to perceive. Indeed, the withdrawal of allele "2" causes the breeding values of the three genotypes to always coincide with their genotypic values due to the absence of dominance interactions (see Table 1). However, statistical dominance interactions occur for this pair in the complete genetic system (see Fig. 1a). They are due to dominance interactions between other pairs of alleles in the same locus, as noted by Yang and Álvarez-Castro (18).

The mismatches between the complete and the reduced models can be interpreted in relation to some features of the theoretical expressions of NOIA. The functional formulation (6) also has a graphical interpretation (17)—a linear regression in which the slope is constrained by the phenotypic difference of the two homozygotes. We have shown how the inverse **S**-matrix of the biallelic functional formulation of NOIA (6) can easily be extended to three alleles (7) in a nested way, without actually modifying the original biallelic matrix. This also holds when extending the functional **S**-matrix instead of its inverse (18). As a consequence, functional models keep their graphical interpretations when withdrawing alleles from them. Conversely, the nested extension of **S**-matrices does not hold for the statistical formulation, in accordance with the mismatches we have just noted. The mismatches between nested models can also be interpreted in connection with orthogonality (see Note 4).

3.2. Diagram

Figure 2 summarizes how QTL mapping and advanced genetic modeling can be combined to perform a comprehensive QTL

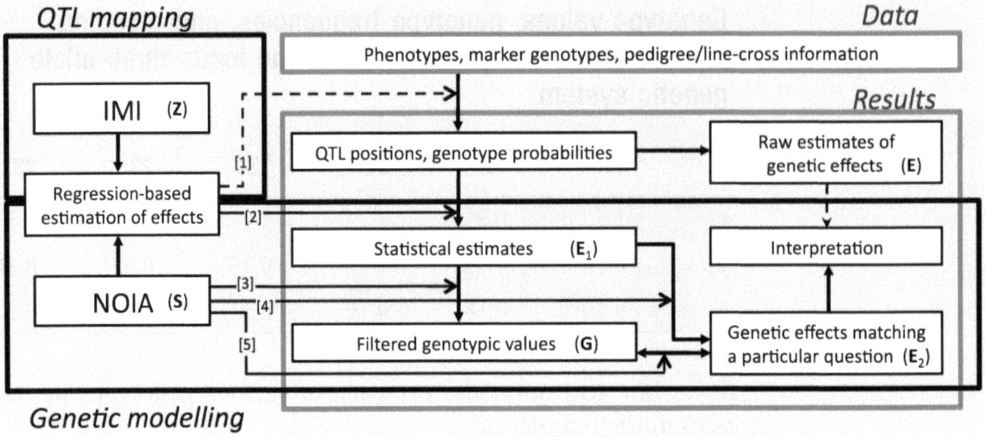

Fig. 2. Diagram representing the use of genetic modeling in QTL analysis. See text for expanded explanations.

analysis. QTL mapping provides genotype probabilities for QTL underlying the trait under study. The box of the regression-based estimation represents the estimation of genetic effects using (3) with the **Z**-matrix of the IMI (as described in Subheading 2.1) and the **S**-matrix of the statistical formulation of NOIA. This **S**-matrix is chosen to fit the experimental population, either for the simple case of a biallelic locus (4) or for multiple alleles and loci (8). The dashed elbow arrow (1) implies that the combined use of IMI and NOIA through (3) has properties that can facilitate this task (recall Note 1).

Whatever method has been used to estimate the positions and genotype probabilities of the significant QTL, it has assumed an underlying model of genetic effects from which estimates of QTL effects, **E**, can be obtained. We refer to these as the raw estimates, as they come directly from whatever procedure has been used in order to map the QTL. As an example, the Haley–Knott regression (32, 33) has been originally implemented with the F_∞ model. Although these raw estimates may allow for some interpretation of the results (vertical dashed arrow), this will be of limited use. Within this diagram, we illustrate the use of flexible genetic modeling strategies to comprehensively address a question of interest. In the forthcoming section, we review some practical examples of this practice.

The solid arrow departing from the box of the regression-based estimation (2) means that this regression provides statistical estimates of genetic effects, which we call $\mathbf{E}_1$. These estimates have a genetic meaning—they provide the heritability and the breeding values of the individuals of the experimental population. They are meant to be fully orthogonal for the population under study (see Subheading 2.1), as noted to be convenient on several occasions (20, 28). In any case, they are the best estimates to initially obtain from the data since they are associated with coherent estimates of genotypic values, **G**, as opposed to other methods in use (29).

The arrow (3) departing from the NOIA box represents the use of a statistical formulation of genetic effects ((3) and (8)) to obtain the vector of genotypic values, **G**. As mentioned above, this vector must be consistent with the particular genetic architecture (marginal and interaction effects) found to be significant after applying appropriate model selection strategies to the data. That architecture is entailed in the vector $\mathbf{E}_1$ and the particular **S**-matrix, $\mathbf{S}_1$, that was used to obtain it. Note that computing genotypic classes as means of individuals with the same genotype is often not possible since some genotypes might be absent from the experimental population. Missing genotypes will often occur when considering genetic networks that involve several alleles and/or loci. But even when all required genotypes are present, the resulting genotype means will involve all levels of epistatic interactions whether they are present in the genetic architecture or not—these will always arise as an artifact of computing the means with finite samples. Therefore, arrow [3] represents how to filter out spurious genetic effects by obtaining the estimates of all (present and absent) genotypic values in accordance with the genetic architecture found to be significant in the QTL mapping experiment.

However, we might be interested in other interpretations from the QTL analysis than just what is associated with the meaning of the estimates in $\mathbf{E}_1$. It will then be necessary to subsequently apply genetic modeling to achieve a more elaborate interpretation of our results. Arrow (4) stands for the use of the transformation tool of NOIA (9) to obtain genetic effects $\mathbf{E}_2$ that give an interpretation of results for a particular question of interest. To address certain questions will require not only transforming the genetic effects but also obtaining the decomposition of the genetic variance for a particular population. Such decompositions are straightforward using NOIA (17). Finally, arrow (5) means that a vector of genotypic values and a vector of genetic effects with a particular meaning are always interchangeable through an appropriate $\mathbf{G} = \mathbf{S} \cdot \mathbf{E}$ formulation. Indeed, they need not come from a QTL mapping experiment but they can, for instance, be designed ad hoc to inspect a particular problem by simulations. In the next section, we review examples of genetic effects that are appropriate to address particular questions of interest.

3.3. Real Data Applications

Most of the routines represented in the diagram above (Fig. 2) have already been applied to real datasets. Álvarez-Castro et al. (34) used NOIA to obtain functional genetic effects by estimating the effects of allele substitutions from the reference of a wild type in order to inspect the role of an interacting pair of epistatic loci in the evolution of growth rate during the domestication process of chicken. Le Rouzic et al. (35) carried out a deeper inspection of this process using an eight-locus genetic network. This study revealed epistatic interactions that cause domestic alleles at any locus of the network to display their positive effects in earlier life stages when domestic alleles are also common at the other loci. In this study, genetic filtering of the raw phenotypic data (see Fig. 2) enabled 6,561 possible genotypic values to be estimated from an experimental population of 800 individuals, based on the network of significant QTL found to affect the trait under study.

Genetic filtering of genotypic values has also proven to be crucial for the study of transgressive segregation. Using this strategy, we have found that hybrid inferiority for growth in chicken (a phenomenon found to consistently emerge in QTL studies of populations as different as wild × domestic and high × low selected line-crosses) is due to epistasis. This study, yet to be published, exemplifies the potential of genetic modeling for dissecting transgressive segregation in general, which could be applied to studying speciation by Dobzhansky–Muller incompatibilities. The flexibility of NOIA for interpreting the results of QTL-mapping experiments—particularly when extended multiple alleles—also makes it applicable to the study of natural populations and in general to studies involving variance component mapping methods, as illustrated by Besnier et al. (36). At the verge of one century after Fisher (1) founded quantitative genetics, advanced models are still being developed that lead to unconventional interpretations of genetic effects that can match any desired empirical situation, particularly involving epistasis.

4. Notes

1. In order to obtain orthogonal estimates of genetic effects, we are interested in the combined use of IMI and NOIA through expression (3). These estimates have a particular meaning in the experimental population, and we deem them to be the appropriate ones from which to eventually obtain estimates of genotypic values and of genetic effects matching additional required meanings. However, it is worth mentioning that orthogonality can be used to assist previous steps of QTL-mapping procedures, particularly by facilitating model selection strategies. This is because estimates of orthogonal estimates remain unchanged in reduced models (29).
2. This definition fits the Kronecker product that is used by default, the left-Kronecker product, which is also the one originally used in genetic modeling by Tiwari and Elston (19). The alternative right-Kronecker product could be used instead. In either case, this product can be used to obtain the scalars in the vectors **G** and **E** and it automatically generates the epistatic

components of the resulting multilocus model of genetic effects. Since the Kronecker product is associative, subsequent loci can be added at any point.

3. Building a multilocus model using the Kronecker product implies assuming that the multilocus genotype frequencies are the products of the single-locus ones. In other words, it assumes random association of alleles between/among loci—in particular, full linkage equilibrium. This constraint does not apply to the functional formulation, in which only one genotype frequency matters at a time—the one of the reference individual genotype, which equals one. When considering environmental effects, an analogous constraint will hold that consists in all genotypes being randomly associated to environments. However, implementing environmental effects is out of the scope of this communication.

4. The mismatches of the reduced cases of the statistical formulation reflect lack of orthogonality (recall Note 1). These mismatches do not occur for the functional formulation although it is the statistical formulation that is intended to be orthogonal. The explanation of this paradox is that the statistical formulation keeps additive and dominance (and epistatic for multiple loci) effects as independent parameters, at the cost of lack of independence among the additive effects of pairs of alleles within each locus.

Acknowledgments

Rong-Cai Yang has contributed to the development of the models of genetic effects that we have reviewed within this book chapter. Carl Nettelblad has extensively worked on the IMI, on which we have also commented. JÁC acknowledges funding by an "Isidro Parga Pondal" contract from the autonomous administration Xunta de Galicia and from project BFU2009-11988 from the Spanish Ministry of Science. ÖC is funded by a EURYI Award from ESF and a Future Research Leader Grant from the Swedish Foundation for Strategic Research. LR recognizes financial support by the Swedish Research Council FORMAS.

References

1. Fisher RA (1918) The correlation between relatives on the supposition of Mendelian inheritance. Trans Roy Soc Edinburgh 52:339–433
2. Edwards AW (2000) The genetical theory of natural selection. Genetics 154:1419–1426
3. Kempthorne O (1997) Heritability: uses and abuses. Genetica 99:109–112

4. Fisher RA (1930) The genetical theory of natural selection. Clarendon, Oxford
5. Wright S (1931) Evolution in Mendelian populations. Genetics 16:93–159
6. Dobzhansky T (1936) Studies on hybrid sterility. II. Location of sterility factors in *Drosophila pseudoobscura* hybrids. Genetics 21:113–135
7. Muller HJ (1942) Isolating mechanisms, evolution, and temperature. Biol Symp 6:71–125
8. Waddington CH (1953) Genetic assimilation of an acquired character. Evolution 7:118–126
9. Kempthorne O (1954) The correlation between relatives in a random mating population. Proc R Soc Lond B Biol Sci 143:102–113
10. Kempthorne O (1957) An introduction to genetic statistics. Wiley, New York
11. Cockerham CC (1954) An extension of the concept of partitioning hereditary variance for analysis of covariances among relatives when epistasis is present. Genetics 39:859–882
12. Cheverud JM, Routman EJ (1995) Epistasis and its contribution to genetic variance components. Genetics 139:1455–1461
13. Cheverud JM (2000) Detecting epistasis among quantitative trait loci. In: Wolf JB, Brodie ED, Wade MJ (eds) Epistasis and the evolutionary process. Oxford University Press, Oxford
14. Mather K, Jinks JL (1982) Introduction to biometrical genetics. Chapman and Hall, London
15. Hansen TF, Wagner GP (2001) Modeling genetic architecture: a multilinear theory of gene interaction. Theor Popul Biol 59:61–86
16. Phillips PC (2008) Epistasis—the essential role of gene interactions in the structure and evolution of genetic systems. Nat Rev Genet 9:855–867
17. Álvarez-Castro JM, Carlborg Ö (2007) A unified model for functional and statistical epistasis and its application in quantitative trait loci analysis. Genetics 176:1151–1167
18. Yang R-C, Álvarez-Castro JM (2008) Functional and statistical genetic effects with multiple alleles. Curr Topics Genet 3:49–62
19. Tiwari HK, Elston RC (1997) Deriving components of genetic variance for multilocus models. Genet Epidemiol 14:1131–1136
20. Yang R-C (2004) Epistasis of quantitative trait loci under different gene action models. Genetics 167:1493–1505
21. Noguera JL, Rodriguez C, Varona L et al (2009) A bi-dimensional genome scan for prolificacy traits in pigs shows the existence of multiple epistatic QTL. BMC Genomics 10:636–648
22. Rönnegård L, Besnier F, Carlborg Ö (2008) An improved method for quantitative trait loci detection of within-line segregation in F2 intercross designs. Genetics 178:2315–2326
23. Wei W-H, Knott SA, Haley CS, de Koning D-J (2010) Controlling false positives in the mapping of epistatic QTL. Heredity 104 (4):401–409
24. Carlborg Ö, Haley CS (2004) Epistasis: too often neglected in complex trait studies? Nat Rev Genet 5:618–625
25. Malmberg RL, Mauricio R (2005) QTL-based evidence for the role of epistasis in evolution. Genet Res 86:89–95
26. Álvarez-Castro JM, Yang RC (2011) Multiallelic models of genetic effects and variance decomposition in non-equilibrium populations. Genetica 139:1119–1134
27. Van der Ween JH (1959) Tests of non-allelic interaction and linkage for quantitative characters in generations derived from two diploid pure lines. Genetica 30:201–232
28. Kao CH, Zeng ZB (2002) Modeling epistasis of quantitative trait loci using Cockerham's model. Genetics 160:1243–1261
29. Nettelblad C, Carlborg Ö, Álvarez-Castro JM (2010) On orthogonal QTL parameter estimates with incomplete genotype information. In: Science GSfA (ed) 10th WCGALP, Leipzig, Germany
30. Fisher RA (1941) Average excess and average effect of a gene substitution. Ann Eugen 11:53–63
31. Bürger R (2000) The mathematical theory of selection, recombination and mutation. Wiley, Chichester
32. Haley CS, Knott SA (1992) A simple regression method for mapping quantitative trait loci in line crosses using flanking markers. Heredity 69:315–324
33. Martínez O, Curnow RN (1992) Estimating the locations and the sizes of the effects of quantitative trait loci using flanking markers. Theor Appl Genet 85:480–488
34. Álvarez-Castro JM, Le Rouzic A, Carlborg Ö (2008) How to perform meaningful estimates of genetic effects. PLoS Genet 4:e1000062
35. Le Rouzic A, Álvarez-Castro JM, Carlborg Ö (2008) Dissection of the genetic architecture of body weight in chicken reveals the impact of epistasis on domestication traits. Genetics 179:1591–1599
36. Besnier F, Le Rouzic A, Álvarez-Castro JM (2010) Applying QTL analysis to conservation genetics. Conserv Genet 11:399–408

Chapter 11

Identifying QTL for Multiple Complex Traits in Experimental Crosses

Samprit Banerjee and Nengjun Yi

Abstract

In this chapter, we consider the problem of jointly analyzing multiple (correlated) complex traits in the context of identifying quantitative trait loci (QTL). The advantages of joint analysis (as opposed independent analysis) is the detection of pleiotropy and improved precision of estimates. The multivariate model is introduced along with a brief description of the setup. The model is evaluated in a Bayesian framework to perform model selection (strategy to identify QTL for each trait). A detailed vignette of a statistical software (R/qtlbim) which uses a Markov Chain Monte Carlo (MCMC) approach to draw samples from the posterior distribution is presented. Strategies of checking MCMC convergence, visualization of posterior samples, model building, and testing pleiotropy with the software are described. Relevant code to perform the analysis on an example (simulated) dataset is also provided.

Key words: QTL, MCMC, Pleiotropy, Joint analysis, Multiple traits

1. Introduction

The broad goal of mapping quantitative trait loci (QTLs) is to shed light on the genetic architecture underlying complex traits. Complex traits are physical expressions of an organism which are controlled by many genes/loci and whose inheritance does not follow simple rules of Mendelian genetics. Over the past few decades, there has been considerable development of statistical methodology to map QTLs for complex traits (brief review can be found in ref. (1)). The biggest challenge in this respect is the vast number of unknown genes, their interactions among themselves and with environmental factors. The focus of this chapter is the simultaneous inference of QTLs for multiple complex traits which has several advantages. First, the chief advantage is detecting pleiotropy, in which action at a single locus leads to variation in a number of traits. For example, one might desire to modify two traits that tend

Scott A. Rifkin (ed.), *Quantitative Trait Loci (QTL): Methods and Protocols*, Methods in Molecular Biology, vol. 871,
DOI 10.1007/978-1-61779-785-9_11, © Springer Science+Business Media New York 2012

to be negatively correlated. If this negative association is due to pleiotropy, it will be very difficult to modify both traits simultaneously. Second, joint analysis increases the power and precision for detecting QTL effects. Among the several methods for joint analysis, refs. (2, 3) are the most comprehensive in terms of software. In this chapter, we describe the methods developed in refs. (3, 4) and the corresponding freely available software R/qtlbim (5).

2. Methods

2.1. Experimental Design

In a backcross design an investigator performing an experiment to identify QTLs chooses two pure-breeding lines that differ in the trait of interest (high (H) or low (L) parental strains). These lines are inbred so that within an inbred strain all individuals are essentially genetically identical and are homozygous at all loci. The low parental line is then mated with the high parental line which forms the first filial generation (or F_1). The F_1 generation gets a copy of the genetic material from each parental line resulting in heterozygous (HL) genotypes. The F_1 progenies are then back-mated with the low parental line resulting in backcross progenies which have two possible genotypes HL or LL. The chromosomes cross-over during meiosis and the idea is to capture these cross-overs or recombination events. Another popular design is the intercross or F_2 design where the progenies of F_1 are mated with themselves or each other to generate the F_2 progenies having three possible genotypes: HH, LH, and LL (see Chapter 10).

2.2. Genetic Model

In order to discern the association between a locus and a phenotype one needs to develop a statistical model to capture this association. Consider the very simple case of one QTL and one trait resulting in the linear model (1).

$$Y_i = \mu + Q_i + e_i \tag{1}$$

Q_i is the effect of the QTL on the *i*th individual which can be modeled using Cockerham's model (6). The key advantage with Cockerham's model is that it leads to orthogonal contrasts so parameter estimates do not depend on the current complexity of the model, allowing testing of nonnested models. For a backcross population with only two segregating genotypes (say, AA and Aa), the contrasts for main effects of AA(Aa) are defined by $\frac{1}{2}(-\frac{1}{2})$. For an F_2 population with three segregating genotypes (say, AA, Aa, and aa), the additive contrasts are defined by 1, 0, and -1, while the dominant contrasts are coded as $-\frac{1}{2}$, $\frac{1}{2}$, and $-\frac{1}{2}$ for AA, Aa, and aa, respectively. The contrasts for dominant effects can be interpreted as deviations from the additive nature of allelic effect, i.e., interactions between the two alleles at a particular locus. The epistatic contrasts are defined by multiplying the contrasts of the corresponding main effects. Note that for an F_2 population there can be four different types of epistatic effects between two loci depending on the nature of main effect at each loci: additive–additive, additive–dominant, dominant–additive, and dominant–dominant interactions. To construct contrasts for G × E interactions one can simply multiply the covariate with the corresponding main effect contrast. As an example, the epistatic model for two loci A and B, each with two alleles (A, a, and B, b) can be presented for a F_2 cross in the following way:

$$Q_i = \mu + \beta_1^{\mathrm{a}} x_{1i}^{\mathrm{a}} + \beta_1^{\mathrm{d}} x_{1i}^{\mathrm{d}} + \beta_2^{\mathrm{a}} x_{2i}^{\mathrm{a}} + \beta_2^{\mathrm{d}} x_{2i}^{\mathrm{d}} + \beta_{12}^{\mathrm{aa}} x_{1i}^{\mathrm{a}} x_{2i}^{\mathrm{a}} + \beta_{12}^{\mathrm{ad}} x_{1i}^{\mathrm{a}} x_{2i}^{\mathrm{d}} + \beta_{12}^{\mathrm{da}} x_{1i}^{\mathrm{d}} x_{2i}^{\mathrm{a}} + \beta_{12}^{\mathrm{dd}} x_{1i}^{\mathrm{d}} x_{2i}^{\mathrm{d}} \quad (2)$$

by defining the coded variables as

$$x_1^{\mathrm{a}} = \begin{cases} 1 & \text{if A is } AA \\ 0 & \text{if A is } Aa \\ -1 & \text{if A is } aa \end{cases}, \quad x_2^{\mathrm{a}} = \begin{cases} 1 & \text{if B is } BB \\ 0 & \text{if B is } Bb \\ -1 & \text{if B is } bb \end{cases}$$

$$x_1^{\mathrm{d}} = \begin{cases} \frac{1}{2} & \text{if A is } Aa \\ -\frac{1}{2} & o.w \end{cases}, \quad x_2^{\mathrm{d}} = \begin{cases} \frac{1}{2} & \text{if B is } Bb \\ -\frac{1}{2} & o.w \end{cases}$$

Note that the superscript a and d correspond to the additive and dominant main effects, while aa, ad, da, and dd correspond to the additive–additive, additive–dominant, dominant–additive, and dominant–dominant interactions.

2.3. Interval Mapping

A QTL associated with a trait might not be located exactly on a particular marker; hence, it is important to look for QTLs between marker intervals. The idea of interval mapping is to search for candidate QTLs between observed marker intervals. This introduces a problem as the genotypes at these putative positions are not observed. One can estimate the genotypes at these candidate loci from the genotypes of the flanking markers and the probability of a recombination event happening between the marker and the putative QTL. A detailed description of this process is given in ref. (7).

2.4. Multivariate Model

The multivariate model is constructed to jointly analyze multiple correlated traits. It is different from a trait-by-trait analysis as it explicitly models the correlation among the traits, which is ignored by the trait-by-trait analysis. Let us consider a very simple case of T correlated traits ($\mathbf{y}_t$, $t = 1, 2, \ldots, T$) and one QTL $\mathbf{Q}$ for a backcross experiment.

$$\mathbf{y}_i = \alpha + \beta \mathbf{Q}_i + \varepsilon_i \quad (3)$$

Here, the subscript i corresponds to the ith individual. It is also assumed that $\varepsilon_i \sim N_T(\mathbf{0}, \Sigma)$ i.e., the residuals for ith individual follow a multivariate (T-variate, the subscript of N and note that

$\mathbf{0}$ is a T-sized vector of zeroes) normal distribution with a covariance matrix Σ. The trait-by-trait analysis is a special case of multivariate analysis when $\Sigma = I$ (where I is the $T \times T$ identity matrix with 1's in the diagonal and 0's elsewhere), and the traits are assumed to be independent.

A simple multivariate model (3) as proposed in Jiang and Zeng (2) answers the question of pleiotropy for a single locus but has several limitations. First, it does not consider the joint effect of several QTLs, and interactions among these QTLs and with environmental factors. Second, it is not practical to assume that the same set of QTLs will be associated with all traits. To address these issues the QTL SUR (seemingly unrelated regression) model of (3) and its extension to include gene–gene and gene–environment interaction (4) is presented here. The idea is to fix a total number of detectable QTLs per trait to an upper bound L (this is described in more detail in Subheading 2.5) and collect the contrasts (described in Subheading 2.2) for main-effects (subscript G), gene–gene (G $\times$ G) interactions (subscript GG), gene–environment (G $\times$ E) interactions (subscript GE), and controlling factors for environmental effects (subscript E) in separate matrices. The resulting model for each trait t is

$$\begin{aligned}\mathbf{y}_t &= \mu_t + \mathbf{X}_{\mathrm{E}}\beta_{\mathrm{tE}} + \mathbf{X}_{\mathrm{tG}}\beta_{\mathrm{tG}} + \mathbf{X}_{\mathrm{tGG}}\beta_{\mathrm{tGG}} + \mathbf{X}_{\mathrm{tGE}}\beta_{\mathrm{tGE}} + \mathbf{e}_t \\ &\equiv \mu_t + \mathbf{X}_t\beta_t + \mathbf{e}_t \end{aligned} \quad (4)$$

where $\boldsymbol{\mu}_t$ is the overall mean for trait t, $\mathbf{X}_{\mathrm{tG}}$ is the matrix of the main-effect predictors of L loci, determined from the genotypes as described in Subheading 2.2, $\mathbf{X}_{\mathrm{tGG}}$, $\mathbf{X}_{\mathrm{tGE}}$, $\mathbf{X}_{\mathrm{E}}$, are the design matrices of the epistatic effects, gene–environment interactions, and environmental effects; $\boldsymbol{\beta}_{\mathrm{tG}}$, $\boldsymbol{\beta}_{\mathrm{tGG}}$, and $\boldsymbol{\beta}_{\mathrm{tGE}}$ are the main effects, G $\times$ G interactions or epistatic effects, and G $\times$ E interactions, respectively, for the tth trait; $\boldsymbol{\beta}_{\mathrm{tE}}$ are the effects of the covariates and $\mathbf{e}_t$ is the trait-specific error term. The residual error vector $\mathbf{e}$ $(e_{ti} : t = 1, \ldots, T,\ i = 1, \ldots, N)$ is assumed to be distributed as $N(\mathbf{0}, \Sigma_{T\times T} \otimes \mathbf{I}_{N\times N})$. Thus, the residual errors are independent among individuals, but are correlated among traits within individuals. Note that design matrices, $\mathbf{X}_{\mathrm{tG}}$, $\mathbf{X}_{\mathrm{tGG}}$, $\mathbf{X}_{\mathrm{tGE}}$, have a subscript t corresponding to the tth trait, which allows each trait to have a separate genetic model. This is a key advantage of the QTL SUR model. The special case $\mathbf{X}_{\mathrm{tG}} = \mathbf{X}_{\mathrm{G}}$ for all t, $\mathbf{X}_{\mathrm{tGG}} = \mathbf{X}_{\mathrm{GG}}$ for all t, $\mathbf{X}_{\mathrm{tGE}} = \mathbf{X}_{\mathrm{GE}}$ for all t is called the "traditional multivariate model" or TMV which considers the same genetic model (same set of QTL main, G $\times$ G, and G $\times$ E interaction effects) for all traits.

2.5. Model Selection

The aim of QTL mapping is to identify the number and location of QTLs affecting a particular trait. A way to solve the unknown QTL location problem is to generate a grid of putative QTL positions across the entire genome. The coarseness or fineness of the grid will depend on the marker density and goals of the study in question. Defining such a grid introduces a problem of unknown QTL genotypes which can be estimated using the interval mapping idea of Subheading 2.3. These genotypes can be updated in the Bayesian framework to produce robust genotypes (please refer to refs. (8–10) for details). Finding the number and combination of QTLs that affects the trait is one of model selection (11). The actual number of detectable QTLs for each trait is usually not too large. One can impose an upper bound, L, on the total number of detectable QTL. The upper bound L is larger than the number of detectable QTL with high probability for a given dataset and can be set based on the initial analyses using conventional mapping methods on each trait (8, 9). One can assign a vector of unobserved indicator variables $\gamma_t = \{\gamma_{t1}, \ldots, \gamma_{tL}\}$ for each trait t to indicate which QTLs are included in $(\gamma_{tj} = 1,\ j = 1, \ldots, L)$ or excluded from $(\gamma_{tj} = 0,\ j = 1, \ldots, L)$ the model. The positions of these L QTLs are stored in the vector $\lambda_t = \{\lambda_{1t}, \ldots, \lambda_{Lt}\}$ for each trait t. Jointly, the vector (λ_t, γ_t) denotes the genetic architecture of the tth trait, i.e., the actual number of QTL $(\sum_j \gamma_{tj})$, their positions, and which traits they affect. To construct the linear model, invoke the QTL SUR model of Subheading 2.4. Two separate SUR models can be considered. The first model is the one that is described above and is named SURd (SUR modeling with different loci used for all traits) and the second is SURs (SUR modeling with same loci used for all traits) which assumes the same location for all QTLs, i.e., $\lambda_1 = \lambda_2 = \cdots = \lambda_T \equiv \lambda$ and hence the same design matrices $\mathbf{X}_1 = \mathbf{X}_2 = \cdots = \mathbf{X}_T \equiv \mathbf{X}$. The design matrix ($\mathbf{X}$) is generically represents $\mathbf{X}_{\mathrm{G}}$, $\mathbf{X}_{\mathrm{GG}}$ and $\mathbf{X}_{\mathrm{GE}}$. It is important to note that the indicator variables (γ_t) are different for each trait, according to the definition of a SUR model. The two common models, the univariate single trait approach (STA) and the traditional multivariate model (TMV), are special cases under the conditions $\Sigma = \mathbf{I}$ and $\gamma_1 = \gamma_2 = \cdots = \gamma_T$. Banerjee et al. (3) provides evidence in favor of the superior performance of the QTL SUR models compared to the TMV.

3. Vignette for Statistical Software

In this section, simultaneous inference of multiple correlated traits to identify QTLs will be discussed using the package R/qtlbim. The package R/qtlbim can be freely downloaded from http://cran.r-project.org or www.qtlbim.com. R/qtlbim depends on certain external R packages, namely, R/qtl, R/coda, R/lattice, R/tools, and R/MASS. The last three packages are included in the default installation of R. However, one needs to install R/coda (12) and

R/qtl (13) to use R/qtlbim. If the packages are not installed R/qtlbim automatically installs them. To invoke the library of functions distributed by R/qtlbim one should type the following command on the R command prompt (represented by ">" in this chapter).

```
> library(qtlbim)
Loading required package: qtl
Loading required package: lattice
Loading required package: coda
Loading required package: tools
Loading required package: MASS
```

It is recommended to have a system with at least 1 GB of RAM and a disk space of at least 10 MB to run R/qtlbim with multiple traits.

3.1. Data Simulation or Real Data Input

R/qtlbim has a built-in function `qb.sim.cross` to simulate a backcross or F_2 dataset of class `cross` (see R/qtl help pages for details). The following chunk of code generates a dataset of 200 individuals (`n.ind=200`) of "backcross" (`type= "bc"`) mating design. These individuals are genotyped for 11 equally spaced markers (`n.mar=11, eq.spacing=TRUE`) on 19 chromosomes each of length 100 cM (`len=rep(100,19)`). Multiple correlated traits can be generated by specifying the option `multiple.trait=TRUE`. Here two correlated traits (`n.pheno=2`) are generated with a correlation (`sigma = rbind(c(1,0.8),c(0.8,1))`) of 0.8 between the traits. There are six QTLs, two on chromosome 1 and 4 and one each on chromosomes 2 and 3. The option `qtl.main` and `qtl.epis` can be used to specify the genetic model, i.e., which QTLs influence the trait and the sizes of their effects. The simulation allows the user to specify different or same genetic model for each trait thereby generating data for a SUR model or a TMV (as described in Subheading 2.4) respectively. Two covariates are generated: a fixed binary covariate with an effect size of 0.5 and a random covariate of five levels whose coefficient are drawn from $N(0, 0.07)$. Gene-by-environment interaction (option `gbye`) are specified with a fixed covariate. Three percent of the genotypes (`missing.geno=0.03`) and 5% of the phenotypes (`missing.pheno=0.05`) were assumed to be missing randomly.

```
> cross <- qb.sim.cross(len = rep(100,19),n.mar = 11, eq.spacing =TRUE,
+   n.ind = 200, type="bc", missing.geno = 0.05, missing.pheno = 0.03,
+   multiple.trait=TRUE,n.pheno=2,sigma=rbind(c(1,0.8),c(0.8,1)),
+   qtl.pos=rbind(qtl.1=c(chr=1,pos=15),
+                 qtl.2=c(1,65),
+                 qtl.3=c(2,12),
```

```
+                      qtl.4=c(3,15),
+                      qtl.5=c(4,23),
+                      qtl.6=c(4,65) ),
+   qtl.main=rbind(main.1=c(ph=1,qtl=1,add=1.5),
+                      main.2=c(1,2,0.7),
+                      main.3=c(1,3,1),
+                      main.4=c(2,3,1),
+                      main4=c(2,4,0.7),
+                      main5=c(2,6,1.2) ),
+   qtl.epis=rbind(epis1=c(ph=1,qtl.a=2,qtl.b=3,aa=-2),
+                        epis2=c(ph=1,1,4,2),
+                        epis3=c(ph=2,2,4,2),
+                        epis4=c(ph=2,1,2,-2)),
+   gbye = rbind(GxE.1=c(ph=1,qtl=1,add=1.5),
+                   GxE.2=c(ph=1,qtl=3,add=-1.5),
+                   GxE.3=c(ph=2,qtl=3,add=-1.5),
+                   GxE.4=c(ph=2,qtl=6,add=1.5)),
+   covariate = c(fix.cov=0.5,ran.cov=0.07))
```

The function `qb.sim.cross` generates an object of class "`cross`." In the case of real datasets, the function `read.cross` of R/qtl can be used to read datasets in a variety of formats and store it as a "`cross`" object. The simulated cross object has an extra element named "`qtl`" which stores the true QTL positions, genotypes and heritability of effects for post-analysis comparison. The summary of this "qtl" element can be viewed as shown below and to get the true parameter values.

```
> names(cross)
[1] "geno"  "pheno" "qtl"

> summary(cross$qtl)
$pos
      chr pos
qtl.1   1  15
qtl.2   1  65
qtl.3   2  12
qtl.4   3  15
qtl.5   4  23
qtl.6   4  65

$herit.main
       pheno qtl        add
main.1     1   1 0.07762380
main.2     1   2 0.06415190
main.3     1   3 0.06415190
main.4     2   3 0.07837382
main.5     2   4 0.07837382
main.6     2   6 0.11285830

$herit.epis
```

```
       pheno qtl.a qtl.b          aa
epis.1     1     2     3 0.06415190
epis.2     1     1     4 0.06415190
epis.3     2     2     4 0.07837382
epis.4     2     1     2 0.07837382

$herit.cov
           fix.cov    ran.cov
Pheno.1 0.01603797 0.01796253
Pheno.2 0.01959345 0.02194467

$herit.gbye
      pheno qtl        add
GxE.1     1   1 0.05196304
GxE.2     1   3 0.05196304
GxE.3     2   3 0.06348279
GxE.4     2   6 0.06348279

$var
        Pheno.1 Pheno.2
Pheno.1     1.0     0.8
Pheno.2     0.8     1.0
```

The summary of the cross object can be viewed by

```
> summary(cross)
    Backcross

    No. individuals:    200

    No. phenotypes:     4
    Percent phenotyped: 98.5 96 96.5 98.5

    No. chromosomes:    19
        Autosomes:      1 2 3 4 5 6 7 8 9 10 11 12 13 14 15 16 17 18 19

    Total markers:      209
    No. markers:         11 11 11 11 11 11 11 11 11 11 11 11 11 11 11 11 11 11
11
    Percent genotyped:  95
    Genotypes (%):      AA:50.7  AB:49.3
```

3.2. Bayesian QTL Analysis

This section describes in greater detail how to generate Markov Chain Monte Carlo (MCMC) samples from the Bayesian posterior to be used for QTL mapping. The function `qb.genoprob` creates a grid of putative QTL positions throughout the entire genome and computes the genotypic probabilities of the same. It would also compute genotypic probabilities for missing markers. By specifying a positive integer value for the option `step`, a grid of putative QTLs can be created across the entire genome at intervals of the size of `step`. The genotypes at these putative loci are unobserved, but the probabilities can be calculated from the observed marker data using the multipoint method (7).

```
> cross <- qb.genoprob(cross,map.func="haldane",
step=1)
```

3.2.1. Specifying the Data

The function qb.data specifies the traits to be analyzed, their underlying distribution, the random and/or fixed covariates and whether to standardize or to use a Box-Cox transformation for nonnormal continuous traits. The traits to be analyzed and the fixed and random covariates are specified by providing the corresponding element of cross$pheno. To jointly analyze multiple traits the option multiple.trait must be turned on. The option multiple.type specifies the type of multivariate model that is to be used. There are two choices, the SUR model or the TMV as described in Subheading 2.4. SUR permits each trait to have a different genetic model while TMV assumes the same model for all traits. Note that the cross object can have several phenotypes some of which could be used as covariates.

```
> data <- qb.data(cross, pheno.col = c(3,4), trait="normal",
multiple.trait=TRUE,fixcov=1, rancov=2,multiple.type="SUR",standardize =
FALSE)
```

3.2.2. Defining the Model

The function qb.model defines the model for the QTL analysis. It specifies (1) whether epistasis is considered, (2) the a priori expected number of main effect QTLs (main.qtl) for each trait, (3) the a priori expected number of total number of QTLs for each trait included in the model through main, epistatic, and gene–environment (G × E) interaction effect (mean.qtl), and (4) the maximum number of QTLs allowed per chromosome (chr.nqtl). The maximum number of QTLs allowed (max.qtl) has a default of $l_0 + 3\sqrt{l_0}$ where l_0 is main.qtl in a nonepistatic and mean.qtl in an epistatic model. The interval (interval) between two flanking QTLs for each chromosome and the fixed covariate(s) interacting with QTLs are also specified. The main.qtl option of the qb.model function refers to the prior number of main effect QTLs. This is obtained generally from a previous rudimentary non-Bayesian analysis for each trait and the maximum among the traits can be considered. For example, R/qtl can be used to analyze this data without epistasis and the number of QTLs detected could be used as the prior number of QTLs. The option intcov can be used to specify which fixed covariates are considered for G × E interaction. If multiple.type = "SUR" in qb.data, the option diff.loc is specified to indicate if different QTL locations are considered for different traits (diff.loc=TRUE) or same set of locations are considered for each trait (diff.loc=FALSE). For more details please refer to (3). The following chunk of code specifies the model for our simulated data:

```
> model <- qb.model(cross, epistasis = TRUE, intcov = 1, main.qtl = 3,
+                   mean.qtl = 6,  interval = rep(5,nchr(cross)),
+                   chr.nqtl = rep(2,nchr(cross)), max.qtl = NULL,
+                   diff.loc = TRUE)
```

3.2.3. Generating MCMC Samples

The function qb.mcmc creates MCMC samples on the data and model specified. The results are saved in a specified directory, default being the current working directory ("."). The genoupdate parameter of the qb.mcmc function should be switched on when there are many missing marker genotypes. When this option is switched off a Haley–Knott regression is performed with expected genotypic values. For our case, we have only 7% of the marker genotypes missing at random; hence, updating genotypes is not imperative. We would be saving 3,000 posterior samples which is the default n.iter. It is worth mentioning that n.iter does not specify the total number samples drawn from the posterior distribution but merely indicates the number of samples that would be saved and used for posterior analysis. The first n.burnin samples are discarded to allow the chain to converge to the posterior distribution, and after that every n.thin sample is saved to reduce serial correlation among consecutive draws resulting in a total of n.burnin + n.iter*n.thin samples drawn.

```
> qbObject <- qb.mcmc(cross, data, model, n.burnin = 5000, n.thin = 20,
+                     n.iter = 3000, genoupdate=FALSE)
qb.mcmc is running 65,000 iterations. The current iterations are saved:
200
400
600
800
1000
1200
1400
1600
1800
2000
2200
2400
2600
2800
3000
MCMC sample has been saved to: ./pheno.normal.1_Nov-15-181148.
Bayesian MCMC took 1.72 minutes.
Warning: Removing external directory ./pheno.normal.1_Nov-15-181148
```

3.2.4. Examining the qb Object

Please note that the plot and summary routines in this package all use the S3 generic method, i.e., an object with a call to qb.xxx is created and then it can be plotted or summarized using the generic plot or summary command. The qbObject is an object of class qb to which we can apply the generic summary or plot routines. We defer plots to later sections. The summary of MCMC posterior samples can be summarized by trait.

```
> summary(qbObject,pheno.col=1)
Bayesian model selection QTL mapping object qbObject on cross object cross
had 3000 iterations recorded at each 20 steps
with 5000 burn-in steps.
MCMC runs saved in qb object.
Traits pheno.normal.1,pheno.normal.2 ( 1,2 ) treated as normal .
Fixed covariate: fix.cov
Random covariate: random.cov
Trait was not standardized.
```

```
Epistasis was allowed.
Prior number of QTL: 3 main, 6 total, with 13 maximum.
Minimum distance between QTL:
 [1] 5 5 5 5 5 5 5 5 5 5 5 5 5 5 5 5 5 5 5 5
Maximum number of QTL:
 [1] 2 2 2 2 2 2 2 2 2 2 2 2 2 2 2 2 2 2 2 2
QTL by environment allowed.
Interacting covariates: 1
Diagnostic summaries:
          nqtl   mean envvar varadd  varaa  envadd  varenv   var
Min.     1.000  8.032 0.9605 0.2748 0.1655 0.01705 -1.8930 0.832
1st Qu.  4.000  9.272 1.3490 0.5303 0.3626 0.22810  0.6967 1.253
Median   5.000  9.571 1.4570 0.6038 0.4230 0.31520  0.8843 1.373
Mean     5.419  9.572 1.4690 0.6110 0.4312 0.36920  0.8500 1.411
3rd Qu.  6.000  9.856 1.5750 0.6821 0.4952 0.43910  1.0440 1.515
Max.    11.000 11.510 2.3490 1.2610 0.8201 2.87200  1.5620 4.112

Percentages for number of QTL detected:
 1  2  3  4  5  6  7  8  9 10 11
 0  2  8 20 25 22 14  6  2  0  0

Percentages for number of epistatic pairs detected:
pairs
 2  3  4  5  6  7
 4 28 36 21  8  2

Percentages for common epistatic pairs:
1:3   1:2   1:7   1:1   1:14  3:9   2:3   2:7   2:12  12:14 1:8   7:14     102
101    90    35     5     4     4     3     2     2     2     2
2:11  4:7   3:13
2     2     1
```

3.2.5. Plotting MCMC History

Convergence of the MCMC algorithm is of critical importance to any Bayesian analysis. The plotting tools in `R/qtlbim` provide a method for visually inspecting the history of the MCMC run. The command `plot(qb.coda(qbObject,phenol.col=1))` shows a default view of the MCMC chain as a time series for a particular trait. Since every iteration of the MCMC algorithm represents a single model for a particular trait; therefore, we can explore the history of the markov chain by plotting them as time series for relevant model features. The time series plotted by `qb.coda` show the sampling histories for:

1. Number of QTLs in each model model (`nqtl`)
2. Mean phenotype according to each model (`mean`)
3. Environmental variability under each model (`envvar`)
4. Variance explained under each model (`var`)

It is possible to plot a different subset of the model characteristics above, by using the optional argument `variables` in the `qb.coda` function. For example, in order to view just the number of QTLs (`nqtl`) and the model means, use the following command. The results of the following command are shown in Fig. 1.

```
>  plot(qb.coda(qbObject,variables=c("nqtl","env-
var"),phenol.col=1))
```

3.2.6. Plot of QTLs by Chromosome

From a biological perspective it is interesting to view the location of possible QTLs along the chromosome. The function `qb.loci` shows a plot of QTLs for each chromosome for a particular trait. The QTLs shown are from single QTL models appearing as posterior samples of the MCMC. In the plot, the actual locations of possible QTLs are jittered slightly in order to give a sense of the density of putative QTLs in the vicinity of each marker. The code

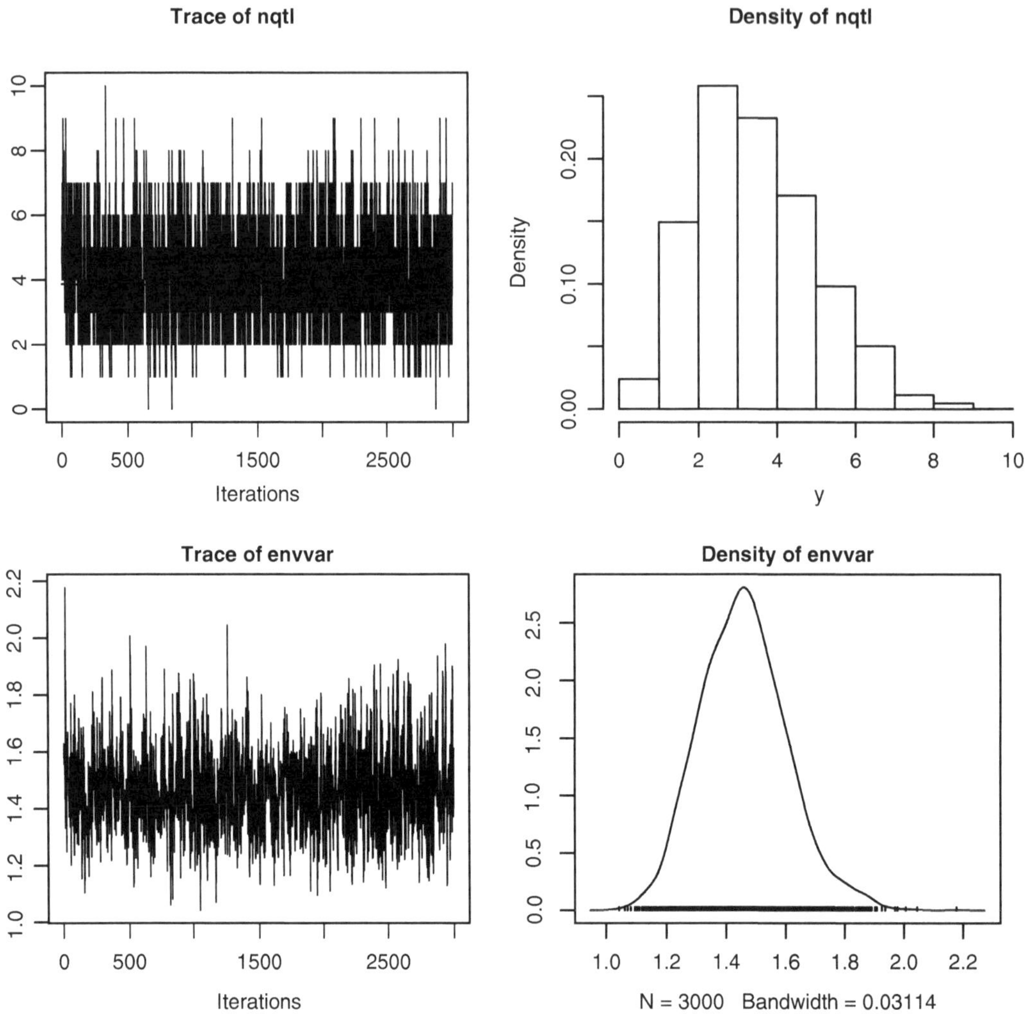

Fig. 1. Diagnostic plot for a MCMC run.

```
> plot(qb.loci(qbObject,pheno.col=1), col = c(all="gray50",main="black",
+                          epistasis="gray80",GxE="gray40",marker="black"))
```

produces a plot shown in Fig. 2 for the first trait with the darker shade of "gray" corresponding to `gray40`.

3.2.7. Summary Plot for Sampled Models

The function `qb.BayesFactor` produces a composite (4-by-2) summary plot of the models sampled by the MCMC chain for a particular trait. These plots are useful as an initial tool for examining the evidence in favor of multiple QTL models and in determining the locations of QTL. Figure 3 shows the plot produced by the command `plot(qb.BayesFactor(qbObject,phenol.col=1),col.prior="gray")`. The interpretation of each of these plots is described below:

1. The plot appearing in the upper-left of the figure represents a plot of the prior distribution for the number of QTLs involved

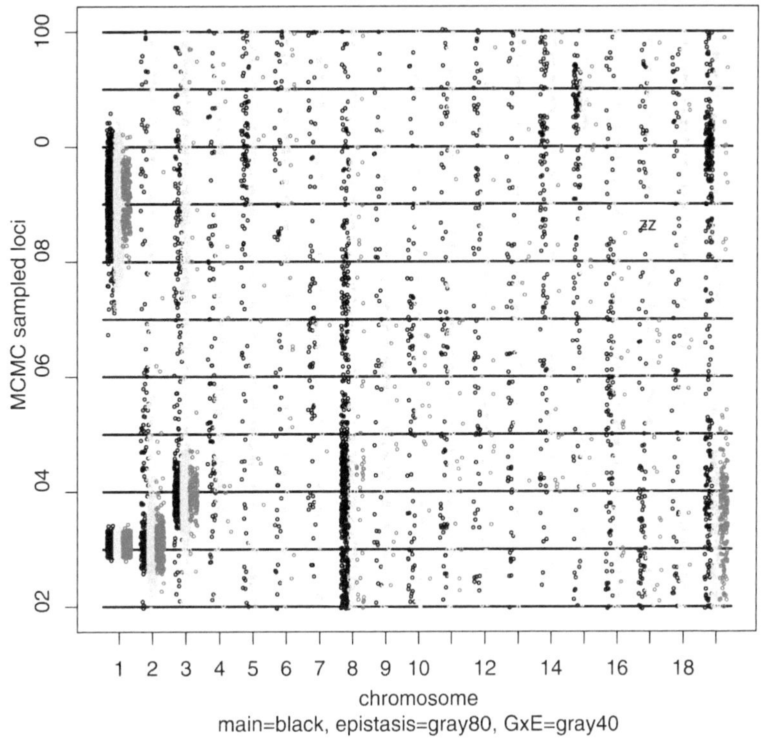

Fig. 2. A jittered plot of QTLs included in the model for the first trait through main, epistatic or G $\times$ E interaction.

in models (shown as a broken grey line) against the corresponding posterior probabilities (shown as a histogram).

2. The plot in the upper-right shows Bayes factor ratios. These are the ratios of posterior probabilities to prior probabilities. For pairs of values along the horizontal axis of this plot, the member of the pair with a larger Bayes factor ratio should be interpreted as more likely. The vertical arrows give an indication of the strength of evidence: weak (BF = 3), moderate (BF = 10), or strong (BF = 30).

3. The second row conveys information in terms of the pattern of chromosomes involved in the models. The third row addresses the frequency of sampling each chromosome. The fourth row shows relative importance of epistatic pairs. Here, the "1:3," or chr 1 by chr 3, epistatic pair is one of the strong effects.

3.3. One Dimensional and Two-Dimensional Genome Scans

In the present context, the term "scan" refers to methods based on constructing one or two dimensional profiles of QTL likelihoods or posterior distributions.

3.3.1. 1D Scan

For every locus in the genome, it is meaningful to examine the chances of this position being a true QTL. In particular, to test

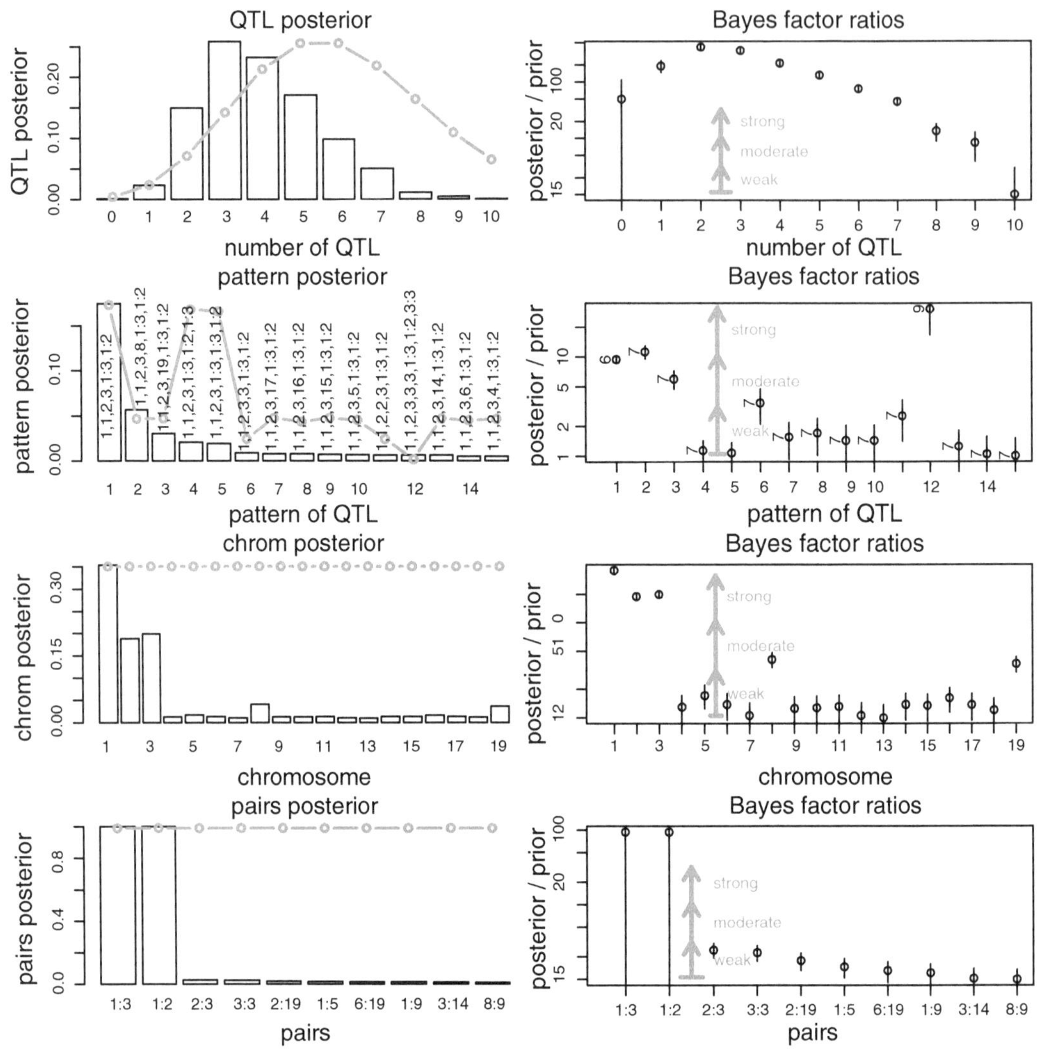

Fig. 3. *Left panels*: Paired plots of posteriors (as *bars*) overlaid by priors (as *grey lines*). *Right panels*: Bayes factor ratios to the least likely model. Models in *right panel* can be compared by vertical separation as scale is geometric. *Grey arrows* on *right panels* indicate weak, moderate, or strong Bayes factors for ratios of 3, 10, or 30, respectively. *Rows* convey information about (1) number of QTL, (2) chromosome pattern of QTL, (3) chromosomes, (4) epistatic pairs.

the *j*th position for each trait t, we can compute the Bayes Factor (BF) as:

$$\mathrm{BF} = \frac{p(\gamma_{tj} = 1|y_t)/p(\gamma_{yj} = 1)}{p(\gamma_{tj} = 0|y_t)/p(\gamma_{yj} = 0)}$$

In practice these marginal posterior probabilities (e.g., $p(\gamma_{tj} = 1|y_t)$) are computed using the idea of model averaging. $p(\gamma_{tj} = 1|y_t)$ is the proportion of sampled models which have included the current position of interest. In essence, we not only consider the one-QTL models with $\gamma_{tj} = 1$ but also any q-QTL model which includes the current position, and hence, we average over different models. Although it might seem paradoxical to compute BF for 1 vs. 0 QTLs in a multiple QTL mapping framework, by virtue of model averaging we can actually control for QTLs elsewhere in the genome. This idea can be extended to investigating contributions in terms of heritability or parameter effects. However, there are some mechanics involved. For instance, scans involving epistasic effects need to consider each pair for both loci. This is termed as a two-dimensional scan.

3.3.2. 2D Scan

A two-dimensional scan involves considering models including a pair of loci (j_1, j_2) to models including either or none. It is important to recall that a locus can be included in the model through its marginal (additive, dominant) and/or epistatic (additive–additive, additive–dominant, dominant–additive, dominant–dominant) effects. BF can be examined for any combination of these effects. One useful hypothesis could be testing the "full" model (marginal + epistatic effects) vs. epistatic effects alone.

3.3.3. Using qb.scan Routines for Multiple Traits

There are two scan routines in R/qtlbim corresponding to a 1D or 2D scan, namely, `qb.scanone` and `qb.scantwo`. They are collectively termed "`qb.scan`" routines. Each iteration of the Monte Carlo output contained in "`qbObject`" represents a single QTL model. The entire Monte Carlo output represents samples from the posterior distribution of all possible models. One simple summary of the MCMC sample is the posterior profile of a particular trait, or the posterior probability of a QTL at each locus for the trait.

```
> one <- qb.scanone(qbObject,type="posterior",pheno.col=1)
> one
posterior of pheno.normal.1 for main,GxE,epistasis,sum

    n.qtl pos m.pos e.pos     main      GxE epistasis     sum
1  2.0000  17    17    17 0.299880 0.299982   0.29934 0.29998
2  1.0675  11    11    11 0.112932 0.111697   0.16639 0.16643
3  1.0745  13    14    13 0.008585 0.010559   0.11452 0.11461
4  0.1186  72    72    74 0.004921 0.000538   0.00152 0.00543
5  0.1083  87    56    87 0.000909 0.000492   0.00257 0.00259
6  0.2042  82    82    94 0.008741 0.001142   0.00293 0.00943
7  0.1003  97     5    97 0.001336 0.000417   0.00303 0.00315
8  0.0759  24    71    85 0.001021 0.000456   0.00200 0.00181
9  0.0712   0    92    29 0.000809 0.000668   0.00150 0.00200
10 0.0695   3    10     2 0.001168 0.000985   0.00167 0.00219
11 0.1758  49    65    49 0.001006 0.000334   0.00686 0.00692
12 0.0685  33    30    53 0.000958 0.000340   0.00200 0.00197
13 0.2727  45    45    41 0.008578 0.000753   0.00204 0.00898
14 0.0755  46    15    46 0.001172 0.000521   0.00209 0.00234
15 0.1197  50    80    50 0.000915 0.000553   0.00497 0.00519
16 0.0849  87    25    87 0.001266 0.000365   0.00182 0.00201
17 0.2253  14    15    26 0.004564 0.001503   0.00225 0.00562
18 0.0816   8     0    18 0.000840 0.000419   0.00153 0.00170
19 0.0702   7    23    81 0.000970 0.000334   0.00167 0.00194
```

Here we show 2 log(BF), or log of the Bayes factor, measuring the strength of evidence (>2.1 is high) for a QTL. In order to examine the effects on chromosomes 1, 2, 3, and 4 more closely, we can plot subsets of chromosomes by using the plot command (Fig. 4).

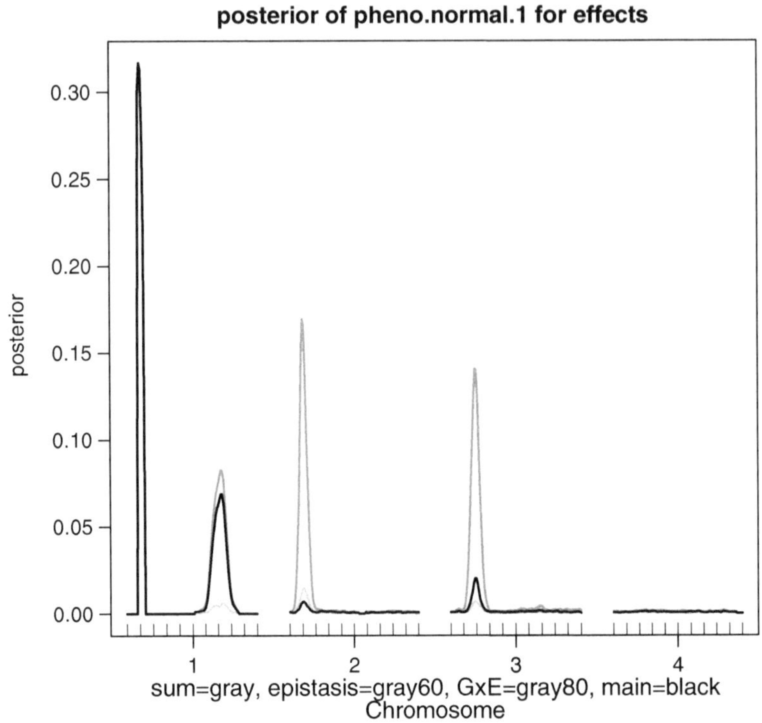

Fig. 4. The qb.scanone results of the first trait for all effects restricted to chromosomes 1, 2, 3 and 4.

```
> one <- qb.scanone(qbObject,type="2logBF",pheno.col=1)
> plot(one,chr=1:4,col=c(sum="gray",main="black",epistasis="gray60",
+       GxE="gray80"))
```

As shown in Fig. 4, the 2 log(BF) profile of the first trait can be obtained for all types of effect, namely, main effect, epistatic and G × E interactions. It might be of interest to look at main effects of all traits simultaneously in a single graphical device. To do that one can run the following chunk of code and get a plot shown in Fig. 5.

```
> plot(qb.scanone(qbObject,type="heritability",pheno.col=1),scan="main",
+              chr=1:4,main="heritability of all traits for main",)
> plot(qb.scanone(qbObject,type="heritability",pheno.col=2),scan="main",
+                      chr=1:4,add=TRUE,col="gray")
> legend("topright",legend=c("pheno.normal.1","pheno.normal.2"),
+           col=c("black","gray"),lty=1)
```

The function qb.scantwo gives a two dimensional scan that allows us to look for possible epistatic effects between putative QTL. We can use qb.scantwo to examine the 2 log(BF) of pair of QTLs for a particular trait (the first trait is shown here) using the following chunk of code.

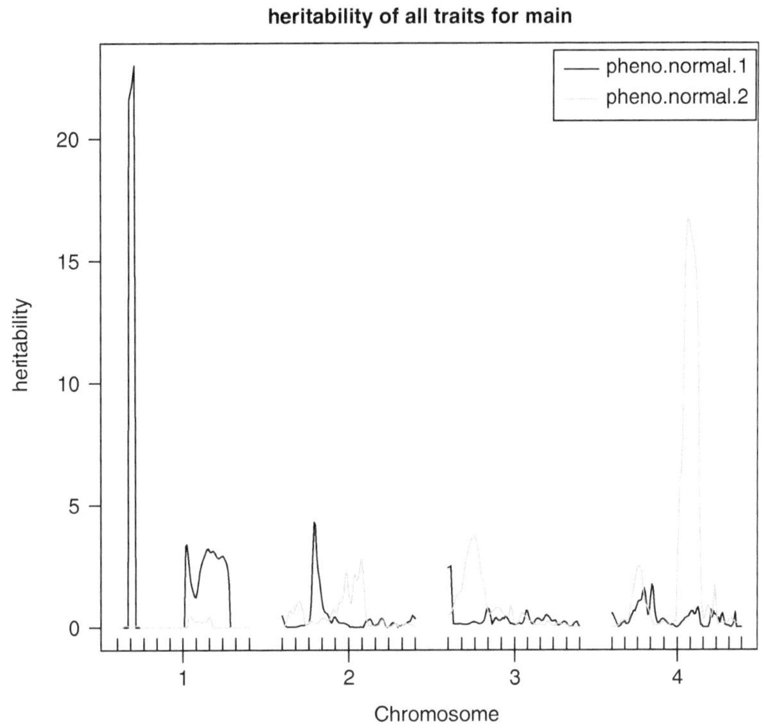

Fig. 5. The qb.scanone results of all traits for main effects restricted to chromosomes 1, 2, 3 and 4. *Grey lines* indicate "heritability" profile for the first trait and *black lines* indicate the same for the second trait.

```
> two <- qb.scantwo(qbObject,type="2logBF",pheno.col=1,verbose=T)
finding all pairs of loci ...

upper: 2logBF of pheno.normal.1 for aa
lower: 2logBF of pheno.normal.1 for add+aa+add.fix.cov

non-epistatic components ...
epistatic components ...
qb.scanone on diagonal with add ...

> plot(two,chr=1:4,col="gray")
```

Figure 6 shows the plot of `qb.scantwo` results. The upper triangle indicates the epistatic effects between pairs of loci for a particular trait and the lower triangle indicates the full model, i.e., main + epistatic + G × E for the corresponding pair influencing a particular trait. As can be seen in Fig. 6, the upper triangle shows two hot spots indicating epistasis between chromosome pair 1 × 2 and 1 × 3.

3.3.4. Types of Scan Summaries

There are several types of scan summaries, illustrated below. These include the following LPD, heritability, variance components, parameter estimates, cell means, posterior probabilities, and Bayes factors. For each type, we can provide a summary scan, and in

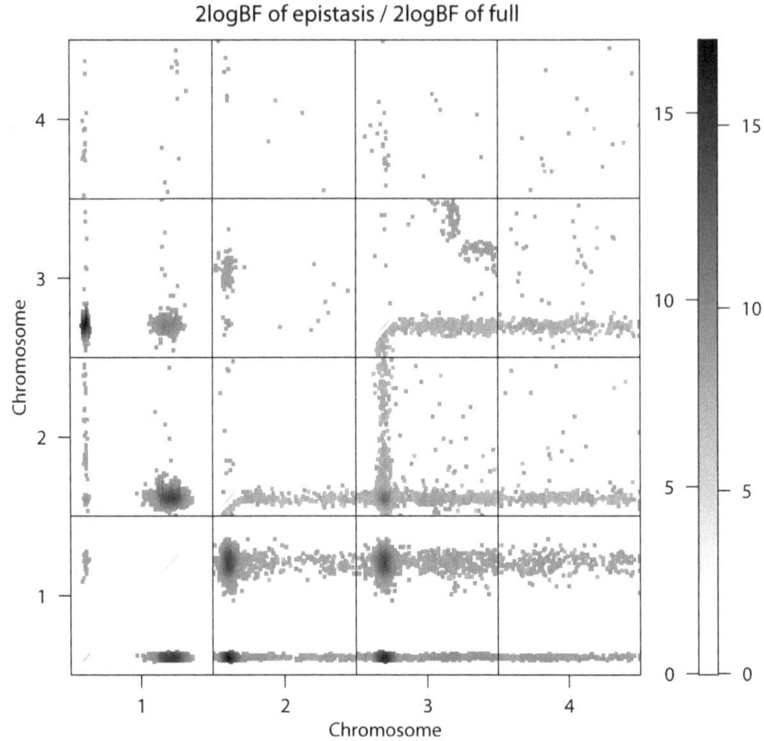

Fig. 6. Plot of qb.scantwo results for the first trait. *Upper triangle* indicates 2 log(BF) for epistatic effects between pairs of loci and *lower triangle* indicates the same for main + epistatic + G × E interaction effects between the pairs of loci.

addition provide detailed broken down by main effects, epistatic effects, and/or G × E (genotype by environment, or genotype by covariate) interactions. These breakdowns can be further divided into Cockerham (6, 14) type effects (additive and dominance for main effects, or the four epistatic interactions of additive–additive (aa), additive–dominant (ad), dominant–additive (da), and dominant–dominant (dd)) if desired.

- `count` gives the count of the number of MCMC samples including this locus. Currently this can be viewed on a log scale using type `log10`.
- `posterior` is the Bayesian posterior probability, basically the `count` divided by the total number of MCMC samples.
- `BF` provides the Bayes factor comparing the model with and without this locus. It is more easily viewed as `2logBF`.
- `estimate` gives model parameter estimates for main effects, epistasis, and GxE interactions.
- `cellmean` provides marginal means at a locus, adjusted for all other model effects from other QTLs and covariates.
- `variance` yields the variance components for QTL effects associated with a particular locus.

- `heritability` is explained variation.
- `LPD` is the log posterior density, adapted from Morton's (15) log odds ratio (LOD) used in human genetics to LOD maps by Lander and Botstein (16). The LPD for QTLs was introduced by Sen and Churchill (17). It tests presence or absence of a QTL at a locus, adjusting for all other possible model effects (other QTL, epistasis, and G × E).
- `detection` is the posterior probability of detection of a QTL at a locus.

3.4. Testing Pleiotropy

It is of considerable biological interest to test if a QTL comaps to more than one trait. This is known as pleiotropy. The function `qb.conjoin` finds the posterior probability (or Bayes Factors) that multiple traits comap to the same locus. The function `qb.conjoin` as default calculates the posterior probability that a particular locus maps to any 1, any 2, . . . all traits. This can be controlled by using the option `set.size`. The following chunk of code illustrates this:

```
> con <- qb.conjoin(qbObject)
> plot(con,size=1,col=c("black","gray"))
```

Figure 7 shows the posterior probability that a QTL maps to exactly one trait (indicated by the option size in the plot

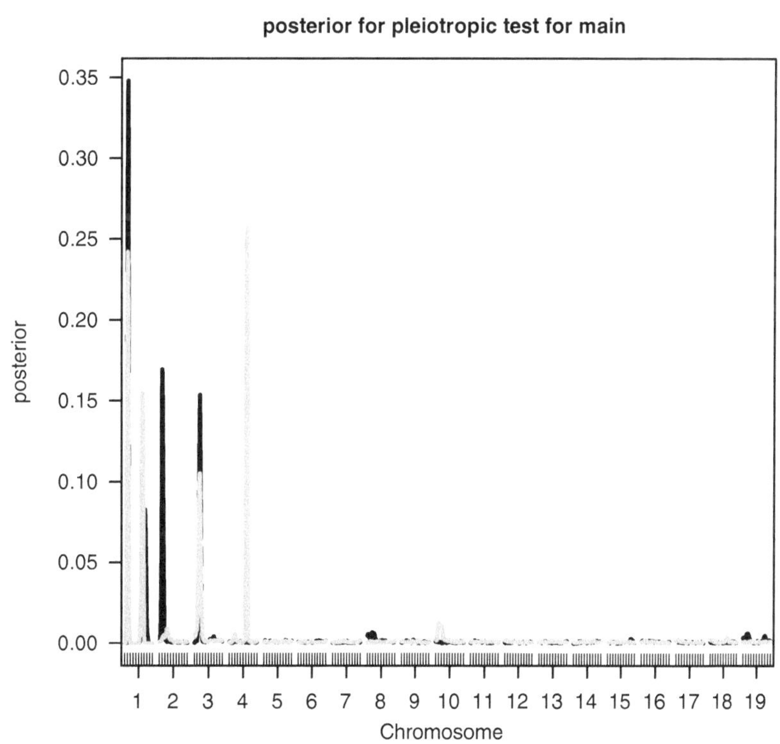

Fig. 7. Posterior profile that a QTL map to exactly one trait. *Black lines* indicate posterior profile for the first trait and *grey lines* indicate the same for the second trait.

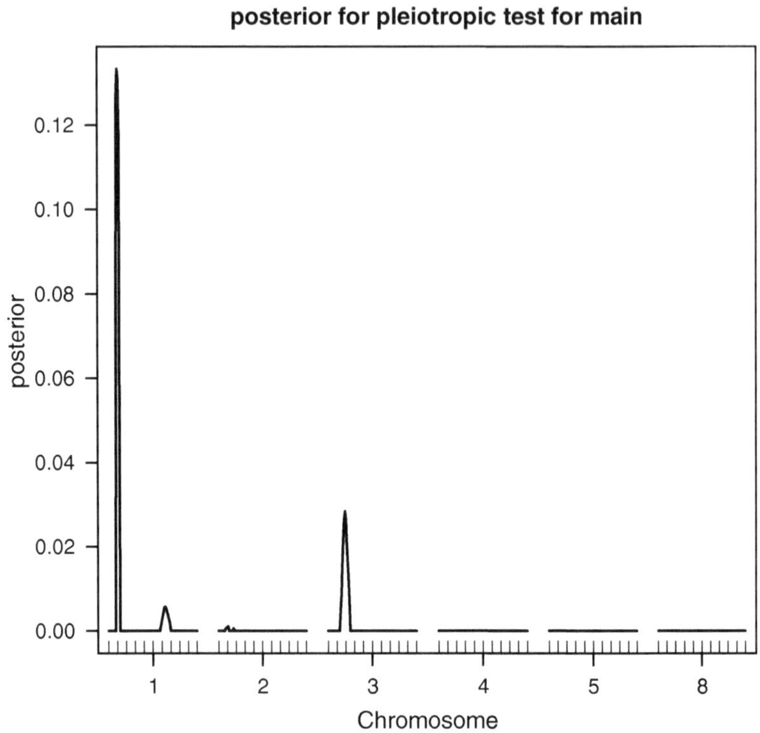

Fig. 8. Posterior profile that a QTL maps to both traits indicating pleiotropy.

command). This is an alternate way of initially examining the MCMC samples. Figure 8 shows the posterior probability that a QTL maps to exactly two traits and hence is a pleiotropic QTL. The can be done by using the same conjoin object and using the following command.

```
>plot(con,size=2,col="black")
```

Figure 8 indicates that chromosome 1 has the strongest pleiotropic QTL. It is worth mentioning that pleiotropic events are rare, and it is recommended to run a longer chain (`n.iter = 10000`) to test pleiotropic effects.

Acknowledgments

We would like to thank Dr. Brian Yandell, University of Wisconsin-Madison, for his immense help in the development of the software, especially the visualization of posterior samples and developing the qb.conjoin routine. SB's work was supported by the NIH Clinical Translational Science Center grant UL1-RR024996 and NY's work was supported by NIH grant 2R01GM069430-06.

References

1. Yi N, Shriner D (2008) Advances in Bayesian multiple quantitative trait loci mapping in experimental crosses. Heredity 100:240–252
2. Jiang C, Zeng ZB (1995) Multiple trait analysis of genetic mapping for quantitative trait loci. Genetics 140:1111–1127
3. Banerjee S, Yandell BS, Yi N (2008) Bayesian quantitative trait loci mapping for multiple traits. Genetics 179:2275–2289
4. Banerjee S, Yandell BS, Yi N (in review) Bayesian genome-wide interacting QTL mapping for multiple traits
5. Yandell BS, Mehta T, Banerjee S et al (2007) R/qtlbim: QTL with Bayesian interval mapping in experimental crosses. Bioinformatics 23:641–643
6. Cockerham CC (1954) An extension of the concept of partitioning hereditary variance for analysis of covariances among relatives when epistasis is present. Genetics 39:859–882
7. Jiang C, Zeng ZB (1997) Mapping quantitative trait loci with dominant and missing markers in various crosses from two inbred lines. Genetica 101:47–58
8. Yi N (2004) A unified Markov chain Monte Carlo framework for mapping multiple quantitative trait loci. Genetics 167:967–975
9. Yi N, Yandell BS, Churchill GA, Allison DB, Eisen EJ, Pomp D (2005) Bayesian model selection for genome-wide epistatic quantitative trait loci analysis. Genetics 170: 1333–1344
10. Yi N, Banerjee S, Pomp D, Yandell BS (2007) Bayesian mapping of genomewide interacting quantitative trait loci for ordinal traits. Genetics 176:1855–1864
11. Broman KW, Speed TP (2002) A model selection approach for the identification of quantitative trait loci in experimental crosses. J R Statist Soc B 64:641–656
12. Plummer M, Best N, Cowles K, Vines K (2006) CODA: convergence diagnosis and output analysis for MCMC. R News 6:7–11
13. Broman KW, Wu H, Sen S, Churchill GA (2003) R/qtl: QTL mapping in experimental crosses. Bioinformatics 19:889–890
14. Kao CH, Zeng ZB (2002) Modeling epistasis of quantitative trait loci using Cockerham's model. Genetics 160:1243–1261
15. Morton NE (1995) LODs past and present. Genetics 140:7–12
16. Lander ES, Botstein D (1989) Mapping mendelian factors underlying quantitative traits using RFLP linkage maps. Genetics 121: 185–199
17. Sen S, Churchill GA (2001) A statistical framework for quantitative trait mapping. Genetics 159:371–387

Chapter 12

Functional Mapping of Developmental Processes: Theory, Applications, and Prospects*

Kiranmoy Das, Zhongwen Huang, Jingyuan Liu, Guifang Fu, Jiahan Li, Yao Li, Chunfa Tong, Junyi Gai, and Rongling Wu

Abstract

Functional mapping is a statistical tool for mapping quantitative trait loci (QTLs) that control the developmental pattern and process of a complex trait. Functional mapping has two significant advantages beyond traditional QTL mapping approaches. First, it integrates biological principles of trait formation into the model, enabling the biological interpretation of QTLs detected. Second, functional mapping is based on parsimonious modeling of mean-covariance structures, which enhances the statistical power of QTL detection. Here, we review the basic theory of functional mapping and describe one of its applications to plant genetics. We pinpoint several areas in which functional mapping can be integrated with systems biology to further our understanding of the genetic and genetic regulatory underpinnings of development.

Key words: Functional mapping, Quantitative trait loci, Developmental trait, Dynamic system, Statistical model

1. Introduction

Many quantitative traits of paramount importance to agriculture, biology, and biomedicine alter their phenotypes over development (1, 2). To map the genetic etiology of these developmental traits in terms of the underlying quantitative trait loci (QTLs), a special analytical approach should be derived by taking into account their dynamic or longitudinal features. Traditionally, dynamic traits are mapped through associating markers with phenotypes for different ages or stages of development and comparing the differences across these stages (3, 4), or by using multiple-trait mapping where the same character is repeatedly measured at different times. These

*The authors Kiranmoy Das and Zhongwen Huang contributed to this work equally.

Scott A. Rifkin (ed.), *Quantitative Trait Loci (QTL): Methods and Protocols*, Methods in Molecular Biology, vol. 871,
DOI 10.1007/978-1-61779-785-9_12, © Springer Science+Business Media New York 2012

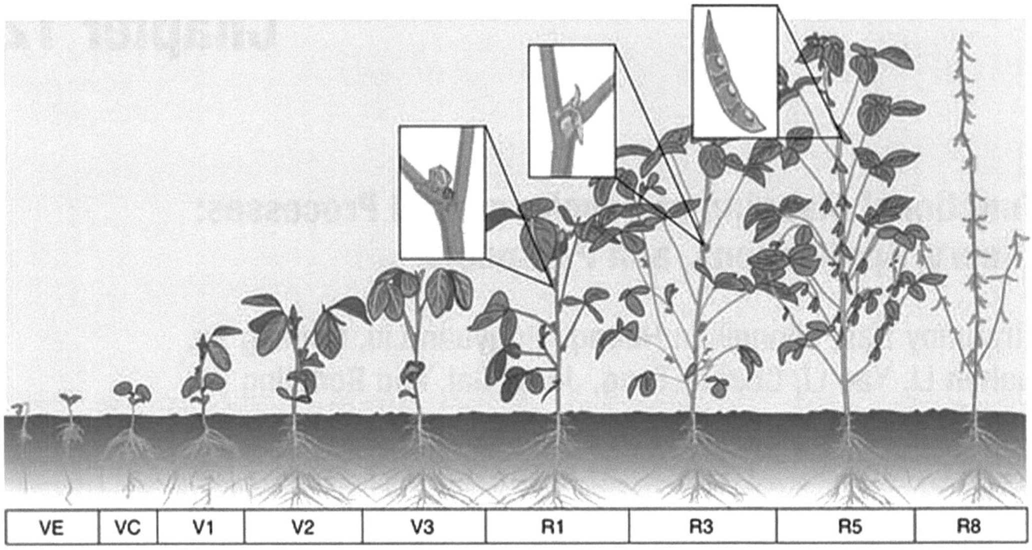

Fig. 1. Different growth stages of a typical soybean plant, including vegetative (V) and reproductive (R) stages. Several vegetative and reproductive developmental milestones are indicated. Adapted from Neeser et al. (53), with permission.

approaches fail to capture the dynamic structure and pattern of the process, which greatly limits the scope of inference about its genetic architecture. To overcome these limitations, a new statistical method, called *functional mapping*, has been developed, which integrates biological mechanisms and processes of the trait into the genetic mapping framework through mathematical and computational models (5–9). While traditional mapping approaches, pioneered by Lander and Botstein (10), are a combination of statistical modeling and classic genetics, functional mapping unifies the strengths of statistics, genetics, and developmental biology, thus facilitating testing the interplay between genetic action and development.

In an example describing the life cycle of a soybean plant (Fig. 1), functional mapping shows tremendous power to map QTLs that control different stages of development from germination to maturity and senescence in this plant. Specifically, the following questions can be addressed:

- How does a specific QTL affect the pattern of development? When is it switched on, when is it switched off, and how long is it expressed?
- Are there different temporal patterns of genetic effects triggered by QTLs in a time course?
- Do QTLs interact with each other and the environment in an interactive network to regulate plant growth and development?
- Do pleiotropic QTLs exist that exert their effects on both vegetative growth and reproductive behavior?

By addressing the questions above, we are in an excellent position to map and characterize the genetic architecture of complex traits and use this knowledge to predict the responses of biological structure, organization, and function to changing internal and external environments.

2. Functional Mapping

2.1. Model Formulation

Functional mapping was proposed in order to dissect the genetic control of QTLs over the length of any developmental stage and any development event. It is based on finite mixture models, a type of density model that is comprised of number of component functions, usually Gaussian. Gaussian mixture models are employed to model genotypic segregation of specific genetic factors that determine dynamic traits. In the discussion below, we use growth curves as an example of a dynamic trait, but the underlying mathematics and the procedures for implementing functional mapping could be applied to any dynamical/longitudinal/functional trait. According to the mixture models, each curve fitted by a finite set of measurements with T time points for individual i, arrayed by $\mathbf{y}_i = (y_i(1), \ldots, y_i(T))$, is assumed to have arisen from one of a known or unknown number of components. Each component is modeled by a multivariate normal distribution density f. Assuming that there are J genotypes contributing to the variation among different curves, such a mixture model is expressed as

$$\mathbf{y}_i \sim p(\mathbf{y}_i|\omega_i, \Psi, \eta) = \omega_{1|i}f_1(\mathbf{y}_i; \Psi_1, \eta) + \cdots + \omega_{J|i}f_J(\mathbf{y}_i; \Psi_J, \eta) \quad (1)$$

where $\omega_i = (\omega_{1|i}, \ldots, \omega_{J|i})$ are the mixture proportions (i.e., QTL genotype frequencies) for individual i which are constrained to be nonnegative and sum to unity, $\Psi = (\Psi_1, \ldots, \Psi_J)$ are the component- (or genotype) specific parameters, with Ψ_j being specific to component j; and $\boldsymbol{\eta}$ are the parameters which are common to all components.

2.2. Model Structure

To solve the functional mapping mixture model (1), we need to do three tasks. First, the frequency of QTL genotype j is derived from the genotypes of the markers that are linked to the QTL. This frequency, expressed as $\omega_{j|i}$, is individual-specific, representing a conditional probability of the QTL genotype given the marker genotype (11). Depending on the nature of the mapping population, $\omega_{j|i}$ can be described in terms of the recombination fraction (linkage mapping for a crossed pedigree) or linkage disequilibrium (association mapping for a natural population).

Second, the mean vector for each QTL genotype in the multivariate normal distribution $f_j(\mathbf{y}_i; \Psi_j, \eta)$, composed of genotypic means at different time points, is fitted by a set of QTL genotype-specific parameters Ψ_j in a parametric, nonparametric, or semiparametric way. If a functional relationship exists between the expectation of an observation and its time of measurements and possibly other covariates, a parametric function can be used. For example, plant height growth may follow a sigmoid or logistic curve (12)

$$g(t) = a(1 + be^{-rt})^{-(k-1)} \tag{2}$$

where a is the asymptotic value when time tends to be infinite, b is the initial growth, r is the relative growth rate, and k is the power at which the metabolic rate of an organ scales as whole-plant biomass. By estimating the mathematical parameters, $\Psi_j = (a_j, b_j, r_j, k_j)$, that define these different curves for individual QTL genotypes j, one can use functional mapping to test for genetic control over developmental patterns of variation for a dynamic trait.

When there is no explicit form for dynamic curves, nonparametric approaches based on B-splines, Legendre polynomials, or kernel estimators can be used to characterize the change of growth over time. A whole life process is composed of two sequential phases, growth and senescence/death. We model the growth phase by the parametric growth law and the death phase by nonparametric Legendre polynomials. This semiparametric approach has been used to successfully identify significant QTLs that control tiller development in rice (13).

Third, models for the covariance structure specify a functional relationship between the variance or covariance of any two observations and the times of their measurements, and possibly other covariates. Robust modeling of longitudinal covariance structure is a prerequisite for appropriate statistical inference of genetic effects on longitudinal traits. The covariance structure can be modeled parametrically by various statistical approaches, such as autoregressive (5), antedependence (14), autoregressive moving average (15), Brownian motion, and Ornstein–Uhlenbeck process. For each of these approaches, it is important to determine the optimal way to model covariance structure. A model selection procedure was proposed to determine the most parsimonious approach.

When no functional relationship exists, nonparametric analogues of parametric modeling can be used (16). Recently, Fan et al. (17) proposed a semiparametric model for the covariance structure of irregular longitudinal data, in which they approached the time-dependent correlation by a parametric function and the time-dependent variance by a nonparametric kernel function. The advantage of this model lies in the combination between the flexibility of nonparametric modeling and parsimony of parametric modeling. The establishment of a robust estimation procedure and asymptotic properties of the estimators will make this semiparametric model useful in the practical estimation of the covariance function.

In many longitudinal trials, data are collected at irregularly spaced time points which may differ between subjects. The efficient estimation of covariance structure in this situation will be a significant concern for detecting the genes that control dynamic traits. Although there are many challenges in modeling the covariance structure of subject-specific irregular longitudinal data, many workers have considered this issue using different approaches. These include nonparametric analysis derived from a two-step estimation procedure (18, 19), a semiparametric approach (20), a penalized likelihood approach (21), and functional data analysis (22, 23).

2.3. Hypothesis Tests

Functional mapping allows one to test for the genetic control of individual growth parameters that define the logistic function (2). Because these parameters describe different biological aspects of growth, such tests are biologically meaningful for understanding the role genes play in regulating a growth process. Also, we can make hypothesis tests based on specific combinations of parameters. For example, the inflection point of a growth curve (2) is the time at which relative growth rate is maximal, calculated by $\ln(b/k-1)/r$. The growth at the inflection point is $ak^{1/(1-k)}$. How genes control the timing and growth at the inflection point can be well understood with functional mapping.

2.4. Genetic Designs

Statistical models developed for mapping complex traits are based on specific genetic populations. Although functional mapping was founded on an experimental cross, its principle can be used in other different designs. Below is a list of commonly used genetic designs for functional mapping.

Experimental crosses: Crossing two inbred strains leads to a backcross or F_2 population, in which different genotypes are generated for each gene (see Chapter 2). Other cross populations include recombinant inbred lines (RILs) (see Chapter 3). An RIL population is generated by continuous inbreeding of the progeny, initiated with two heterozygous founders, for an adequately large number of generations that leads to the disappearance of any heterozygote. Linkage analysis in terms of the recombination fraction between different loci establishes the foundation for genetic mapping with experimental crosses.

Multigenerational families: In humans, adequate numbers of progeny cannot be generated from a single family nor is it possible to make controlled crosses. For this species, a nuclear family with multiple successive generations is often used in order to accumulate a sufficient number of progeny for genetic mapping. The recombination fraction and identical-by-decent (IBD) coefficient are the key for genetic mapping with multigenerational families.

Natural populations with unrelated individuals: The genetic mapping of complex traits can be conducted by sampling a collection of unrelated individuals at random from a natural population. In a population, different loci are genetically associated, with the extent described by a parameter called the linkage disequilibrium (LD). LD-based mapping is meritorious in terms of its simple sampling scheme (especially suitable for humans) and high-resolution dissection of a QTL into a narrow genomic region.

Natural populations with unrelated families: Although LD mapping has tremendous potential to fine map functional genes for a complex trait, it may provide a spurious estimate of LD in practice when the association between genes is due to evolutionary forces, such as mutation, drift, selection, population structure, and admixture. A mapping strategy that samples unrelated families (composed of parents and offspring) from a natural population is helpful for overcoming the limitations of LD mapping by simultaneously estimating the linkage and linkage disequilibrium.

Natural populations with related families: Genetic studies of some complex traits require a mapping population to be derived from multiple related families. For such a genetic design, the recombination fraction, IBD, and linkage disequilibrium will all need to be estimated, tracing the cotransmission of alleles from parents to their offspring. This design is powerful, for example, for studying the evolution of genes that control drug response.

2.5. Applications

Functional mapping has been used for mapping dynamic QTLs in poplars (24), jujubes (25), soybeans (26), rice (13), maize (27), yeast (15), oysters (C.F. Tong, R.L. Wu, unpublished data), mice (28), humans (29), and drug response (30, 31). We use a real example for soybeans to demonstrate the practical application of functional mapping. The mapping population includes 184 recombinant inbred lines (RILs) derived from two cultivars, Kefeng No. 1 and Nannong 1138-2, and was genotyped for 488 markers to construct a linkage map covering 4,151.2 cM of the genome with 25 linkage groups (32). The plants and their parents were grown in a simple lattice design with two replicates at Jiangpu Soybean Experiment Station, Nanjing Agricultural University, China. Ten serial plants in the second row of a plot were randomly selected for testing plant height for every time in the whole growing season. After 20 days of seedling emergence, plant heights (from the ground to the terminal bud of the plant) were measured once every 5–10 days until most plants stopped height growth. A total of 6–8 measurements were taken for the RILs studied.

By scanning the genome of soybean, the model identified three significant QTLs ($P < 0.05$) that were responsible for growth trajectories of plant heights. These three height QTLs are located at 48.1 cM between markers GMKF082c and GMKF168b on linkage

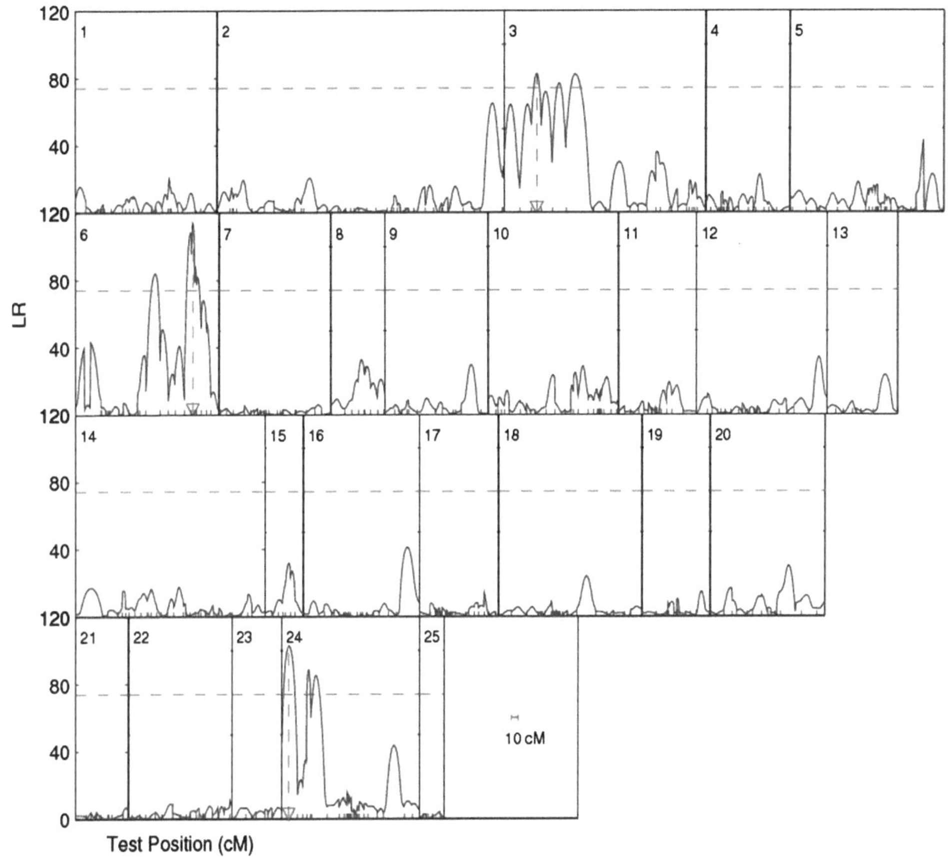

Fig. 2. The profiles of the log-likelihood ratios (LR) between the full model (there is a QTL) and reduced model (there is no QTL) for soybean height growth trajectories throughout the soybean genome composed of 25 linkage groups The genomic position corresponding to the peak of the curve is the maximum-likelihood estimate of the QTL location. *Tick marks* on the *x*-axis represent the positions of microsatellite markers on each chromosome (bar, 10 cM). The critical thresholds for acclaiming the genome-wide existence of a QTL are obtained from permutation tests. The 95th percentile (indicated at *horizontal lines*) of the distribution of the maximum LR values obtained from 200 permutation tests is used as an empirical critical value to declare genome-wide existence of a QTL at the 5% significance level.

group 3, 176.3 cM between markers GMKF059a and satt319 on linkage group 6, and 11 cM between markers sat_231 and LE23T on linkage group 24, respectively (Fig. 2).

An important advantage of functional mapping is its ability to characterize the temporal patterns of the genetic control of a dynamic trait by providing a platform for testing several biologically meaningful questions, such as how each QTL affects developmental trajectories and when a QTL starts to affect growth process. Figure 3 illustrates two different growth curves for each QTL detected. If two growth curves affected by a QTL have different ages and/or growth at the inflection point, this indicates that the inflection point is under the determination of the QTL. Because the inflection point represents the point at which a soybean plant

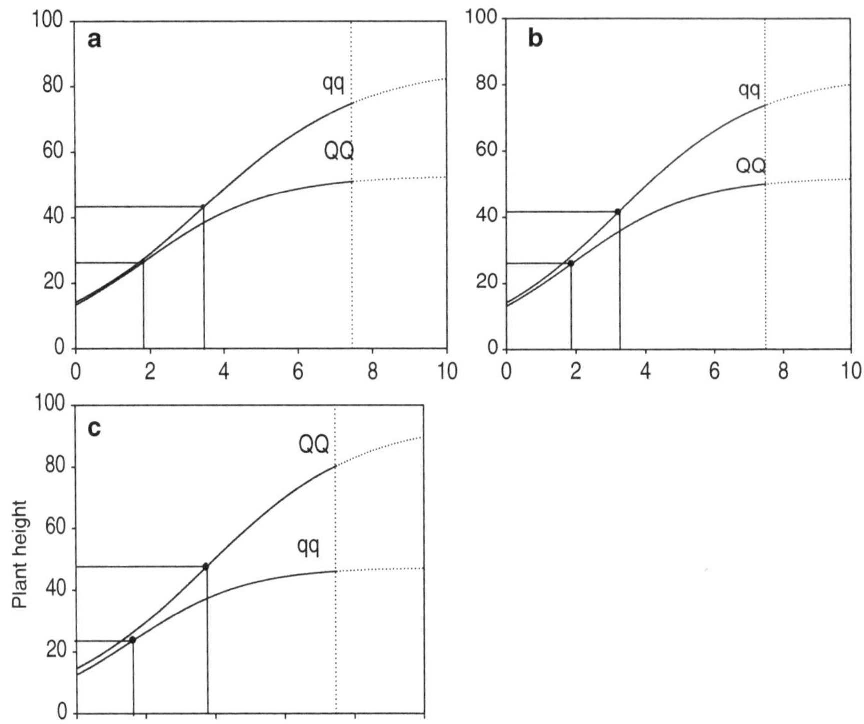

Fig. 3. Growth curves of two different QTL genotypes for each of three QTLs detected on linkage group 3 (**a**), 6 (**b**), and 24 (**c**). The coordinates of the inflection point for each curve are indicated by the *horizontal* and *vertical lines*. The differentiation patterns of growth curves beyond the maximum observed age (75 days after seedling emergence) affected by the QTL are represented by *dotted lines*. Two genotypes at a QTL are denoted by QQ (with alleles inherited from Kefeng No. 1) and qq (with alleles inherited from Nannong 1138-2), respectively.

has a maximum rate of plant height growth, the genetic control of the inflection point suggests that the growth trajectory can be genetically modified to increase soybean's capacity to compete with other plants or weeds. All three QTLs detected trigger strong genetic effects on the inflection point (Fig. 3).

The dynamic patterns of additive effects on plant height growth, triggered by each QTL, were tested using the functional mapping approach. Additive effects of the three detected QTLs for plant height changing with growth period are shown in Fig. 4. Of the three QTLs detected in our experiment, the additive effect of a QTL in linkage group 24 is positive and the other two are negative, which shows that the two QTLs controlling plant height in linkage groups 3 and 6 are contributed by parent Kefeng No. 1 and the other one is contributed by parent Nannong 1138-2. Notice that the additive effects for each QTL increase with age (Fig. 4).

2.6. Software Development of Functional Mapping

We developed a web-based user interface, *FunMap*, designed to map QTL affecting dynamic traits or infinite-dimensional traits in well-structured pedigrees or natural populations (http://statgen.

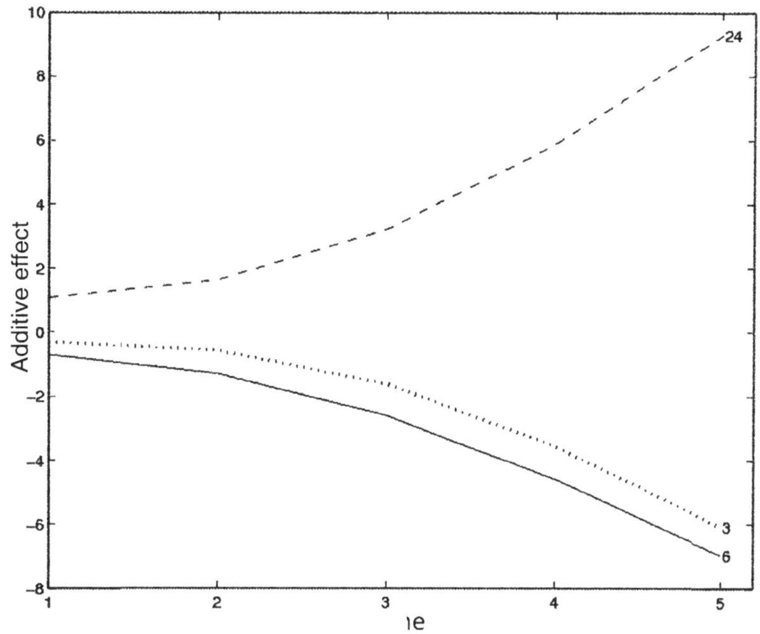

Fig. 4. Estimated additive effect curves for the QTLs at on linkage groups 3, 6, and 24.

psu.edu/software.html). User input includes three files: longitudinal trait data, marker genotypes and/or a linkage map. This software allows a systematic genome-wide scan and significance tests of QTL throughout the map. The dynamic change of QTL effects during the time course of growth is automatically drawn, from which specific biological hypotheses regarding the genetic control mechanisms of growth and development can be tested. The description of this software was published in Ma et al. (33).

More recently, we have extended functional mapping to the genetic dissection of dynamic traits in a full-sib family derived from two heterozygous parents (34). A full-sib family has been widely used as a mapping population for outcrossing species in which it is impossible to inbred lines but a controlled cross may generate a sufficiently large progeny. In such an outcrossing family, there are many different types of markers or QTLs: (1) testcross loci that are heterozygous in parent one but homozygous in parent two (expressed as $ab \times aa$), (2) testcross loci that are homozygous in parent one but heterozygous in parent two (expressed as $aa \times ab$), (3) intercross loci that are heterozygous in both parents that share the same system of alleles (expressed as $ab \times ab$), and (4) intercross loci that are heterozygous in both parents between which at least one allele is different (expressed as $ab \times ac$ or $ab \times cd$). In our newly developed software *3FunMap* (34), linkage analysis using all these different types of markers has been incorporated into functional mapping. A model selection procedure has also been implemented to detect an optimal number of QTL genotypes that are segregating in the full-sib family, allowing precise mapping of dynamic traits for outcrossing species.

3. Functional Mapping Meets Systems Biology

3.1. Systems Biology

Traditional statistical models for functional mapping are designed to directly link DNA-based polymorphisms with a phenotype (Fig. 5), ignoring the biochemical pathways from DNA to high-order phenotypes. The "black box" that lies between genotype and phenotype limits our inference of causal networks of interacting genes and our long-term goal of explaining genetic variation for complex phenotypes in terms of the underlying genes, the alteration of their allelic effects over different genetic backgrounds and a range of environments, their pleiotropic effects on multiple developmentally related traits, and the molecular and functional basis of their genetic effects (35).

The recent completion of genome sequencing projects for humans and many other species, along with the increasing availability of global gene expression, proteomic and metabolomic data, has stimulated our need to integrate genotype–phenotype relationships across multiple levels of biological organization so that we can uncover genetic pathways involved in the variation of complex traits.

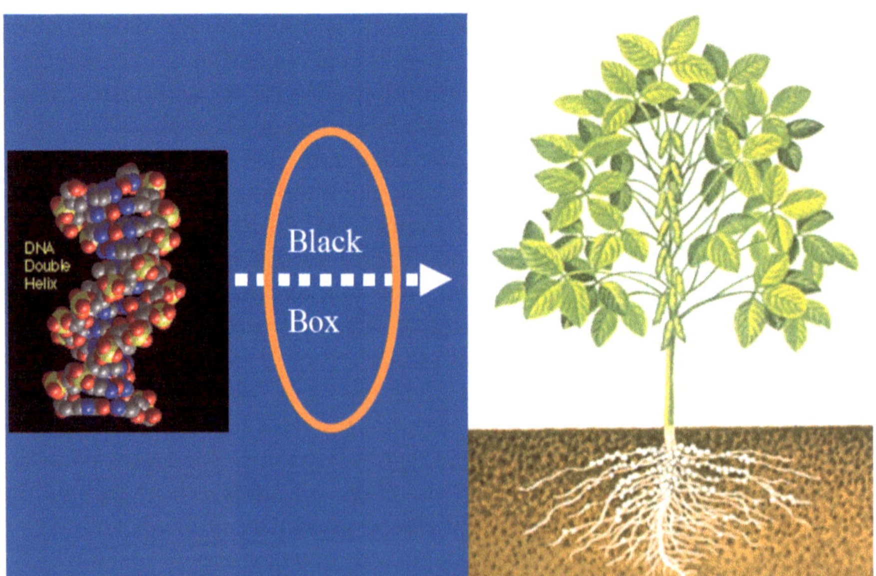

Fig. 5. Traditional genetic mapping linking DNA variants (at the *left*) to the phenotype (at the *right*). This approach does not consider the biochemical steps from DNA to the phenotype. The "black box" that exists between genotype and phenotype affects our ability to address the biological complexity of phenotypic formation and development.

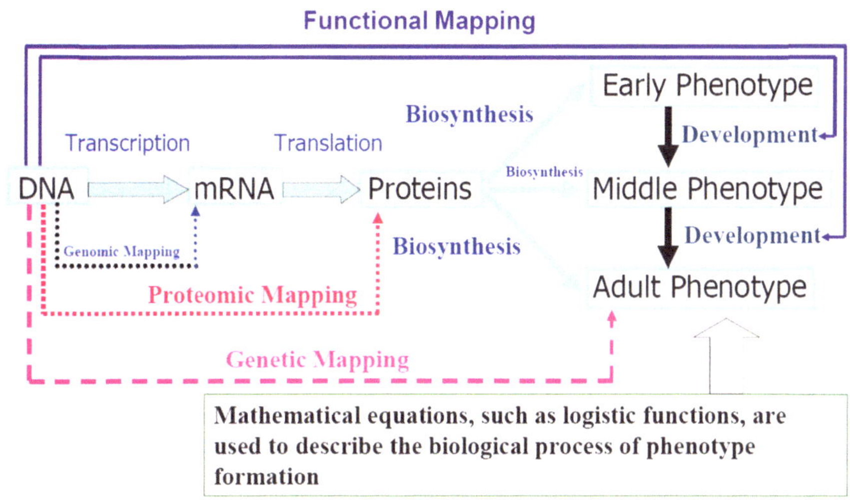

Fig. 6. Biological networks of the phenotypic formation and development of a trait. Genetic mapping is moving from a direct genotype–phenotype correspondence (Fig. 5) to regulatory networks that underlies the formation of a phenotypic trait.

Such integration, as part of systems genetics (35), needs the development of powerful statistical and computational models which can identify specific genes and their interactions for complex traits. It is our hope that the results from these models will ultimately facilitate a comprehensive understanding of biological, pathological, and developmental mechanisms involved in complex traits or diseases.

The development of any trait can be modeled as a dynamical system consisting of various biological parts (expressed at different levels of organization) which coordinate to determine a final phenotype through genetic regulation (36). The "Central Dogma" of biology (Fig. 6), subject to continuous addendums and modifications in the recent past, is a fundamental rule for the formation and control of every aspect of a living system. The behavior and outcome of this system can be changed by altering the pathways of one or more parts. This will need our profound understanding of how different parts are coordinated and organized into a whole system and what are the genetic roots of the function of these parts.

3.2. Modeling Regulatory Networks

Highly parallel technology makes it now possible to measure multiple features of complex systems at various levels of biological organization from the cell to the whole organism within a defined, fully delineated framework. The challenge is to determine how this information is decoded according to the physiological function of the system (37).

To measure a system, even at the single-cell level, an understanding of how gene, protein, metabolic and physiological events are expressed in time course is crucial. Attempts to correlate gene expression data with proteomic and metabolomic data have been made by using classic correlation methods or multivariate statistics. However, they have often proved to be unsatisfactory even for simple systems such as yeasts (38) in large part because the timescales of various biological control functions are either very different or simply unknown.

To understand the true quantitative relationship between the variation in activity of every one of the thousands of gene–protein couples or protein–metabolite couples in a cellular system, it is important to consider several critical factors, that is, the time displacement of the genetic and protein synthetic and posttranslational events, their different timescales and their half-lives. Differential equations (DE) that model electronic networks in engineering have been proposed to describe regulatory networks of a biological system (39–44). These DE methods were applied to model the a regulatory network of *Halobacterium salinarum*, suggesting that the model could predict mRNA levels of 2,000 out of a total 2,400 genes found in the genome (a network with 1,431 predicted regulatory influences controlling 459 biclusters that represent 85% of the genes in the genome) (45). A similar application was made to model human regulatory networks (mediating TLR-5-mediated stimulation of macrophages) and several other microbial networks (42). The accuracy and precision of a regulatory network can be increased when the model is combined with environmental and genetic perturbations by incorporating the principle of functional mapping.

3.3. Functional Mapping of Regulatory Networks with Differential Equations

The quantitative relationships between genes and proteins determine the morphological or physiological behavior of a complex trait. For example, the molecular clock is determined by oscillations in both mRNA and protein levels of the basic gene c-hairy1 (46). The coexpression of mRNA and protein levels can be described by a system of differential equations (DE). We can use a system of delay differential equations to specify the dynamic behavior of the clock, expressed as

$$\begin{aligned} \frac{\mathrm{d}M}{\mathrm{d}t} &= \frac{r_{\mathrm{m}}}{1+(P/k)^{n}} - q_{\mathrm{m}}M \\ \frac{\mathrm{d}P}{\mathrm{d}t} &= r_{\mathrm{p}}M(t-\tau)^{m} - q_{\mathrm{p}}P \end{aligned} \tag{3}$$

where M and P are the relative concentration of mRNA and the effective protein measured at a particular time t, respectively, r_{m} is the scaled mRNA production rate constant, r_{p} is the protein production rate constant, q_{m} and q_{p} are the mRNA and protein degradation rate constants, respectively, n is the Hill coefficient, m is the exponent of the nonlinearity in the protein production cascade, τ is the total duration of protein production from mRNA, and k is a scaling constant. Equation (3) constructs an unperturbed (free-running) system of the intracellular rhythm generator that is defined by seven parameters (n, m, τ, r_{m}, r_{p}, q_{m}, q_{p}). The behavior of this system can be determined and predicted by the change of these parameter combinations.

By integrating (3) into functional mapping, we can characterize specific QTLs that control and regulate the emergent properties of the dynamic system. Specifically, by testing the genetic control of DE parameters individually or jointly per their biological meanings, functional mapping can identify the genetic mechanisms for key biochemical pathways that lead to the final performance of the system. For example, with a time delay that characterizes the total duration of protein production from mRNA, model (3) captures a negative molecular feedback loop to produce circadian oscillations. We have studied the dynamic behavior of this system in terms of local stability and Hopf bifurcation analysis. A linear analysis for the system of DE (3) near the equilibrium shows that under certain conditions for the parameters of the system, there is a critical time delay τ_0, and the equilibrium changes stability from asymptotically stable for $\tau < \tau_0$ to unstable for $\tau > \tau_0$. At $\tau = \tau_0$, a Hopf bifurcation, which is the birth of a limit cycle from an equilibrium, occurs. We also found the conditions for the parameters under finitely many stability switches can occur for the system before final instability. We have further derived an explicit formula for determining the directions of the Hopf bifurcations and the stability of bifurcating periodic solutions using the theory of normal form and center manifold. The influences of all parameters on the period and amplitude of oscillations have been examined.

Integration of functional mapping with dynamic modeling of the system is critically reliant upon the mathematical tools to solve differential equations. There is a pressing need for the involvement of mathematicians in genetic mapping dynamical systems.

3.4. Functional Mapping of Regulatory Networks by Integrating Protein–Protein Interactions

The interactions between proteins play an important role in numerous biological functions. Signals from the exterior of a cell are communicated to the inside of that cell by protein–protein interactions of signaling molecules. This process, called signal transduction, affects many biological processes. Proteins might interact for a long time to form part of a protein complex, a protein may be carrying another protein, or a protein may interact briefly with another protein just to modify it. Goldbeter (47), for example, presented an excellent example of the role protein–protein interactions play in regulating circadian rhythms.

Based on the negative control exerted by the PER protein on the expression of per, a molecular model governed by a set of five ordinary differential equations was derived (47–49). The per gene is first expressed in the nucleus and transcribed into per mRNA. The latter is transported into the cytosol, where it is translated into the PER protein, P_0, and degraded. The PER protein undergoes multiple phosphorylation, from P_0 into P_1 and from P_1 into P_2. These modifications, catalyzed by a protein kinase, are reverted by a phosphatase. The fully phosphorylated form of the protein is marked up for degradation and transported into the nucleus in a reversible manner. The nuclear form of the protein (P_N) represses the transcription of the gene. In the model, the temporal variation of the concentrations of mRNA (M) and of the various forms of the regulatory protein—cytosolic (P_0, P_1, P_2) or nuclear (P_N)—is governed by the following system of kinetic equations:

$$\begin{aligned}
\frac{dM}{dt} &= v_s \frac{K_I^n}{K_I^n + P_N^n} - v_m \frac{M}{K_m + M} \\
\frac{dP_0}{dt} &= k_s M - V_1 \frac{P_0}{K_1 + P_0} + V_2 \frac{P_1}{K_2 + P_1} \\
\frac{dP_1}{dt} &= V_1 \frac{P_0}{K_1 + P_0} - V_2 \frac{P_1}{K_2 + P_1} - V_3 \frac{P_1}{K_3 + P_1} + V_4 \frac{P_2}{K_4 + P_2} \\
\frac{dP_2}{dt} &= V_3 \frac{P_1}{K_3 + P_1} - V_4 \frac{P_2}{K_4 + P_2} - v_d \frac{P_2}{K_d + P_2} - k_1 P_2 + k_2 P_N \\
\frac{dP_N}{dt} &= k_1 P_2 - k_2 P_N
\end{aligned} \tag{4}$$

where per mRNA (M) is synthesized in the nucleus and transfers to the cytosol (where it accumulates at a maximum rate v_d) and it is degraded by an enzyme of maximum rate v_m and Michaelis constant K_m, and the rate of synthesis of the PER protein, proportional to M, is characterized by an apparent first-order rate constant k_s. Parameters $V_1, \ldots, V_4$ and $K_1, \ldots, K_4$ denote the maximum rate and Michaelis constant of the kinase(s) and phosphatase(s) involved in the reversible phosphorylation of P_0 into P_1 and P_3 into P_2, respectively. The fully phosphorylated form (P_2) is degraded by an enzyme of maximum rate v_d and Michaelis constant K_d, and transported into the nucleus at a rate characterized by the apparent first-order rate constant k_1. Transport of the nuclear, bisphosphorylated form of PER (P_N) into the cytosol is characterized by the apparent first-order rate constant k_2. The negative feedback exerted by nuclear PER on per transcription is described by an equation of the Hill type, in which n denotes the degree of cooperativity, and K_I denotes the threshold constant for repression.

When a regulatory network has a complex structure, differential equations with high dimensions can be used or derived. By accounting for the effect of light on the circadian system induced by the degradation of the timeless (or TIM) protein, an extended, ten-variable model was proposed in which the negative regulation is exerted by a complex of proteins formed by PER and TIM (50). In mammals, the role of TIM as a partner for PER is played by the cryptochrome (CRY) protein, and light operates by inducing gene expression rather than protein degradation as in Drosophila (51, 52). An extended model governed by a system of 16 kinetic equations was constructed by Leloup and Goldbeter (49).

Mathematical methods for a high-dimensional group of differential equations can be incorporated into statistical models. A series of hypothesis tests can be generated and addressed about the genetic effects of QTLs on the coordination of biological parts involved in a complex dynamic system (54).

4. Concluding Remarks

Currently, we are in the midst of a genomic revolution. As the cost of methods for measuring mRNA, protein and other indicators continues to fall, it becomes reasonable to design experiments that capture the dynamic processes of phenotypic formation across timescales. With these data, the respective systems disciplines arise from the study of the transcriptome (the set of RNA transcripts) and the metabolome (the entire range of metabolites taking part in a biological process). Other -omes (sets) that may also be of interest include: the interactome (complete set of interactions between proteins or between these and other molecules), the localizome (localization of transcripts, proteins, etc.), or even the phenome (complete set of phenotypes) of a given organism. There is a daunting need on the reconstruction of biological networks by relating interactomes, localizomes, and phenomes to final phenotypes.

In particular, functional mapping coupled with rigorous mathematical modeling will come to play an increasingly important means of studying developmental events from morphogenesis to pattern formation through mapping the underlying transcriptional, proteomic, and metabolomic QTLs and interaction networks among these different types of QTLs. Functional mapping allows us to test what are the most important pathways that cause final phenotypes and how genes control these pathways. Such an understanding will yield insights that are important for predicting disease risk and individual therapeutic treatments in human populations, for accelerating selective breeding programs in agriculturally important plants and animals, and for predicting adaptive evolution and speciation in nature.

Acknowledgments

The preparation of this manuscript is partially supported by grants from NSF (0540745), National Natural Science Foundation of China (09-95671 and 30230300), National Key Basic Research Program of China (2009CB1184 and 2010CB1259), the Changjiang Scholars Award, and "One-thousand Person" Award.

References

1. Tosh D, Slack J (2002) How cells change their phenotype. Nat Rev Mol Cell Biol 3:187–194
2. Rice S (2008) Theoretical approaches to the evolution of development and genetic architecture. Ann N Y Acad Sci 1133:67–86
3. Emebiri LC, Devey ME, Matheson AC et al (1998) Age-related changes in the expression of QTLs for growth in radiata pine seedlings. Theor Appl Genet 97:1053–1061
4. Wu RL, Bradshaw HD, Stettler RF et al (1998) Developmental quantitative genetics of growth in *Populus*. Theor Appl Genet 97:1110–1119
5. Ma C, Casella G, Wu RL (2002) Functional mapping of quantitative trait loci underlying the character process: a theoretical framework. Genetics 161:1751–1762
6. Wu RL, Ma C, Lou Y et al (2003) Molecular dissection of allometry, ontogeny and plasticity: a genomic view of developmental biology. Bioscience 53:1041–1047
7. Wu RL, Lin M (2006) Functional mapping—how to map and study the genetic architecture of dynamic complex traits. Nat Rev Genet 7:229–237
8. Li Y, Wu RL (2010) Functional mapping of growth and development. Biol Rev 85:207–216
9. He Q, Berg A, Li Y et al (2010) Modeling genes for plant structure, development and evolution: functional mapping meets plant ontology. Trends Genet 26:39–46
10. Lander ES, Botstein D (1989) Mapping Mendelian factors underlying quantitative traits using RFLP linkage maps. Genetics 121: 185–199
11. Wu RL, Ma C, Casella G (2007) Statistical genetics of quantitative traits: linkage, maps, and QTL. Springer, New York
12. West GB, Brown JH, Enquist BJ (2001) A general model for ontogenetic growth. Nature 413:628–663
13. Cui Y, Zhu J, Wu RL (2006) Functional mapping for genetic control of programmed cell death. Physiol Genomics 25:458–469
14. Zhao W, Chen Y, Casella G et al (2005) A nonstationary model for functional mapping of complex traits. Bioinformatics 21:2469–2477
15. Li N, McMurry T, Berg A et al (2010) Functional clustering of periodic transcriptional profiles through ARMA(p, q). PLoS One 5(4):e9894
16. Yap J, Fan J, Wu RL (2009) Nonparametric modeling of covariance structure in functional mapping of quantitative trait loci. Biometrics 65:1068–1077
17. Fan J, Huang T, Li R (2007) Analysis of longitudinal data with semiparametric estimation of covariance function. J Am Stat Assoc 35: 632–641
18. Fan J, Zhang J (2000) Two-step estimation of functional linear models with applications to longitudinal data. J Roy Stat Soc B 62: 303–322
19. Wu W, Pourahmadi M (2003) Nonparametric estimation of large covariance matrices of longitudinal data. Biometrika 90:831–844
20. Fan J, Li R (2004) New estimation and model selection procedures for semiparametric modeling in longitudinal data analysis. J Am Stat Assoc 99:710–723
21. Huang J, Liu N, Pourahmadi M et al (2006) Covariance selection and estimation via penalized normal likelihood. Biometrika 93:85–98
22. Yao F, Müller H, Wang J (2005) Functional data analysis for sparse longitudinal data. J Am Stat Assoc 100:577–590
23. Yao F, Müller H, Wang J (2005) Functional regression analysis for longitudinal data. Ann Statist 33:2873–2903
24. Zhang B, Tong C, Yin T et al (2009) Detection of quantitative trait loci influencing growth trajectories of adventitious roots in *Populus* using functional mapping. Tree Genet Genom 5:539–552
25. Tong CF, Shen LY, Pang XM et al (2010) A conceptual model for structural mapping of complex phenotypes. Front Biosci (in press)
26. Li H, Huang W, Wu S et al (2007) A conceptual framework to mapping quantitative trait loci governing ontogenetic allometry. PLoS One 2(8):1245
27. Coelho WuS, Li Y et al (2007) Identification of quantitative trait loci that affect endo reduplication in *Zea mays* endosperm. Theor Appl Genet 115:1147–1162
28. Liu T, Wu R (2009) A Bayesian algorithm for functional mapping of dynamic traits. Algorithms 2:667–691
29. Li N, Das K, Wu R (2009) Functional mapping of human growth trajectories. J Theor Biol 261:33–42
30. Lin M, Aqvilonte C, Johnson J (2005) Sequencing drug response with HapMap. Pharmacogenomics J 5:149–156
31. Lin M, Hou W, Li H et al (2007) *Modeling* sequence-sequence interactions for *drug response*. Bioinformatics 23:1251–1257
32. Zhang W, Wang Y, Luo G et al (2004) QTL mapping of ten agronomic traits on the

soybean (*Glycine max* L. Merr.) genetic map and their association with EST markers. Theor Appl Genet 108:1131–1139
33. Ma C, Wu RL, Casella G (2004) FunMap: functional mapping of complex traits. Bioinformatics 20:1808–1811
34. Tong CF, Wang Z, Zhang B et al (2011) 3FunMap: full-sib family functional mapping of dynamic traits. Bioinformatics 27:2006–2008
35. Mackay T, Stone E, Ayroles J (2009) The genetics of quantitative traits: challenges and prospects. Nat Rev Genet 10:565–577
36. De Hoog C, Mann M (2004) Proteomics. Annu Rev Genomics Hum Genet 5:267–293
37. Nicholson J, Holmes E, Lindon J et al (2004) The challenges of modeling mammalian biocomplexity. Nat Biotechnol 22:1268–1274
38. Gygi S, Rochon Y, Franza B et al (1999) Correlation between protein and mRNA abundance in yeast. Mol Cell Biol 19:1720–1730
39. Gardner T, Bernardo D, Lorenz D et al (2003) Inferring genetic networks and identifying compound mode of action via expression profiling. Science 301:102–105
40. Tegner J, Yeung M, Hasty J et al (2003) Reverse engineering gene networks: integrating genetic perturbations with dynamical modeling. Proc Natl Acad Sci U S A 100:5944–5949
41. Yeung M, Tegner J, Collins J (2002) Reverse engineering gene networks using singular value decomposition and robust regression. Proc Natl Acad Sci U S A 99:6163–6168
42. Gilchrist M, Thorsson V, Li B et al (2006) Systems biology approaches identify ATF3 as a negative regulator of Toll-like receptor 4. Nature 441:173–178
43. Bonneau R, Facciotti M, Reiss D et al (2007) A predictive model for transcriptional control of physiology in a free living cell. Cell 131: 1354–1365
44. Bonneau R, Reiss D, Shannon P et al (2006) The Inferelator: an algorithm for learning parsimonious regulatory networks from systems-biology data sets de novo. Genome Biol 7:R36
45. Bonneau R (2008) Learning biological networks: from modules to dynamics. Nat Chem Biol 4:658–664
46. Feng P, Navaratna M (2007) Modelling periodic oscillations during somitogenesis. Math Biosci Eng 4:661–673
47. Goldbeter A (1995) A model for circadian oscillations in the *Drosophila* period protein (PER). Proc R Soc Lond B Biol Sci 261: 319–324
48. Goldbeter A (1996) Biochemical oscillations and cellular rhythms: the molecular bases of periodic and chaotic behaviour. Cambridge University Press, Cambridge
49. Leloup J, Goldbeter A (2003) Toward a detailed computational model for the mammalian circadian clock. Proc Natl Acad Sci U S A 100:7051–7056
50. Leloup J, Goldbeter A (1998) A model for circadain rhythms in *Drosophila* incorporating the formation of a complex between the PER and TIM proteins. J Biol Rhythms 13:70–87
51. Reppert S, Weaver D (2002) Coordination of circadian timing in mammals. Nature 418: 935–941
52. Goldbeter A (2002) Computational approaches to cellular rhythms. Nature 420:238–245
53. Neeser C, Dille JA, Krishnan G et al (2004) WeedSOFT®: a weed management decision support system. Weed Sci 52:115–122
54. Fu G, Luo J, Berg A et al (2010) A dynamic model for functional mapping of biological rhythms. J Biol Dyn 4:1–10

Chapter 13

Statistical Models for Genetic Mapping in Polyploids: Challenges and Opportunities

Jiahan Li, Kiranmoy Das, Jingyuan Liu, Guifang Fu, Yao Li, Christian Tobias, and Rongling Wu

Abstract

Statistical methods for genetic mapping have well been developed for diploid species but are lagging in the more complex polyploids. The genetic mapping of polyploids, where genome number is higher than two, is complicated by uncertainty about the genotype–phenotype correspondence, inconsistent meiotic mechanisms, heterozygous genome structures, and increased allelic (action) and nonallelic (interaction) combinations. According to their meiotic configurations, polyploids can be classified as bivalent polyploids, in which only two chromosomes pair during meiosis at a time, and multivalent polyploids, where multiple chromosomes pair simultaneously. For some polyploids, these two types of pairing occur at the same time, leading to a mixed category. This chapter reviews several challenges due to the complexities of linkage analysis in polyploids and describes statistical models and algorithms that have been developed for linkage mapping based on their distinct meiotic characteristics. We discuss several issues that should be addressed to better understand the genome structure and organization of polyploids and the genetic architecture of complex traits for this unique group of plants.

Key words: Linkage, QTL, Polyploidy, Bivalent, Multivalent, Statistical model

1. Introduction

Many of domesticated plant taxa (75%) are polyploid (1). In agriculture, polyploids are among the most important crops; alfalfa, banana, canola, coffee, cotton, potato, soybean, strawberry, sugarcane, sweet potato, and wheat are excellent examples. Several current comparative mapping studies using molecular markers reveal that some crop species traditionally considered as diploids, such as maize and modern species of Brassica, are actually polyploids, whereas for others such as cotton, the level of ploidy is higher than originally recognized (2). Polyploidy is also recognized as an important evolutionary force in flowering plants (3–9). An estimate

Scott A. Rifkin (ed.), *Quantitative Trait Loci (QTL): Methods and Protocols*, Methods in Molecular Biology, vol. 871,
DOI 10.1007/978-1-61779-785-9_13,

from fossil plants suggests that as much as 70% of all angiosperms have experienced one or more episodes of polyploidization (10). Several genetic and genomic attributes of polyploids have been thought to be the key for their tremendous success of broad adaptation to extreme environments (reviewed in (11)).

Polyploids have been classified as either *allopolyploids* derived from the chromosome combination of distinct genomes and subsequent chromosome doubling, or *autopolyploids*, originated from the chromosome doubling of genetically similar genomes by fusion of unreduced gametes (12). Allopolyploids are generally disomic because only strictly homologous chromosomes can pair, whereas autopolyploids are often polysomic due to chromosome pairings among all homologues (13). However, there are many exceptions. For example, it is not absolutely impossible that allopolyploids display polysomic inheritance in some polyploid taxa (14, 15), while autotetraploid potato and alfalfa are thought to be virtually predominantly disomic (16, 17). In real life, there exist many intermediate types between the two extremes of disomic and polysomic inheritance (18), in which both disomic and polysomic inheritance can occur simultaneously during meiosis. Even for extreme disomic polyploids, chromosome pairing is not necessarily limited between homologous chromosomes (19). The complexity of polyploid types is recognized to represent necessary steps in plant evolution (5, 20, 21).

Recent advances in molecular genotyping techniques have enabled geneticists to study the origin, inheritance, and genetic architecture of polyploids using multilocus marker data. Statistical methods for analyzing the segregation and transmission of polyploid molecular markers and their association with quantitative traits are qualitatively different from those developed for diploids (e.g., (22, 23)). This is due to several complexities of inheritance in polyploids, i.e.: (1) there are many uncertainties on the genotype-phenotype correspondence for partially informative markers, (2) meiotic mechanisms vary, depending on the type of polyploids, (3) there are heterozygous genome structures owing to outcrossing behavior, and (4) allelic (action) and nonallelic (interaction) combinations increase exponentially with the number of alleles. Despite these complexities, several statistical models have been developed for linkage analysis in polyploids (24–26). Although early models were mostly based on the assumption of disomic inheritance, more advanced methods have now been developed to take into account polysomic inheritance (27–35). To facilitate linkage analysis modeling, Wu and colleagues classified polyploids into the bivalent type, in which only two chromosomes pair during meiosis, although more similar chromosomes have a higher pairing probability than less similar ones (30, 32), multivalent type, where four chromosomes pair simultaneously at meiosis, leading to double reduction (29, 33, 35), and a mixed type with both bivalent and multivalent pairings occurring at the same time (28, 31). In this chapter, we review and discuss existing statistical models for polyploid mapping. We first pinpoint the complexities of linkage mapping in this group of species and then provide statistical resolution on overcoming these complexities by incorporating the cytological behavior of meioses for different types of polyploids.

2. Complexities of Polyploid Inheritance

2.1. Genotype-Phenotype Correspondence Uncertainties

In polyploids, the genotype-phenotype correspondence cannot always be inferred simply from the genotype segregation in a progeny. This uncertainty may be due to unknown dosage of a restriction fragment visualized as a band on autoradiographs. For example, in tetraploids, the presence of a band may be due to AAAA (quadruple-dose fragment—quadruplex), AAAa (triple-dose fragment—triplex), AAaa (double-dose fragment—duplex), or Aaaa (simple-dose fragment—simplex). For some polyploid species, such as sugarcane (37), unknown ploidy levels increase the complexity still further. The presence of a band in such polyploids of unknown ploidy level may result from any one of many possible genotypes composed of four from tetraploids, six from hexaploids, eight from octoploids, and ten from dexaploids.

2.2. Unknown Meiotic Configurations

Unlike diploids, polyploids may undergo either bivalent or multivalent formation, or both. For the bivalent formation, identical or at least fully homologous genomes can occur in pairs, but different pairs of genome (homoeologous) have a strong pairing barrier (15, 36). Strong cytological evidence suggests that homologous chromosomes preferentially pair over homoeologous chromosomes (e.g., (20, 38–40)). The difference between the two types of homologous and homoeologous pairings is expressed as *the preferential pairing factor* (41). In many proven autotetraploids, such as *Tradescantia*, *Dactylis*, *Hyoscyamus*, and *Solanum* species, estimates of the preferential pairing factor that were significantly greater than zero were obtained using different cytological models (19, 38, 40), pointing to considerable preferential pairing in some of the sets of four chromosomes.

Multivalent formation may occur when all homologous chromosomes have equal opportunities to pair at meiosis (15, 18, 42, 43). Multivalent formation typical of polysomic polyploids can result in *double reduction*, a phenomenon in which two sister chromatids of a single chromosome move into the same gamete (44–47). Figure 1 shows the cytological process of double reduction formation in a multivalent tetraploid. Experiments aimed at estimating the frequency of double reduction in autotetraploids have yielded values ranging from 0 to almost 0.30 (48–53).

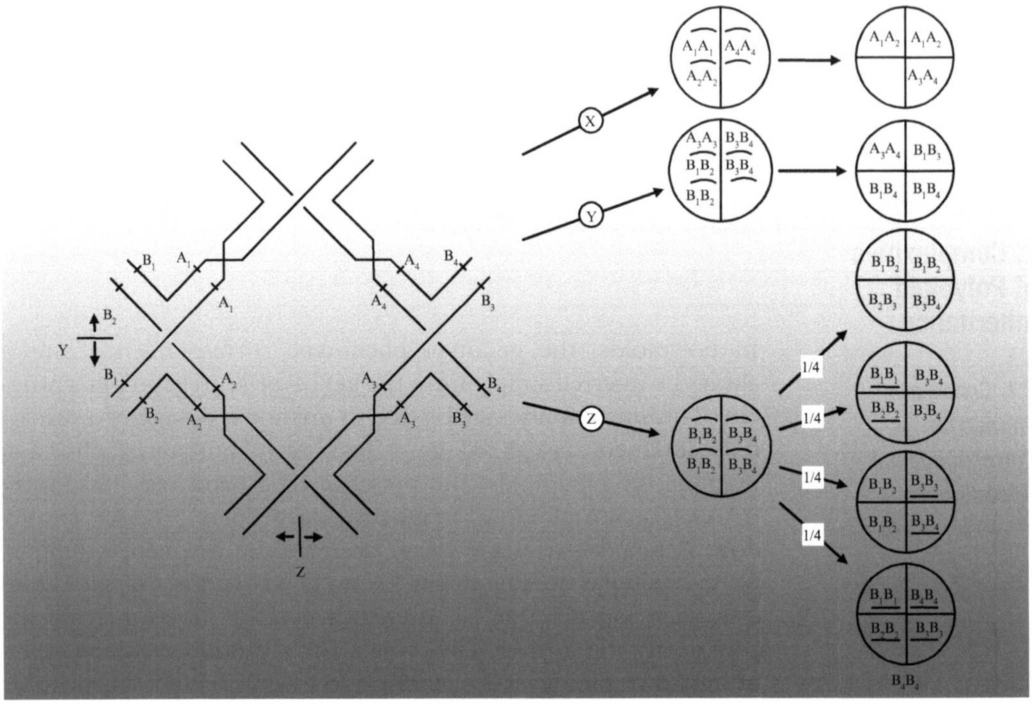

Fig. 1. A diagram for the segregation patterns of loci A and B during meiosis in an autopolyploid. Locus A having no crossover with the centromere undergoes path X of reductional separation (no double reduction), whereas locus B displaying a crossover with the centromere undergoes either path Y of equational separation with no double reduction or path Z of equational separation with double reduction. Gametes having undergone double reductions are underscored. Adapted from (29).

From a genetic viewpoint, the occurrence and frequency of double reduction are expected to affect the pattern of gene segregation and, therefore, linkage mapping in polysomic polyploids.

2.3. Complexity of Genome Structure

Polyploids generally display high levels of heterozygosity owing to the combination of different genomes (reviewed in (11)). For example, assuming simple tetrasomic segregation, selfing of a heterozygous autotetraploid of genotype aabb is expected to produce progeny in the ratio of 1aaaa:34 heterozygotes (of various genotypes):1bbbb, a huge increase over expectations for a diploid with disomic inheritance (i.e., 1aa:2ab:1bb).

In addition, increased heterozygosity in polyploids makes the generation of homozygous inbred lines much more difficult as compared to the generation of homozygous inbred diploid lines. For a mapping progeny derived from non-inbred lines, linkage analysis is considerably complicated due to increased combination of different marker types (dominant vs. codominant, fully informative vs. partially informative, or diallelic vs. multiallelic) and by unknown linkage phases between different markers (30). Although the use of a pseudo-backcross test strategy can partially solve this problem (37, 54), this strategy can only characterize part of the genome which is heterozygous in one parent and null in the other. To characterize the entire genome of polyploids, linkage phases should be characterized prior to the estimation of linkage.

2.4. Increased Number of Gene Actions and Interactions

As can be imagined, increased allelic or nonallelic combinations due to multiple alleles result in complex gene actions and interactions at QTL in polyploids. Currently, there are only a few quantitative genetic models that have been developed to characterize gene effects and gene interactions of various orders in polyploids (32, 35, 55, 56). These limited models are based on simplified gene effects, especially simplified gene interactions, although no justification has been provided for such a simplification.

3. Multilocus Linkage Analysis

3.1. Existing Problems

During the past two decades, a number of genome studies have been launched to conduct linkage mapping in a variety of polyploids ranging from potato (tetraploid) to sugarcane (octoploid) (37, 54, 57–63). Currently, there are two basic approaches for linkage mapping in polyploids: (1) the use of diploid relatives to address polyploid questions; for example, the genetic maps of wheat and potato were built using closely related diploid species (64, 65) and (2) the development of specific statistical methods for polyploids (24–26, 66). While the first approach is limited due to a lack of diploid relatives, the second approach has been based on a number of restrictive simplifying assumptions. Two of the most important assumptions include random pairings of chromosomes during meiosis and no double reduction—each chromosome will segregate from its pair at meiosis into a different gamete. The use of these two assumptions blurs the distinction of different polyploid origins, allo- vs. autopolyploids, and different meiotic behaviors, disomic vs. polysomic polyploids, and may perhaps lead to erroneous inference about linkage in polyploids.

A prerequisite for linkage analysis is the segregation of distinguishable genotypes in a progeny population. In usual diploids, segregation patterns of marker genotypes can be predicted based on marker phenotypes. However, for polyploids, many factors complicate the inference of the genotype of a progeny from its phenotype or of gamete formation from gamete genotype.

3.2. Recent Developments

Three kinds of models have been developed for bivalent and multivalent polyploids and their mixed type. In each kind of model, we examine the influences of meiotic configurations on the estimation of linkage and build up a unified statistical framework to simultaneously estimate the dose of restriction fragment, ploidy levels, and linkage phases.

The bivalent model. A unified framework is designed to simultaneously estimate the dose of fragment, ploidy level (denoted by x), the preferential pairing factor, linkage and linkage phases in disomic polyploids. In our earlier work, each of these parameters was estimated separately (28, 30).

Consider a tetraploid, in which there are four sets of chromosomes. If chromosomes 1 and 2 are homologous, as are chromosomes 3 and 4, there are three different combinations for the bivalent pairing. One of the three pairs β_1 is between homologues, and the other two β_2 and β_3 are between homoeologues, which are complete homoeologous pairings. If the preferential pairing factor is denoted as p, the frequencies of β_1, β_2, and β_3 are $b_1 = 1/3 + p$, $b_2 = 1/3 - 1/2p$, and $b_3 = 1/3 - 1/2p$, respectively.

Let us consider two of the markers M_1 and M_2 which are both heterozygous in parent P but homozygous in parent Q. These two markers are assumed to be fully informative, each with four different marker alleles assigned to the four homologous chromosomes of the heterozygous parent P. The four alleles of this parent are labeled by P_1^1, P_1^2, P_1^3 and P_1^4 at marker M_1 and by P_2^1, P_2^2, P_2^3 and P_2^4 at marker M_2. The four alleles at each marker are identical in parent Q. The recombination fraction between the two markers is denoted by θ. For the heterozygous parent P, there are possibly a total of 24 nonallelic configurations or linkage phase arrangements between the two markers, which are not known *a priori*. Assume that the two markers have a linkage phase arrangement, schematically expressed as

$$\frac{P_1^1}{P_2^1}\Bigg|\frac{P_1^2}{P_2^2}\Bigg|\frac{P_1^3}{P_2^3}\Bigg|\frac{P_1^4}{P_2^4}\Bigg| \times \frac{Q_1}{Q_2}\Bigg|\frac{Q_1}{Q_2}\Bigg|\frac{Q_1}{Q_2}\Bigg|\frac{Q_1}{Q_2}\Bigg|\frac{Q_1}{Q_2}\Bigg|, \quad (1)$$

where lines indicate the individual homologous chromosomes on which the two markers are located. The recombination fraction θ is estimated on the basis of the segregation of the two-marker genotypes observed in the pseudo-test backcross family. However, for a disomic tetraploid, the observations of the marker genotypes are confounded by different chromosome pairings β_1, β_2, and β_3 for a given nonallelic configuration.

For bivalent pairings, parent P generates 36 diploid gametes at the two markers, whose genotypes are arrayed by

$$2G_2^{\beta}=\left(P_1^1P_1^2\ P_1^1P_1^3\ P_1^1P_1^4\ P_1^2P_1^3k\ P_1^2P_1^4\ P_1^3P_1^4\right)^{T}\left(P_2^1P_2^2\ P_2^1P_2^3\ P_2^1P_2^4\ P_2^2P_2^3\ P_2^2P_2^4\ P_2^3P_2^4\right),$$

where T denotes the transpose of a vector. The frequencies of these gametes depend on the preferential pairing factor and recombination fraction (30). Based on different doses assumed for each marker, the gamete genotypes in this array can be collapsed into a small number of distinguishable groups from which a unified model can be framed and used to provide simultaneous estimation of different parameters of interest.

The multivalent model. Based on a theoretical model proposed by Fisher (48), Wu et al. (29) have developed a maximum likelihood-based method to estimate the linkage between fully informative markers under multivalent formation based on a pseudobackcross design. This method has been extended to include any type of markers in a full-sib family. A unified framework needs to be developed by simultaneously estimating the dose of fragment, ploidy level, the frequency of double reduction, linkage, and linkage phases in multivalent polyploids.

Unlike bivalent pairings, quadrivalent pairings will cause each parent to generate 100 diploid gametes, which are categorized into four types each with a different cytological behavior: (1) double reductions for both markers, (2) double reductions for marker M_1, (3) double reductions for marker M_2, (4) random chromosomal pairings (with no double reduction). Gametes due to double reductions are derived from two sister chromatids of a single chromosome, whereas those due to random pairings result from two sister chromatids each from one of two different chromosomes. These four types of gametes under quadrivalent pairings for parent P are, respectively, arrayed by

$$
\begin{aligned}
{}_1G_1^Q &= \left(P_1^kP_1^k\ P_2^kP_2^k\ P_3^kP_3^k\ P_4^kP_4^k\right)^T\left(P_1^lP_1^l\ P_2^lP_2^l\ P_3^lP_3^l\ P_4^lP_4^l\right),\\
{}_1G_2^Q &= \left(P_1^kP_1^k\ P_2^kP_2^k\ P_3^kP_3^k\ P_4^kP_4^k\right)^T\left(P_1^lP_2^l\ P_1^lP_3^l\ P_1^lP_4^l\ P_2^lP_3^l\ P_2^lP_4^l\ P_3^lP_4^l\right),\\
{}_2G_1^Q &= \left(P_1^kP_2^k\ P_1^kP_3^k\ P_1^kP_4^k\ P_2^kP_3^k\ P_2^kP_4^k\ P_3^kP_4^k\right)^T\left(P_1^lP_1^l\ P_2^lP_2^l\ P_3^lP_3^l\ P_4^lP_4^l\right),\\
{}_2G_2^Q &= \left(P_1^kP_2^k\ P_1^kP_3^k\ P_1^kP_4^k\ P_2^kP_3^k\ P_2^kP_4^k\ P_3^kP_4^k\right)^T\\
&\quad\left(P_1^lP_2^l\ P_1^lP_3^l\ P_1^lP_4^l\ P_2^lP_3^l\ P_2^lP_4^l\ P_3^lP_4^l\right),
\end{aligned}
$$

whose diploid gamete frequencies are expressed in terms of the frequencies of double reduction and linkage (see refs. (29, 33) for the derivation of the EM algorithm for estimating the unknown parameters).

The mixed polyploid model. The bivalent and multivalent models are combined to simultaneously estimate the dose of fragment, ploidy level, the preferential pairing factor, the frequency of double reduction, linkage, and linkage phase in a general polyploid system. A general polyploid model has been developed for simultaneous estimation of the preferential pairing factor, the frequency of double reduction, and linkage in a tetraploid species (31).

For an arbitrary tetraploid, the genotypes of all possible two-marker diploid gametes for parent P are expressed by a 10×10 matrix

$$
G = \begin{bmatrix} {}_1G_1 & {}_1G_2 \\ {}_2G_1 & {}_2G_2 \end{bmatrix} = \begin{bmatrix} 0 & 0 \\ 0 & {}_2G_2^{\beta} \end{bmatrix} + \begin{bmatrix} {}_1G_1^Q & {}_1G_2^Q \\ {}_2G_1^Q & {}_2G_2^Q \end{bmatrix}, \quad (2)
$$

where ${}_1G_1$, ${}_1G_2$, and ${}_2G_1$ are derived from only quadrivalent pairings, and ${}_2G_2$ from both bivalent and quadrivalent pairings. The mixed frequencies of two-marker diploid gametes under both bivalent and quadrivalent pairings for parent P

$$\left|\begin{array}{c|c} P^k_{r_1} & P^k_{r_2} \\ P^l_{s_1} & P^l_{s_2} \end{array}\right| \quad r_1, r_2, s_1, s_2 = 1, \ldots, 4 \tag{3}$$

can be written in matrix notation **H**. For each of the three bivalent pairings β_1–β_3, a total of 16 two-marker gametes are generated, which are classified into three types: (1) four gametes with no recombinant, (2) eight gametes with one recombinant, and (3) four gametes with two recombinants. The first and last types of gametes are duplicated among the three bivalent pairings. Thus, the frequencies of these duplicated gametes should be summed over two of the three bivalent pairings. Based on these classifications, the matrix $\mathbf{H}^{\beta}$ for the frequencies of diploid gametes at markers M^k and M^l derived from bivalent pairings can be expressed, under Expression 3, as

$$\mathrm{H}^{\beta} = \begin{array}{c} \\ P^l_1P^l_1 \\ P^l_2P^l_2 \\ P^l_3P^l_3 \\ P^l_4P^l_4 \\ P^l_1P^l_2/P^l_2P^l_1 \\ P^l_1P^l_3/P^l_3P^l_1 \\ P^l_1P^l_4/P^l_4P^l_1 \\ P^l_2P^l_3/P^l_3P^l_2 \\ P^l_2P^l_4/P^l_4P^l_2 \\ P^l_3P^l_4/P^l_4P^l_3 \end{array} \begin{array}{cccccccccc} P^k_1P^k_1 & P^k_2P^k_2 & P^k_3P^k_3 & P^k_4P^k_4 & P^k_1P^k_2 & P^k_1P^k_3 & P^k_1P^k_4 & P^k_2P^k_3 & P^k_2P^k_4 & P^k_3P^k_4 \\ 0 & 0 & 0 & 0 & 0 & 0 & 0 & 0 & 0 & 0 \\ 0 & 0 & 0 & 0 & 0 & 0 & 0 & 0 & 0 & 0 \\ 0 & 0 & 0 & 0 & 0 & 0 & 0 & 0 & 0 & 0 \\ 0 & 0 & 0 & 0 & 0 & 0 & 0 & 0 & 0 & 0 \\ 0 & 0 & 0 & 0 & \frac{1}{2}(1-\theta)^2 b_2 & \frac{1}{4}\theta(1-\theta)b_2 & \frac{1}{4}\theta(1-\theta)b_2 & \frac{1}{4}\theta(1-\theta)b_2 & \frac{1}{4}\theta(1-\theta)b_2 & \frac{1}{2}\theta^2 b_2 \\ 0 & 0 & 0 & 0 & \frac{1}{4}\theta(1-\theta)b_2 & \frac{1}{4}(1-\theta)^2(b_1+b_2) & \frac{1}{4}\theta(1-\theta)b_1 & \frac{1}{4}\theta(1-\theta)b_1 & \frac{1}{4}\theta^2(b_1+b_2) & \frac{1}{4}\theta(1-\theta)b_2 \\ 0 & 0 & 0 & 0 & \frac{1}{4}\theta(1-\theta)b_2 & \frac{1}{4}\theta(1-\theta)b_1 & \frac{1}{4}(1-\theta)^2(b_1+b_2) & \frac{1}{4}\theta^2(b_1+b_2) & \frac{1}{4}\theta(1-\theta)b_1 & \frac{1}{4}\theta(1-\theta)b_2 \\ 0 & 0 & 0 & 0 & \frac{1}{4}\theta(1-\theta)b_2 & \frac{1}{4}\theta(1-\theta)b_1 & \frac{1}{4}\theta^2(b_1+b_2) & \frac{1}{4}(1-\theta)^2(b_1+b_2) & \frac{1}{4}\theta(1-\theta)b_1 & \frac{1}{4}\theta(1-\theta)b_2 \\ 0 & 0 & 0 & 0 & \frac{1}{4}\theta(1-\theta)b_2 & \frac{1}{4}\theta^2(b_1+b_2) & \frac{1}{4}\theta(1-\theta)b_1 & \frac{1}{4}\theta(1-\theta)b_1 & \frac{1}{4}(1-\theta)^2(b_1+b_2) & \frac{1}{4}\theta(1-\theta)b_2 \\ 0 & 0 & 0 & 0 & \frac{1}{2}\theta^2 b_2 & \frac{1}{4}\theta(1-\theta)b_2 & \frac{1}{4}\theta(1-\theta)b_2 & \frac{1}{4}\theta(1-\theta)b_2 & \frac{1}{4}\theta(1-\theta)b_2 & \frac{1}{2}(1-\theta)^2 b_2 \end{array}$$

where the chromosomes carrying alleles P^k_1 and P^k_2 at marker M^k are assumed to be homologous, and the same for the chromosomes carrying P^k_3 and P^k_4 at marker M^k, θ is the recombination fraction between the two markers, and $b_1 = 1/3 + p$, $b_2 = 1/3 - 1/2p$, and $b_2 = 1/3 - 1/2p$.

The theory for two-point analysis in each polyploid model will be extended to multilocus linkage analysis and phase analysis for ordering markers on a linkage group. Several approaches have been suggested to perform multilocus linkage analysis in model systems (22) and outcrossing species. The multilocus approach takes into account the cosegregation of genes at several linked markers simultaneously based on a hidden Markov model (HMM) (34).

4. QTL Mapping

4.1. A General Framework

Based on marker and map analyses, a general statistical framework for QTL mapping will be developed for each polyploid model, **bivalent, multivalent, or mixed**. The genetic mapping of QTL in polyploids will be based on the mixture model, a model widely used in statistical genetic research (23). In one version of a mixture model, each observation y is assumed to have arisen from one of k (k possibly unknown but finite) components, each component being modeled by a density from the parametric family f:

$$p(y|\pi, \varphi, \eta) = \pi_1 f(y; \varphi_1, \eta) + \cdots + \pi_k f(y; \varphi_k, \eta), \tag{4}$$

where $\pi = (\pi_1, \ldots, \pi_k)$ are the mixture proportions which are constrained to be nonnegative and sum to unity; $\varphi = (\varphi_1, \ldots, \varphi_k)$ are the component specific parameters, with φ_j being specific to component j; and η is a parameter which is common to all components.

A genetic mapping project built upon a mixture model contains two major tasks: (1) deriving the mixture proportions $(\pi_1, \ldots \pi_k)$, denoted as the frequencies of QTL genotypes, the density functions specified by gene effects of putative QTL $(\varphi_1, \ldots, \varphi_k)$ and the common residual variance (σ^2), and (2) estimating unknown QTL parameters included in the mixture model. The first task, called *genetic modeling*, is relevant to experimental designs, marker types, meiotic configurations, population structures, reproductive behaviors, and genetic effects. Genetic effects specified by Eq. (4), for a tetraploid are contained in the normal distribution density. The second task relies upon extensive computer simulations and statistical/computational algorithms and is thus called *statistical modeling*.

4.2. Genetic Modeling

The genetic models for QTL identification should take into account the cytological properties of polyploids. For example, the preferential pairing factor (for the bivalent polyploid model), the frequency of double reduction (for the multivalent polyploid model), or both (for the mixed polyploid model), should be incorporated into a map construction strategy to estimate the linkage of markers (measured by the recombination fraction) and their order. QTL identification based on the linkage map includes an additional dimension, i.e., the quantitative genetic properties of QTL, their number, their gene actions and interactions, and their relationships with the environment.

4.3. Statistical Algorithms

Mixture models for QTL mapping are commonly analyzed by the maximum likelihood (ML) method (23) and increasingly by the Bayesian approach (67–69).

Maximum likelihood method. The ML approach to parameter estimation in mixture models obtains point estimates $(\hat{\pi}, \hat{\varphi}, \hat{\sigma}^2)$ of the parameters $\Omega = (\pi, \varphi, \sigma^2)$ by maximizing the likelihood. The maximum likelihood estimates (MLEs) of the unknown parameters Ω under the mixture QTL model can be computed by implementing an EM algorithm (70, 71). Based on Eq. (4), the log-likelihood of a mapping population of size N is given by

$$\log\ell(\Omega) = \sum_{i=1}^{N} \log\left[\sum_{j=1}^{k} \pi_j f_j(y_i)\right], \tag{5}$$

where, to ease notation, we write $f_j(y_i) = f(y_i; \varphi_j, \eta)$. The derivatives of the log-likelihood are

$$\begin{aligned}\frac{\partial}{\partial\Omega_\varphi}\log\ell(\Omega) &= \sum_{i=1}^{N}\sum_{j=1}^{k}\frac{\pi_j\frac{\partial}{\partial\Omega_\varphi}f_j(y_i)}{\sum_{j=1}^{k}\pi_j f_j(y_i)}\\ &= \sum_{i=1}^{N}\sum_{j=1}^{k}\frac{\pi_j f_j(y_i)}{\sum_{j=1}^{k}\pi_j f_j(y_i)}\frac{\partial}{\partial\Omega_\psi}\log f_j(y_i),\\ &= \sum_{i=1}^{N}\sum_{j=1}^{k}\Pi_{ij}\frac{\partial}{\partial\Omega_\varphi}\log f_j(y_i)\end{aligned} \tag{6}$$

where we define

$$\Pi_{ij} = \frac{\pi_j f_j(y_i)}{\sum_{j=1}^{k}\pi_j f_j(y_i)},$$

which could be thought of as a posterior probability that individual i has a QTL genotype j. We then implement the EM algorithm with the expanded parameter set $\{\Omega, \Pi\}$, where $\Pi = \{\Pi_{ij}, j = 1,\ldots,k, i = 1,\ldots,N\}$. Conditional on Π, we solve for the zeros of $(\partial/\partial\Omega_\varphi)\log l(\Omega)$ to get our estimates of Ω (the M step). The estimates are then used to update Π (the E step), and the process is repeated until convergence. The values at convergence are the maximum likelihood estimates (MLEs).

However, there can sometimes be problems when ML is used for QTL mixture models. First, for some choices of parametric families, f, the likelihood is unbounded. Second, in complex situations the likelihood function can have many local maxima, each of which may give different (and possibly reasonable) plug-in estimates for quantities of interest. In these cases, it could be difficult to choose one of these point estimates of the parameters over the others.

Third, and most importantly, when a QTL mapping strategy incorporates population and quantitative genetic properties of genes, as proposed here, it will encounter a much higher dimensional space for the unknown parameters than traditional QTL modeling strategies. Although the mere existence of a high-dimensional parameter space is not necessarily detrimental, extra care must be taken in searching for the ML estimator. An extra complication (not only of ML) is that the uncertainty about the actual number of QTL for a quantitative trait results in extra difficulty in model fitting and selection.

The Bayesian method. Although ML will be perfectly reasonable in a number of situations, we also want to investigate the use of a Bayesian approach which can avoid many of the problems described above. In ML, the unknown parameters are treated as unknown variables (unobservables), and the likelihood function is maximized in these variables. In the Bayesian paradigm, each unobservable parameter is given a prior distribution, and we then infer the posterior distribution of each unobservable conditional on the data (the observables). The summary statistics of the posterior distribution, e.g., the mean, the mode or the median, can be regarded as Bayesian estimates of unobservables (72). The interval estimate can be obtained simply by examining the posterior distribution. Let us denote the observables by a vector y (the data vector) and unobservables by a parameter vector $\Omega = (\pi, \varphi, \eta)$. The posterior distribution is

$$p(\Omega|y) = \frac{p(y,\Omega)}{p(y)} = \frac{p(y|\Omega)p(\Omega)}{p(y)} \propto p(y|\Omega)p(\Omega),$$

where $p(*)$ is a generic expression for a probability density, $p(y|\Omega)$ is the likelihood and $p(\Omega)$ is the prior probability distribution of the unobservables. Because the denominator is just the probability density of y, not a function of the parameters, it can be ignored. We partition the vector Ω into $\Omega = [\Omega_j \, \Omega_{-j}]$, where Ω_j is a single element of the unobservables and Ω_{-j} is the rest of the unobservables that exclude Ω_j. The marginal posterior distribution of Ω_j is expressed by

$$p(\Omega_j|y) = \int p(\Omega_j, \ \Omega_{-j}|y)\mathrm{d}\Omega_{-j} \propto \int p(y|\Omega_j, \Omega_{-j})p(\Omega_j, \Omega_{-j})\mathrm{d}\Omega_{-j}.$$

The mean of this marginal posterior distribution is a candidate Bayesian estimator of Ω_i. This marginal distribution rarely has an explicit form, and numerical integration is often prohibited because the dimensionality of Ω_{-i} may be high. However, a Markov chain Monte Carlo (MCMC) algorithm can be used to simulate the sample from the joint posterior distribution. The potential of the Bayesian approach implemented with the Gibbs sampler or Metropolis–Hastings algorithm for genome mapping has been explored for several relatively simple genetic designs (67–69). In particular, because we are now able to examine the entire posterior distribution of each parameter, we will be better able to deal with problems such as multimodality of the likelihood function.

As an illustration, the EM algorithm described above can be thought of as an average of a completed-data EM algorithm as follows: For $i = 1, \ldots, N$, define the augmented variable Z_i to satisfy

$$\Upsilon_i|Z_i = j' \sim f_{j'}(y), \quad P(Z_i = j') = \gamma_i^{(j')}.$$

Then, Eq. (5) is the observed data log-likelihood, with the complete-data log-likelihood given by

$$\log \ell(\Omega|\Upsilon, Z) = \sum_{i=1}^{N} \log f_{Z_i}(y_i). \quad (7)$$

We could now estimate Ω using a Gibbs sampler that generates $\Omega|Z$ from Eq. (7), and $Z|\Omega$ from

$$P(Z_i = j'|\Omega) = \frac{\gamma_i^{(j')} f_{j'}(y_i)}{\sum_{j=1}^{k} \gamma_i^{(j)} f_j(y_i)}.$$

The posterior modes obtained from the Gibbs sampler are the MLEs of the EM algorithm, as Π_{ij} of Eq. (6) satisfies $\Pi_{ij} = P(Z_i = j|\Omega)$. But here we are not limited to just looking at posterior modes—examination of the entire posterior distribution of each parameter will give us information on both its precision of estimation and shape of distribution.

5. Special Considerations

5.1. Marker Informativeness

Because crosses in most polyploid species do not employ inbred lines, the pattern of marker segregation varies from one locus to the next. Some markers are codominant, whereas others are dominant. Some markers are more informative, while others are less informative. In diploids, such variable segregation patterns lead to a high degree of complexity for linkage analysis, phase analysis, and QTL identification (73). With no doubt, this issue is much more complicated in polyploid analysis, but must be addressed for more precise and useful mapping.

For a full-sib family initiated with two outbred tetraploid parents, there are up to eight different alleles observed for a given marker locus. These alleles are denoted by *a*, *b*, *c*, and *d* for parent P and *e*, *f*, *g*, and *h* for parent Q. For dominant markers, dominant alleles are indicated by the presence of bands on a gel and recessive alleles (denoted by *o*) are indicated by the absence of bands. For each parent (say P), there are a total of 16 possible phenotypes that can be classified into five different phenotypes in terms of the number of bands observed: four bands (one genotype *abcd*), three bands (four genotypes *abcc*, *abbc*, *aabc*, and *abco*), two bands (six genotypes *abbb*, *aabb*, *aaab*, *abbo*, *aabo*, and *aboo*), one band (four genotypes

Table 1
Types of diploid gametes derived from an autotetraploid with different genotypes

A1	Ten gametes with formation proportion $1(aa):1(bb):1(cc):1(dd):1(ab):1(ac):1(ad):1(bc):1(bd):1(\mathrm{cd})$ for genotype abcd.
A2	Seven gametes with formation proportion $1(oo):1(ab):1(ac):1(bc):2(a\_):2(b\_):2(c\_)$ for genotype abco.
A3	Six gametes with formation proportion $1(aa):1(bb):1(ab):2(ac):2(bc):3(cc)$ for genotype *abcc*, $1(aa):1(cc):1(ac):2(ab):2(bc):3(bb)$ for genotype *abbc*, or $1(bb):1(cc):1(bc):2(ab):2(ac):3(aa)$ for genotype *aabc*.
A4	Four gametes with formation proportion$1(oo):2(a_):2(ab):5(b_)$ for genotype *abbo* or$1(oo):2(ab):2(b_):5(a_)$ for genotype *aabo*.
A5	Four gametes with formation proportion $1(ab):3(oo):3(a\_):3(b\_)$ for genotype *aboo*.
A6	Three gametes with formation proportion $1(aa):3(ab):6(bb)$ for genotype *abbb* or$1(bb):3(ab):6(aa)$ for genotype *aaab*.
A7	Three gametes with formation proportion $3(aa):3(bb):4(ab)$ for genotype *aabb*.
A8	Two gametes with formation proportion $1(oo):9(a\_)$ for genotype *aaao*
A9	Two gametes with formation proportion $3(oo):7(a\_)$ for genotype *aaoo*
A10	Two gametes with formation proportion $4(a\_):6(oo)$ for genotype *aooo*
A11	One gamete *aa* for genotype *aaaa* and *oo* for genotype *oooo*.

aaaa, *aaao*, *aaoo*, and *aooo*), and no band (one genotype *oooo*). These 16 phenotypes can be classified into 11 different types based on the number of the gamete phenotypes generated and the relative proportions of gamete formations (30) (Table 1):

It should be noted that the gamete types derived from the process of double reduction (44, 46, 47) are considered in these classifications. For example, for type A1, genotype *abcd* produces double reduction-type gametes *aa*, *bb*, *cc*, and *dd*. Similar classifications can also be made for the second parent Q with alleles denoted by *e*, *f*, *g*, *h*, and *o*. For one parent, the markers of type A1 are fully informative because all of the ten gamete types can be phenotypically distinguished based on their genotypes, whereas the markers of types A2–A10 are partially informative, because some of the gamete types have identical phenotypes. The markers from A11 are noninformative given its single gamete phenotype.

5.2. Higher-Ploidy Model

We will also derive statistical methods for genome mapping in hexaploid, octoploid, and dexaploid species. These derivations are not difficult in principle, but they will be much more tedious technically than what can be done for tetraploids. For a hexaploid plant, triploid gametes are generated at meiosis. Theoretical models of a general hexaploid based on random pairings propose three different modes for the formation of triploid gametes in hexaploids: (1) hexavalent pairing, (2) quadrivalent + bivalent pairing, and (3) bivalent pairing, with the respective frequencies 8/15, 6/15, and 1/15 (28, 42). But empirical data do not support such a prediction for the frequencies of chromosome pairings (74). As in the general tetraploid model, each of the three modes is affected by preferential pairings, and also the first two modes undergo double reduction because of multivalent pairings at meiosis. The occurrence of preferential pairing results in lower multivalent pairing than predicted on the basis of a random pairing (75), which should be considered in model derivations. As in a general tetraploid, an additional constant parameter is required for characterizing the frequency of double reduction at a QTL in a general hexaploid. But for a general octoploid and dexaploid, two such additional parameters are required. Statistical genomic methods developed for polyploids of any level of ploidy will be broadly useful for understanding the effects of ploidy on genetic architecture and evolution in plants.

6. Notes

Multilocus molecular data sets are particularly useful for the understanding of evolutionary processes (76) and the development of superior varieties in plant species (77). Detailed genetic linkage maps constructed from molecular markers can be used to compare the differentiation of genome structure, organization and function among species and identify genes or quantitative trait loci (QTL) responsible for economically important traits in plants. There are also many efforts to employ marker-based maps in both evolutionary and breeding studies of polyploids (58, 78), but significant challenges confront successful application to each due to a serious lack of statistical genetic methods for analyzing the polyploid data. The statistical methods developed for linkage analysis in normal diploid species (e.g., (22, 23)) cannot be directly adapted to perform linkage mapping in polyploids because polyploids have complicated cytological peculiarities that are qualitatively different from diploids.

The development of statistical methods that associate molecular marker and phenotypic information should be based on the cytological properties of polyploids. Statistical methodologies have been developed under three different polyploid models, bivalent, multivalent, and mixed. Both the maximum likelihood and Bayesian approaches should be developed to provide estimates of linkage maps and QTL parameters. With the availability of a massive amount of marker and phenotype data in polyploid species being collected, these tools can help molecular geneticists, quantitative geneticists, evolutionary geneticists, or plant breeders from both academic institutions and industrial sectors to unravel the genetic base of quantitative traits in polyploids and, ultimately, develop genetically productive varieties of crop species.

Acknowledgment

This work is supported through the Office of Sciences (BER), US Department of Energy, Interagency Agreement no. DE-A102-07ER64453.

References

1. Hilu KW (1993) Polyploidy and the evolution of domesticated plants. Am J Bot 80:1491–1499
2. Leitch IJ, Bennett MD (1997) Polyploidy in angiosperms. Trends Plant Sci 2:470–476
3. Stebbins GL (1971) Chromosomal evolution in higher plants. Addison-Wesley, Reading, MA
4. Grant V (1981) Plant speciation, 2nd edn. Columbia University Press, NY
5. Bever JD, Felber F (1992) The theoretical population genetics of autopolyploidy. Oxford Surv Evol Biol 8:185–217
6. Ramsey J, Schemskem DW (1998) Pathways, mechanisms, and rates of polyploid formation in flowering plants. Annu Rev Ecol Syst 29:467–501
7. Soltis DE, Soltis PS (1993) Molecular data and the dynamic nature of polyploidy. Crit Rev Plant Sci 12:243–273
8. Soltis DE, Soltis PS (1999) Polyploidy: recurrent formation and genome evolution. Trends Ecol Evol 14:348–352
9. Otto SP, Whitton J (2000) Polyploid incidence and evolution. Annu Rev Genet 2000 (34):401–437
10. Masterson J (1994) Stomatal size in fossil plants—evidence for polyploidy in majority of angiosperms. Science 264:421–424
11. Soltis PS, Soltis DE (2000) The role of genetic and genomic attributes in the success of polyploids. Proc Natl Acad Sci USA 97:7051–7057
12. Stebbing GL (1950) Variation and evolution in plants. Columbia University Press, NY
13. Peloquin SJ (1981) In: Frey KJ (ed) Plant breeding. Iowa State University Press, Ames, IA, pp 117–150
14. Sarvella P (1958) Multivalent formation and genetic segregation in some allopolyploid gossypium hybrids. Genetics 43:601–619
15. Sybenga A (1996) Chromosome pairing affinity and quadrivalent formation in polyploids: do segmental allopolyploids exist? Genome 39:1176–1184
16. Swaminathan MS, Howard HW (1953) The cytology and genetics of the potato (*Solanum tuberosum*) and related species. Bibliogr Genet 16:1–192
17. Bingham ET, McCoy TJ (1988) Cytology and cytogenetics of alfalfa. In: Hanson AA (ed) Alfalfa and alfalfa improvement. Agron. Monogr. 29 ASA, CSSA and SSSA, Madison, WI, pp 737–776
18. Jackson RC, Jackson JW (1996) Gene segregation in autotetraploids: prediction from meiotic configurations. Am J Bot 83:673–678
19. Sybenga A (1984) Preferential pairing estimates from multivalent frequencies in tetraploids. Genome 37:1045–1055
20. Allendorf FW, Danzmann RG (1997) Secondary tetrasomic segregation of MDH-B and prefer-ential pairing of homeologues in rainbow trout. Genetics 145:1083–1092
21. Fjellstrom RG, Beuselinck PR, Steiner JJ (2001) RFLP marker analysis supports tetrasomic inheritance in *Lotus corniculatus* L. Theor Appl Genet 102:718–725
22. Lander ES, Green P (1987) Construction of multilocus genetic linkage maps in human. Proc Natl Acad Sci 84:2363–2367
23. Lander ES, Botstein D (1989) Mapping Mendelian factors underlying quantitative traits using RFLP linkage maps. Genetics 121:185–199

24. Hackett CA, Bradshaw JE, Meyer RC et al (1998) Linkage analysis in tetraploid species: a simulation study. Genet Res 71:143–154
25. Ripol MI, Churchill GA, da Silva JAG et al (1999) Statistical aspects of genetic mapping in autopolyploids. Gene 235:31–41
26. Luo ZW, Hackett CA, Bradshaw JE et al (2001) Construction of a genetic linkage map in tetraploid species using molecular markers. Genetics 157:1369–1385
27. Luo ZW, Zhang Z, Leach L et al (2006) Constructing genetic linkage maps under a tetrasomic model. Genetics 172:2635–2645
28. Wu RL, Gallo-Meagher M, Littell RC et al (2001) A general polyploid model for analyzing gene segregation in outcrossing tetraploid species. Genetics 159:869–882
29. Wu SS, Wu RL, Ma CX et al (2001) A multivalent pairing model of linkage analysis in autotetraploids. Genetics 159:1339–1350
30. Wu RL, Ma CX, Casella G (2002) Abivalent polyploid model for linkage analysis in outcrossing tetraploid species. Theor Pop Biol 62:129–151
31. Wu RL, Ma CX, Casella G (2004) A mixed polyploid model for linkage analysis in tetraploids. J Comput Biol 11:562–580
32. Wu RL, Ma CX, Casella G (2004) A bivalent polyploid model for mapping quantitative trait loci in outcrossing tetraploids. Genetics 166:581–595
33. Wu RL, Ma CX (2005) A general framework for statistical linkage analysis in multivalent tetraploids. Genetics 170:899–907
34. Leach LJ, Wang L, Kearsey MJ et al (2010) Multilocus tetrasomic linkage analysis using hidden Markov chain model. Proc Natl Acad Sci USA 107:4270–4274
35. Li JH, Das K, Fu GF et al (2010) EM algorithm for mapping quantitative trait loci in multivalent tetraploids. Int J Plant Genom 2010:216547
36. Hickok LG (1978) Homoeologous chromosome pairing: frequency difference in inbred and intraspecific hybrid polyploid ferns. Science 202:982–984
37. Ming R, Liu SC, Lin YR et al (1998) Detailed alignment of *Saccharum* and *Sorghum* chromosomes: comparative organization of closely related diploid and polyploid genomes. Genetics 150:1663–1682
38. Lenz EM, Grane CF, Sleper DA et al (1983) An assessment of preferential chromosome pairing at meiosis in *Dactylis glomerata*. Can J Genet Cytol 25:222–232
39. Haynes KG, Potts WE, Camp MJ (1991) Estimation of preferential pairing in tetraploid × diploid hybridizations. Theor Appl Genet 81:504–508
40. Matsubayashi M (1991) Phylogenetic relationships in the potato and related species. In: Tsuchiya T, Gupta PK (eds) Chro-mosome engineering in plants: genetics, breeding, evolution. Part B. Elsevier, Amsterdam, pp 93–118
41. Sybenga A (1988) Mathematical models for estimating preferential pairing and recombination in triploid hybrids. Genome 30:745–757
42. Jackson RC, Casey J (1982) Cytogenetic analysis of autopolyploids: models and methods for triploids to octoploids. Am J Bot 69:487–501
43. Hauber DP, Reeves A, Stack SM (1999) Synapsis in a natural autotetraploid. Genome 42:936–949
44. Darlington CD (1929) Chromosome behaviour and structural hybridity in the *Tradescantiae*. J Genet 21:207–286
45. Haldane JBS (1930) Theoretical genetics of autopolyploids. Genetics 22:359–372
46. Mather K (1935) Reductional and equational separation of the chromosomes in bivalents and multivalents. J Genet 30:53–78
47. Mather K (1936) Segregation and linkage in autotetraploids. J Genet 32:287–314
48. Fisher RA (1947) The theory of linkage in polysomic inheritance. Philos Trans Roy Soc Ser B 233:55–87
49. Fisher RA (1949) The theory of inbreeding. Hafner, NY
50. Welch JE (1962) Linkage in autotetraploid maize. Genetics 47:367–396
51. Tai GCC (1982) Estimation of double reduction and genetic parameters of autotetraploids. Heredity 49:63–70
52. Tai GCC (1982) Estimation of double reduction and genetic parameters in autotetraploids based on $4x$-$2x$ and $4x$-$4x$ matings. Heredity 49:331–335
53. Haynes KG, Douches DS (1993) Estimation of the coefficient of double reduction in the cultivated tetraploid potato. Theor Appl Genet 85:857–862
54. Brouwer DJ, Osborn TC (1997) Molecular marker analysis of the approach to homozygosity by selfing diploid alfalfa. Crop Sci 37: 1326–1330
55. Rowe DE, Hill RR (1984) Theoretical improvement of autotetraploid crops: interpopulation and intrapopulation selection. USDA Tech Bull No. 1689: 32 pp****

56. Wricke G, Weber WE (1986) Quantitative genetics and selection in plant breeding. Walter de Gruyter and Co., Berlin
57. Wu KK, Burnquist W, Sorrells ME et al (1992) The detection and estimation of linkage in polyploids using single-dose restriction fragments. Theor Appl Genet 83:294–300
58. Yu KF, Pauls KP (1993) Segregation of random amplified polymorphic DNA markers and strategies for molecular mapping in tetraploid alfafa. Genome 36:844–851
59. da Silva J, Sorrells ME, Burnquist WL et al (1995) RFLP linkage map and genome analysis of *Saccharum spontaneum*. Genome 36:782–791
60. Grivet L, D'Hont A, Roques D et al (1996) RFLP mapping in cultivated sugarcane (*Saccha-rum* spp.): genome organization in a highly polyploid and aneuploid interspecific hybrid. Genetics 142:987–1000
61. Meyer RC, Milbourne D, Hackett CA et al (1998) Linkage analysis in tetraploid potato and association of markers with quantitative resistance to late blight (*Phytophthora infestans*). Mol Gen Genet 259:150–160
62. Hoarau JY, Offmann B, D'Hont A et al (2001) Genetic dissection of a modern sugarcane cultivar (*Saccharum* spp.). I. Genome mapping with AFLP markers. Theor Appl Genet 103:84–97
63. Rajapakse S, Byrne DH, Zhang L et al (2001) Two genetic linkage maps of tetraploid roses. Theor Appl Genet 103:575–583
64. Kam-Morgan LNW, Gill BS, Muthukrishnan S (1989) DNA restriction fragment length polymorphisms: a strategy for genetic mapping of D genome of wheat. Genome 32:724–732
65. O'Donoughue LS (1992) An RFLP-based map of oat on a cross between two diploid taxa (*Avena atlantica* × *A. hirtula*) Genome 35:765–771
66. Doerge RW, Craig BA (2000) Model selection for quantitative trait locus analysis in polyploids. Proc Natl Acad Sci USA 97:7951–7956
67. Satagopan JM, Yandell YS, Newton MA et al (1996) A Bayesian approach to detect quantitative trait loci using Markov chain Monte Carlo. Genetics 144:805–816
68. Sillanpaa MJ, Arjas E (1999) Bayesian mapping of multiple quantitative trait loci from incomplete outbred offspring data. Genetics 151:1605–1619
69. Xu SZ, Yi NJ (2000) Mixed model analysis of quantitative trait loci. Proc Natl Acad Sci USA 97:14542–14547
70. Dempster AP, Laird NM, Rubin DB (1977) Maximum likelihood from incomplete data via EM algorithm. J Roy Stat Soc Ser B 39:1–38
71. Meng XL, Rubin DB (1993) Maximum likelihood estimation via the ECM algorithm—A general framework. Biometrika 80:267–278
72. Carlin BP, Louis TA (1998) Bayes and empirical byes methods for data analysis. Chapman and Hall, London
73. Wu RL, Ma CX, Painter I et al (2002) Simultaneous maximum likelihood estimation of linkage and linkage phases in outcrossing species. Theor Pop Biol 61:349–363
74. Khawaja HIT, Ellis JR, Sybenga J (1995) Cytogenetics of natural autohexaploid *Lathyrus palustris*. Genome 38:827–831
75. Sybenga A (1995) Meiotic pairing in autohexaploid Lathyrus: a mathematical model. Heredity 75:343–350
76. Rieseberg LH, Linder CR (1999) Hybrid classification: insights from genetic map-based studies of experimental hybrids. Ecology 80:361–370
77. Wu RL, Zeng Z-B, McKeand SE et al (2000) The case for molecular mapping in forest tree breeding. Plant Breed Rev 19:41–67
78. Solti DE, Riesberg LH (1986) Autopolyploidy in *Tolmeica menziesii* (*Saxifragaceae*): genetic insight from enzyme electrophoresis. Am J Bot 73:310–318

Part IV

Case Studies

Chapter 14

eQTL

Lun Li, Xianghua Zhang, and Hongyu Zhao

Abstract

The goal of mapping expression quantitative trait loci (eQTLs) is to identify genomic regions regulating gene expression traits, which can be gathered through microarrays, RNA-Seq, or related methods. Because thousands of expression traits are analyzed simultaneously, eQTL analysis can help elucidate regulatory networks and provide valuable insights into the molecular mechanisms underlying complex traits. Numerous eQTL studies have been conducted to delineate regulatory networks in various organisms, and they have led to many significant findings. In this chapter, we provide a step-by-step protocol for genome-wide eQTL mapping and downstream analysis.

Key words: Coexpression network, eQTL, Microarray, Multiple-marker test, Single nucleotide polymorphism, Single-marker test, Systems biology

1. Introduction

Quantitative trait locus (QTL) mapping methods have been widely applied to various species to identify chromosomal regions and genetic variants affecting a wide range of traits, and these efforts have led to the discoveries of variants associated with many phenotypes, such as hair colors, height, and lipid levels (1–3). With the advance of microarray technologies, the expression levels of tens of thousands of genes can be measured simultaneously, and the genomic regions regulating these expression levels can be detected in the same manner as traditional QTL mapping. In this context, the genetic loci associated with the expression traits are termed eQTLs (expression quantitative trait loci). Recently, eQTL studies have been performed in numerous species ranging from model organisms to humans (4–6) to reveal gene expression regulation networks. Because a large set of genes are analyzed systematically, it is informative for pathway and network analysis. Moreover, it can provide great insight into molecular mechanisms underlying complex traits and has been found to be a valuable source of

Scott A. Rifkin (ed.), *Quantitative Trait Loci (QTL): Methods and Protocols*, Methods in Molecular Biology, vol. 871,
DOI 10.1007/978-1-61779-785-9_14, © Springer Science+Business Media New York 2012

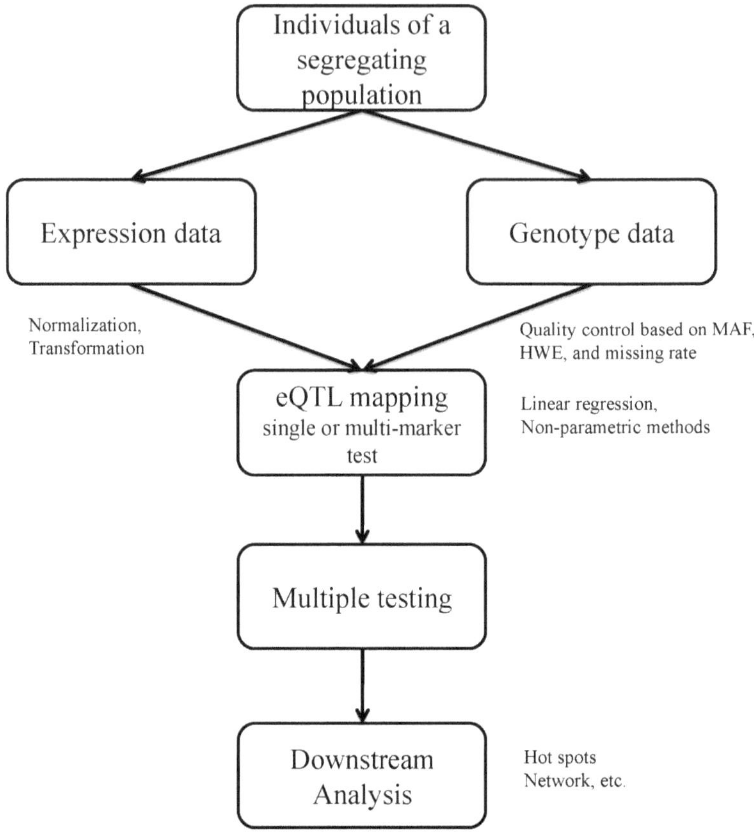

Fig. 1. Flow chart of eQTL analysis.

information to understand the genetic architecture underlying complex phenotypes compared to traditional genetic analysis solely based on phenotypic traits.

In this chapter, we provide a step-by-step guide for genome-wide eQTL mapping and downstream analysis (Fig. 1). To illustrate the statistical methods employed in such analysis, we use a publicly available eQTL dataset from Hapmap II derived from EBV-transformed B cells (7).

2. Data

Data for genome-wide eQTL mapping analysis consist of high-density SNP genotype data and microarray expression data measured on the same group of individuals in a segregating population. It is conceivable that, in the future, sequencing methods will replace microarrays to both quantify gene expression levels and infer genotypes. We focus on microarray data in this chapter and note that the general analysis principle applies to the sequencing data as well. Usually, the sample size for eQTL studies varies from tens to hundreds. The power of identifying *trans*-eQTLs depends on the allele frequencies and effect size (8) and a larger sample size (>200) is normally required (9). In this chapter, we use a publicly available eQTL dataset from HapMap to illustrate the analysis methods. For this dataset, expression profiling was performed on EBV-transformed B cells in 270 individuals, and their genotypes were collected through HapMap II with Illumina HumanRef-6 v1 Expression BeadChips (7). The expression data can be downloaded from GEO (GSE6536), and the phase II HapMap data together with SNP annotations can be downloaded from the HapMap Website (10). This expression dataset has a total of 47,297 probes and the expression levels have already been normalized. The phase II HapMap genotype data contain nearly four million markers. The gene annotation file can be downloaded from Refseq.

Throughout this chapter, a relatively small sample set, comprising 60 unrelated Caucasian individuals, is used for illustration purpose. We note that it would be desirable to have a larger size of samples for eQTL analysis if resources are available to obtain them. As for gene expression data, only the top 25% most differentially expressed transcripts (10,048 in total) are analyzed. We consider genetic markers on the 22 autosomes.

2.1. Expression Data

Microarray data need be normalized first to correct for potential biases due to systematic variations in microarray experiments, so that the expression levels of different samples are comparable. Quantile-normalization is a robust, fast and commonly used normalization procedure. This method orders probe intensities per sample and then replaces the intensity by the mean of measurements at that rank in all the samples (11). This normalization method can be easily conducted by the "normalize.quantiles" function in the Bioconductor "Affy" package (12). Depending on the methods applied to the eQTL dataset, additional normalization steps may be necessary. For example, the expression data in the sample dataset have been quantile-normalized, but a large number of outliers are still observed. If linear regression is applied in eQTL mapping, these outliers could lead to false positives or negatives results (13). In this case, the expression data need be further transformed to ensure the normality (14). For example, the expression levels for transcript i across the individuals can be transformed through the following steps: first the mean μ_i and variance σ_i^2 are calculated across all the individuals for this transcript, and then the j-th observation is replaced by the $r_j/(n + 1)$ quantile of $N(\mu_i, \sigma_i^2)$, where r_j is the rank of this observation and n is the total number of observations. This procedure will ensure that the expression data follow a normal distribution with their mean and variance the same as those in the original observations.

Table 1
Example of a PED file containing two SNPs

NA06985	NA06985	0	0	2	1	C	C	G	G
NA06993	NA06993	0	0	2	1	C	C	G	G
NA11995	NA11995	0	0	2	1	0	0	G	G

2.2. Genotype Data

Genotype data should be pre-processed with a rigorous quality control (QC) process to ensure that the called genotypes are of high quality in order to avoid false positives due to genotyping errors. First, samples with a large proportion of untyped SNPs should be removed (e.g., more than 5%) as the DNA of these samples may be of low quality. Then the missing rate of each SNP needs to be calculated based on the remaining samples, and SNPs with a relatively large missing rate (e.g., 5%) need to be filtered out because there may be many uncertainties for the called genotypes of these SNPs. Thereafter, SNPs whose genotype frequencies do not follow the Hardy–Weinberg equilibrium (e.g., HWE p-value <0.001) need to be removed because empirical data have suggested that large deviations of genotype frequencies from HWE probably mostly likely result from genotyping errors. Finally, SNPs with minor allele frequencies (MAF) less than a prespecified threshold (e.g., 0.05) are discarded from further analysis, since statistical power of SNPs with low MAF is not sufficient for detecting eQTLs and genotyping errors are more likely to occur for low MAF SNPs.

In our analysis presented here, QC is performed using PLINK (15), which can process large-scale genotyping data rapidly and filter the SNPs based on the above criteria. PLINK requires a special white-space (space or tab) delimited format for genotype and SNPs annotation files, referred as to PED and MAP files, respectively. In PED files, the first six columns are required (Table 1): family ID (FID), individual ID (IID), parental ID, maternal ID, sex, and phenotype. For the data consisting of only unrelated individuals, FIDs are set equal to IIDs, and both paternal and maternal IDs are set as missing, by default 0. In the fifth column, 1 stands for male, 2 for female and otherwise unknown. The sixth column is the phenotype column in the PED file. If more than one phenotype is to be analyzed, an alternative phenotype file needs to be specified (discussed later). Starting from the seventh column, every two columns represent the biallelic genotypes of a marker. The genotypes can be coded as any letters or numbers defined by users (e.g., A, C, G, T or 1, 2, 3, 4). A missing genotype is represented by "0" by default, and if the genotype of a marker is untyped, both of the alleles must be "0" in the PED file.

Table 2
Example of SNPs annotation file in PLINK format (referred to as MAP file)

Chromosome	SNP ID	Genetic distance	Position
1	rs123456	0	1234555
1	rs4030303	0	72434
1	rs4030300	0	72515

A SNP annotation file (MAP file) is required in PLINK together with a PED file. MAP files are also while-space delimited, in which each line represents a single marker and contains four columns (Table 2). Genetic distance may not be necessary and can be set as zeros. The markers in the MAP file should follow the same order as in the PED file. Here, the PED and MAP files are named as "ceu.ped" and "ceu.map" respectively.

We use the following command to perform QC.

```
plink --file ceu --mind 0.05 --geno 0.05 --maf 0.05 --
hwe 0.001 --recode --out ceuQC
```

Where the "file" flag is to specify the genotype data, the "mind" and "geno" options are to remove the individuals with at least 5% SNPs untyped and SNPs with larger than 5% missing rate, the "maf" and "hwe" flags are to specify exclusion thresholds for MAF and the Hardy–Weinberg equilibrium, "recode" makes PLINK generate a new dataset (including a PED file and a MAP file), and the "out" option specifies file name for it. In this data set, no individuals are removed and ~190,000 SNPs are left and exported to ceuQC.ped and ceuQC.map.

To avoid false positives due to population stratification, we apply EIGENSTRAT to the new genotype data to detect individuals whose genotypes do not fall into the general population of study and to correct for population stratification (16). EIGENSTRAT is a widely used program for population heterogeneity detection and correction based on principal component analysis (PCA) of the genotype data. And the following command is used, where "-i", "-a" and "-b" parameters specify the genotype file, SNP file and individual file in EIGENSTRAT format or PLINK genotype files, respectively; the number of components to output is set by "-k" option; "-o", "-p", "-e" and "-l" flags are to set the output file of principal components, prefix of output plot files of top two principal components, output file of all eigenvalues, and the log file respectively; and "-m" is to specify the maximum outliers of removal. In this sample dataset, no individuals are reported as outliers.

```
smartpca.perl --i ceuQC.ped -a ceuQC.map -b ceuQC.map -
k 60 -o ceuQC.pca -p ceuQC.plot -e ceuQC.eval -l ceuQC.
log -m 5
```

3. eQTL Mapping

eQTL mapping is to identify the genetic markers affecting expression traits. Many statistical methods are available to test for associations between SNPs and expression traits. The simplest method is to regress each expression trait on each single marker using a linear regression (single-marker test) model. For a pair of transcript *i* and marker *j* in the dataset, this simple model can be denoted as:

$$\Upsilon_{ik} = \alpha_i + \beta_{ij} X_{ik} + \in_{ij},$$

where Υ_{ik} is the expression value, X_{jk} is the genotype data coded as the number of minor alleles (0, 1 or 2) of the *k*-th individual, β_{ij} is the slope of the regression, and $\in_{ij}$ is the error term following $N(0, \sigma^2)$. Based on this regression model, a *p*-value can be derived to indicate the degree of statistical evidence against the null hypothesis $H_0 : \beta_{ij} = 0$. Nonparametric methods such as Spearman rank sum correlation (7, 17) can also be used. They are not sensitive to outliers in the gene expression data but may have reduced power compared when the above model assumption holds. In addition, nonparametric methods can be computationally more intensive for genome-wide eQTL datasets, which usually contain tens of thousands of markers and transcripts and including hundreds of samples.

A number of software packages are available for this association analysis. Among them, PLINK is a free, open source, computationally efficient toolset, developed especially for large-scale data analysis, but only implements parametric methods for association studies. R is a comprehensive statistical program, but it is computationally slow dealing with large-scale datasets. Here, we use PLINK to perform single-marker analysis as an example.

As mentioned in the last section, when more than one phenotype is tested, an alternative phenotype file is needed. Therefore, expression data need to be converted to the PLINK phenotype file format (Table 3), which is also white-space delimited, and requires the first two columns as FIDs and IIDs, and third column onward is the phenotype. The converted file is named as "lcl.pheno".

The association between each pair of marker and transcript is calculated using the *assoc* option of PLINK.

```
plink --file ceuQC --pheno lcl.pheno --all-pheno --
assoc --pfilter 0.01
```

The "pheno" option is for specifying the phenotype file, and the "all-pheno" flag will make PLINK test all the phenotypes listed

Table 3
Example of phenotype file format

FID	IID	GI_21070955-A	GI_4505876-A	GI_23238255-A
NA06985	NA06985	8.624491	9.279807	7.564693
NA06993	NA06993	9.583381	8.374762	8.656823
NA06994	NA06994	9.329642	9.001222	7.913402

Table 4
Result file for plink.GI_4505876_A.qassoc

CHR	SNP	BP	NMISS	BETA	SE	R^2	T	P
1	rs12562034	808311	60	0.2964	0.1104	0.1105	2.685	0.009446
1	rs819980	1510967	58	0.5105	0.1248	0.2302	4.092	0.0001386
1	rs6690515	1532592	60	0.4511	0.1122	0.218	4.021	0.0001697

in the files, and for each phenotype the statistics of all markers tested will be exported to a *qassoc* file(e.g., "plink.GI_4505876-A.qassoc", see Table 4). "pfilter" option is added so that only results with *p*-value smaller than the threshold are reported.

4. Multiple Testing Adjustments

Because more than one billion pairwise comparisons would be performed if every transcript-SNP pair was considered, the multiple testing problem is very severe for eQTL analysis. There may be many false positives if the statistical significance level is not appropriately controlled. There are several methods for accounting for multiple testing. The most straightforward and widely used method is Bonferroni correction, in which *p*-value for each detected eQTL is adjusted by the total number of tests performed in analysis. Bonferroni adjustments can be overly conservative in the context of eQTL mapping, since the tests are not independent due to the correlation structure (linkage disequilibrium) in the genome and correlated expression levels among genes.

Another approach is to calculate the empirical *p*-values through permutations (18). In this procedure, the observed expression levels for each gene expression are permuted 1,000–10,000 times. In each permutation run, the sample labels are shuffled between individuals. Thereafter all the markers are re-tested on the new data and the minimum p-value is recorded. The empirical p-value is the fraction of permutations where the observed p-value is larger than the permuted minimum p-value. In PLINK, permutation p-values can be calculated with the "perm" or "maxT" parameters. Typically, an empirical p-value less than 0.001 is deemed significant, but this cutoff is still arbitrary. To estimate the false discovery rate (FDR) for such a threshold (19), for gene expression trait m, the most significant marker associated is detected and a corresponding permutation p-value p_m is then derived. If a significant threshold of permutation p-value is specified as α, the FDR is denoted as: $\mathrm{FDR} = \frac{M_\alpha}{|m:p_m \leq \alpha|}$.

These permutation-based multiple testing correction approaches are extremely time-consuming. To reduce the computational cost, a common null distribution can be derived by merging test statistics from all the permuted traits (20). In this manner, a large number of tests are conducted (~1 million) for each permutation run, so the empirical null distribution is very stable and three permutation runs are reported to be sufficient to estimate FDR correctly. With a threshold of α, the FDR is defined as the proportion of the average number of significant eQTLs in the permuted datasets to the number of eQTLs identified in the original data.

eQTLs can be categorized as local eQTLs (*cis*-acting) and distal eQTLs (*trans*-acting) based on the distance to the target gene. A *cis*-eQTL is typically within 1 Mb (or less) from the target gene; otherwise, it is a *trans*-eQTL. *cis* and *trans* associations should be corrected for multiple testing separately because the number of tests for *trans* associations is thousands of times more than that for *cis* associations, and more statistical penalties should be put on *trans*-regulations for multiple correction. In this sample dataset, three permutations are done to estimate the null distribution, and then an FDR computation is performed separately for *cis* and *trans* association to estimate the nominal p-value cutoffs with FDR <10%. This results in a threshold of 1.1×10^{-4} for *cis*- and 5×10^{-8} for *trans* eQTLs, respectively.

5. Single-Marker Analysis Results

After multiple testing corrections, 14,086 *cis* associations and 6,644 *trans* associations are detected (Table 5, Fig. 2). Among the top associations, the probe GI_32306519-S corresponding to FLT1 expression (vascular endothelial growth factor), is *trans*-regulated by rs10876864 (chromosome 13:54687352) and GI_18426974-S, the probe for HLA.DQA1 expression (major histocompatibility complex), is *cis*-regulated by rs9272346 (chromosome 6:32713214). As shown in Fig. 3, some loci on the genome regulate a large number of transcripts (termed as hot

Table 5
Summary result when the FDR is controlled to be below 0.1

Category	Significant associations	eSNPs	Transcripts identified	Unique genes
Cis	14,086	13,293	1,062	1,040
Trans	6,644	4,902	718	716

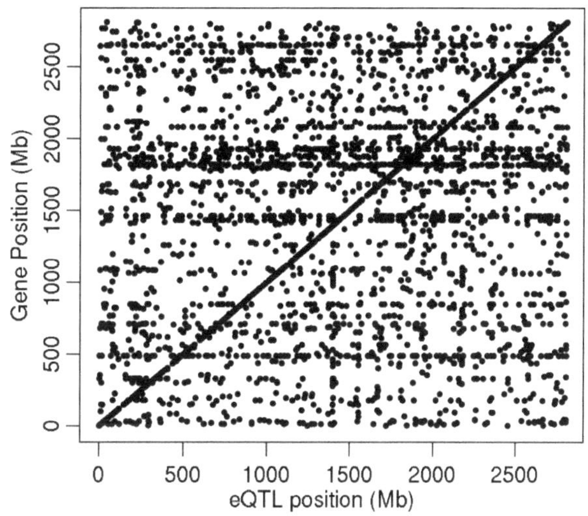

Fig. 2. Genome-wide eQTL mapping. Each *dot* represents a significant eQTL, with the gene position on the *y*-axis and the QTL position on the *x*-axis. The *dots* on the diagonal are the *cis*-eQTLs, otherwise are *trans*.

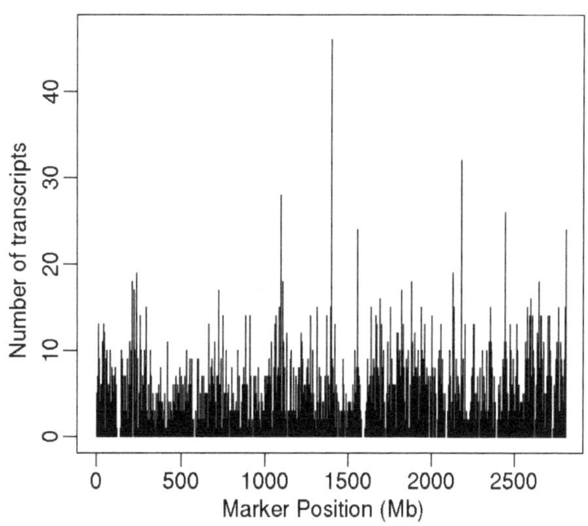

Fig. 3. Histogram of significant eQTLs in a 5 Mb window across the autosomal genome.

spots), for example, the SNP rs1771417 (chromosome 13:97115831) is linked to 29 unique transcripts. In particular, rs4425194 (chromosome 22:47895589) is linked to a group of 14 genes (FOXM1, MCM7, STMN1, DAZAP1, CDC20, CDCA3, KIF11, BRRN1, TRIP, KIF2C, CDCA2, AURKB, MPHOSPH1, HMGB2), and the functional annotation enrichment analysis conducted by DAVID, a popular Web-based functional annotation tool (21), shows that those genes are significantly enriched in biologic processes of cell cycle (GO:0007049) with a p-value of 7.5×10^{-7} and M phase (GO:0000279) with a p-value equal to 3.1×10^{-6}.

6. Coexpression Network

Recent studies have shown that *trans*-eQTLs form hot spots, where expression levels of some genes across the genome show linkage to the same genetic locus. These genes tend to coordinate with each other to perform a shared function and are often expressed simultaneously, called co-expression. Thus, studying the co-expression pattern and their relationships with genotypes at eQTLs is of great interest.

Several methods have been proposed for co-expression analysis. Usually, a gene co-expression network is constructed from microarray gene expression profiles based on some correlation measure. Nodes in the network correspond to genes, and edges with weights between nodes indicate the strength of the coexpression. Coexpression networks can be further divided into gene modules, which are sets of highly correlated genes that form subnetworks.

In the eQTL context, in addition to testing if the modules are enriched for functional annotations, we can also identify *trans*-eQTLs hot spots, which are indicative of coregulation, perhaps by a transcriptional regulator within a hot spot.

Weighted gene coexpression network (WGCN) analysis, a commonly used method in gene expression network analysis, is adopted here to reconstruct the human coexpression network (22) based on the observed expression data. The R package WGCNA provides a set of R functions to perform the analysis based on this method, and it can be downloaded from CRAN (http://cran.r-project.org/web/packages/). WGCN uses a soft-threshold instead of a hard-threshold method to construct the coexpression network and uses topological overlap to detect gene modules, which leads to better performance. In what follows, we give a brief description of the construction process of the WGCN. See ref. (22) for more details.

Initially, the construction of the coexpression network involves the calculation of pair-wise Pearson correlation of all gene pairs to obtain a similarity matrix, the element of which is calculated as:

$$s_{ij} = \mathrm{cor}(x_i, x_j),$$

Here, x_i and x_j are expression profiles of gene i and j, respectively.

Then, an adjacency matrix is obtained by employing a power function to the similarity matrix:

$$a_{ij} = |s_{ij}|^{\beta},$$

The adjacency matrix defines the weighted coexpression network, in which gene i and gene j are linked by an edge with weight a_{ij}. The selection of the power β is based on the scale-free criterion such that the resulting network is approximately scale-free and previous studies have shown that the method is robust to different β. The scale free fitness property of each network given a specific β can be measured by R^2 index, which can be calculated using WGCNA package. Usually, the smallest β giving an R^2 index larger than 0.8 is chosen. In our analysis, the β is set as 8.

The next step is to group highly coexpressed genes into modules, which is equivalent to extracting subnetworks with highly connected nodes from the co-expression network. The adjacency matrix is further transformed into a topological overlap matrix, which captures the direct interaction as well as the indirect interactions through all the other genes between any gene pairs. Hierarchical clustering, combined with a dynamic programming procedure, is used to group genes into modules based on the topological overlap measure.

As mentioned before, coexpressed genes tend to be coregulated and possibly have similar functions. Therefore, genes in the same module are expected to be enriched in some special functional categories and may share the same eQTLs, especially *trans*-eQTLs. Every module is also tested for the enrichment of eQTL-regulated genes using a Fisher's exact test.

In the sample dataset, ~4,000 transcripts with variance larger than 0.1 are used to construct the WGCN, and 17 coexpression modules are detected, among which are 13 modules enriched in *trans*-eQTLs and 12 enriched in *cis*-eQTLs. Among different modules, one module harboring ~30 *trans*-eQTLs are enriched in immune GO terms, such as response to virus, response to biotic stimulus and response to other organisms.

7. Alternative Mapping: Gene Based

Due to the large number of tests in eQTL studies, a single marker, carrying the true regulatory signal, may not pass the multiple testing threshold if its signal is moderate or weak. Therefore, multiple SNPs in a gene region may be jointly considered to enhance the statistical power in association analysis (23–26). The method using the first few principal components is reported to have relatively good performance among other methods (27). For this method, the genotype matrices of genes are obtained by combining the genotypes of SNPs located in or near (e.g., less than 10 kb) the gene. PCA is then applied to genes' genotype matrix, and the components that explain at least 85% of the variation are used in the multiple regression (17) to test the association of the trait and a gene.

For our sample dataset, 984,081 SNPs are mapped to 23,808 known genes based on RefSeq annotations from NCBI, and 18,836 genes containing at least two SNPs are analyzed. Missing values are removed. We use "prompc" function in R to perform PCA. A number of new eQTLs are detected by this method. For example, expression levels of HBE1 (located on chromosome 12, probe GI_28302129-S) is found significantly *trans*-regulated by GABRA5 (located on chromosome 15) with a p-value of 9.73×10^{-25}, whereas no SNPs are found linked to this probe by single-marker mapping methods.

8. Conclusions

In this chapter, we describe a step-by-step protocol for detecting eQTLs and associated module and network analysis. First, careful data pre-processing is needed both for microarray expression and genotype data measured on the same group of individuals from a segregating population. Microarray expression levels should be normalized to adjust systematic variations, and low quality markers and samples need to be filtered out based on a number of filtering criteria, such as missing rate, MAF, and HWE. After data pre-processing, the genomic locations associated with expression traits can be identified using either single-marker or multi-marker analysis. For single-marker tests, the genotypes of a marker are correlated with the expression values of a particular gene using parametric or nonparametric methods, while in multimarker tests, multiple SNPs in a gene region may be jointly considered to enhance the statistical power in association analysis. Due to the large number of tests performed, eQTL mapping analysis needs to have stringent multiple comparison corrections, in which different corrections are made for *cis* and *trans* associations separately. After eQTLs have been detected, downstream analysis may include the detection of eQTL hot spots as well as the correlating the coexpression patterns with these hot spots. In addition, functional annotation enrichment analysis can be conducted to interpret the results. As eQTL data are information rich, many more sophisticated methods (28–30) have been developed to more effectively analyze these data.

Although it is beyond the scope to discuss these methods in detail in this chapter, interested readers can refer to these more advanced papers for the detailed statistical methods.

Acknowledgments

Supported in part by fellowship awards from the China Scholarship Council and NIH grant GM 59507.

References

1. Falchi M, Andrew T, Snieder H, Swaminathan R, Surdulescu G, Spector T (2005) Identification of QTLs for serum lipid levels in a female sib-pair cohort: a novel application to improve the power of two-locus linkage analysis. Hum Mol Genet 14:2971–2979
2. Lettre G, Jackson AU, Gieger C, Schumacher FR, Berndt SI, Sanna S, Eyheramendy S, Voight BF, Butler JL, Guiducci C, Illig T, Hackett R, Heid IM, Jacobs KB, Lyssenko V, Uda M, Boehnke M, Chanock SJ, Groop LC, Hu FB, Isomaa B, Kraft P, Peltonen L, Salomaa V, Schlessinger D, Hunter DJ, Hayes RB, Abecasis GR, Wichmann HE, Mohlke KL, Hirschhorn JN (2008) Identification of ten loci associated with height highlights new biological pathways in human growth. Nat Genet 40:584–591
3. Weedon MN, Lango H, Lindgren CM, Wallace C, Evans DM, Mangino M, Freathy RM, Perry JRB, Stevens S, Hall AS, Samani NJ, Shields B, Prokopenko I, Farrall M, Dominiczak A, Johnson T, Bergmann S, Beckmann JS, Vollenweider P, Waterworth DM, Mooser V, Palmer CNA, Morris AD, Ouwehand WH, Caulfield M, Munroe PB, Hattersley AT, McCarthy MI, Frayling TM (2008) Genome-wide association analysis identifies 20 loci that influence adult height. Nat Genet 40:575–583
4. Brem RB, Yvert G, Clinton R, Kruglyak L (2002) Genetic dissection of transcriptional regulation in budding yeast. Science 296:752–755
5. Morley M, Molony CM, Weber TM, Devlin JL, Ewens KG, Spielman RS, Cheung VG (2004) Genetic analysis of genome-wide variation in human gene expression. Nature 430:743–747
6. Schadt EE, Monks SA, Drake TA, Lusis AJ, Che N, Colinayo V, Ruff TG, Milligan SB, Lamb JR, Cavet G, Linsley PS, Mao M, Stoughton RB, Friend SH (2003) Genetics of gene expression surveyed in maize, mouse and man. Nature 422:297–302
7. Stranger BE, Nica AC, Forrest MS, Dimas A, Bird CP, Beazley C, Ingle CE, Dunning M, Flicek P, Koller D, Montgomery S, Tavare S, Deloukas P, Dermitzakis ET (2007) Population genomics of human gene expression. Nat Genet 39:1217–1224
8. Grundberg E, Kwan T, Pastinen TM (2010) Analysis of the impact of genetic variation on human gene expression. Methods Mol Biol 628:321–339
9. Breitling R, Li Y, Tesson BM, Fu J, Wu C, Wiltshire T, Gerrits A, Bystrykh LV, de Haan G, Su AI, Jansen RC (2008) Genetical genomics: spotlight on QTL hotspots. PLoS Genet 4:e1000232
10. Frazer K, Ballinger D, Cox D, Hinds D, Stuve L, Gibbs R, Belmont J, Boudreau A, Hardenbol P, Leal S, Pasternak S, Wheeler D, Willis T, Yu F, Yang H, Zeng C, Gao Y, Hu H, Hu W, Li C, Lin W, Liu S, Pan H, Tang X, Wang J, Wang W, Yu J, Zhang B, Zhang Q, Zhao H, Zhou J, Gabriel S, Barry R, Blumenstiel B, Camargo A, Defelice M, Faggart M, Goyette M, Gupta S, Moore J, Nguyen H, Onofrio R, Parkin M, Roy J, Stahl E, Winchester E, Ziaugra L, Altshuler D, Shen Y, Yao Z, Huang W, Chu X, He Y, Jin L, Liu Y, Sun W, Wang H, Wang Y, Xiong X, Xu L, Waye M, Tsui S, Xue H, Wong J, Galver L, Fan J, Gunderson K, Murray S, Oliphant A, Chee M, Montpetit A, Chagnon F, Ferretti V, Leboeuf M, Olivier J, Phillips M, Roumy S, Sallée C, Verner A, Hudson T, Kwok P, Cai D, Koboldt D, Miller R, Pawlikowska L, Taillon-Miller P, Xiao M, Tsui L, Mak W, Song Y, Tam P, Nakamura Y, Kawaguchi T, Kitamoto T, Morizono T, Nagashima A, Ohnishi Y, Sekine A, Tanaka T, Tsunoda T, Deloukas P, Bird C, Delgado M, Dermitzakis E, Gwilliam R, Hunt S, Morrison J, Powell D, Stranger B, Whittaker P, Bentley D, Daly M, de Bakker P, Barrett J, Chretien Y, Maller J, McCarroll S, Patterson N, Pe'er I, Price A,

Purcell S, Richter D, Sabeti P, Saxena R, Schaffner S, Sham P, Varilly P, Stein L, Krishnan L, Smith A, Tello-Ruiz M, Thorisson G, Chakravarti A, Chen P, Cutler D, Kashuk C, Lin S, Abecasis G, Guan W, Li Y, Munro H, Qin Z, Thomas D, McVean G, Auton A, Bottolo L, Cardin N, Eyheramendy S, Freeman C, Marchini J, Myers S, Spencer C, Stephens M, Donnelly P, Cardon L, Clarke G, Evans D, Morris A, Weir B, Mullikin J, Sherry S, Feolo M, Skol A, Zhang H, Matsuda I, Fukushima Y, Macer D, Suda E, Rotimi C, Adebamowo C, Ajayi I, Aniagwu T, Marshall P, Nkwodimmah C, Royal C, Leppert M, Dixon M, Peiffer A, Qiu R, Kent A, Kato K, Niikawa N, Adewole I, Knoppers B, Foster M, Clayton E, Watkin J, Muzny D, Nazareth L, Sodergren E, Weinstock G, Yakub I, Birren B, Wilson R, Fulton L, Rogers J, Burton J, Carter N, Clee C, Griffiths M, Jones M, McLay K, Plumb R, Ross M, Sims S, Willey D, Chen Z, Han H, Kang L, Godbout M, Wallenburg J, L'Archevêque P, Bellemare G, Saeki K, An D, Fu H, Li Q, Wang Z, Wang R, Holden A, Brooks L, McEwen J, Guyer M, Wang V, Peterson J, Shi M, Spiegel J, Sung L, Zacharia L, Collins F, Kennedy K, Jamieson R, Stewart J, Consortium IH (2007) A second generation human haplotype map of over 3.1 million SNPs. Nature 449:851–861

11. Bolstad B, Irizarry R, Astrand M, Speed T (2003) A comparison of normalization methods for high density oligonucleotide array data based on variance and bias. Bioinformatics 19:185–193
12. Gentleman RC, Carey VJ, Bates DM, Bolstad B, Dettling M, Dudoit S, Ellis B, Gautier L, Ge Y, Gentry J, Hornik K, Hothorn T, Huber W, Iacus S, Irizarry R, Leisch F, Li C, Maechler M, Rossini AJ, Sawitzki G, Smith C, Smyth G, Tierney L, Yang JY, Zhang J (2004) Bioconductor: open software development for computational biology and bioinformatics. Genome Biol 5:R80
13. Motulsky H, Brown R (2006) Detecting outliers when fitting data with nonlinear regression—a new method based on robust nonlinear regression and the false discovery rate. BMC Bioinformatics 7:123
14. Lai Y, Wu B, Chen L, Zhao H (2004) A statistical method for identifying differential gene-gene co-expression patterns. Bioinformatics 20:3146–3155
15. Purcell S, Neale B, Todd-Brown K, Thomas L, Ferreira M, Bender D, Maller J, Sklar P, de Bakker P, Daly M, Sham P (2007) PLINK: a tool set for whole-genome association and population-based linkage analyses. Am J Hum Genet 81:559–575
16. Kendziorski C, Wang P (2006) A review of statistical methods for expression quantitative trait loci mapping. Mamm Genome 17:509–517
17. Ballard D, Abraham C, Cho J, Zhao H (2010) Pathway analysis comparison using Crohn's disease genome wide association studies. BMC Med Genomics 3:25
18. Churchill G, Doerge R (1994) Empirical threshold values for quantitative trait mapping. Genetics 138:963–971
19. Benjamini Y, Hochberg Y (1995) Controlling the false discovery rate: a practical and powerful approach to multiple testing. J R Stat Soc Series B Stat Methodol 57:289–300
20. Schadt E, Molony C, Chudin E, Hao K, Yang X, Lum P, Kasarskis A, Zhang B, Wang S, Suver C, Zhu J, Millstein J, Sieberts S, Lamb J, GuhaThakurta D, Derry J, Storey J, Avila-Campillo I, Kruger M, Johnson J, Rohl C, van Nas A, Mehrabian M, Drake T, Lusis A, Smith R, Guengerich F, Strom S, Schuetz E, Rushmore T, Ulrich R (2008) Mapping the genetic architecture of gene expression in human liver. PLoS Biol 6:e107
21. da Huang W, Sherman BT, Tan Q, Collins JR, Alvord WG, Roayaei J, Stephens R, Baseler MW, Lane HC, Lempicki RA (2007) The DAVID gene functional classification tool: a novel biological module-centric algorithm to functionally analyze large gene lists. Genome Biol 8:R183
22. Zhang B, Horvath S (2005) A general framework for weighted gene co-expression network analysis. Stat Appl Genet Mol Biol 4: Article17
23. Gauderman W, Murcray C, Gilliland F, Conti D (2007) Testing association between disease and multiple SNPs in a candidate gene. Genet Epidemiol 31:383–395
24. Wang T, Elston R (2007) Improved power by use of a weighted score test for linkage disequilibrium mapping. Am J Hum Genet 80:353–360
25. Wang K, Abbott D (2008) A principal components regression approach to multilocus genetic association studies. Genet Epidemiol 32:108–118
26. Chapman J, Cooper J, Todd J, Clayton D (2003) Detecting disease associations due to linkage disequilibrium using haplotype tags: a class of tests and the determinants of statistical power. Hum Hered 56:18–31
27. Ballard DH, Cho J, Zhao H (2010) Comparisons of multi-marker association methods to detect association between a candidate region and disease. Genet Epidemiol 34:201–212

28. Zhang W, Zhu J, Schadt EE, Liu JS (2010) A Bayesian partition method for detecting pleiotropic and epistatic eQTL modules. PLoS Comput Biol 6:e1000642
29. Veyrieras JB, Kudaravalli S, Kim SY, Dermitzakis ET, Gilad Y, Stephens M, Pritchard JK (2008) High-resolution mapping of expression-QTLs yields insight into human gene regulation. PLoS Genet 4:e1000214
30. Zhu J, Zhang B, Smith EN, Drees B, Brem RB, Kruglyak L, Bumgarner RE, Schadt EE (2008) Integrating large-scale functional genomic data to dissect the complexity of yeast regulatory networks. Nat Genet 40:854–861

Chapter 15

Genetic Mapping of Quantitative Trait Loci for Disease-Related Phenotypes

Marcella Devoto and Mario Falchi

Abstract

Quantitative variation underlies normal as well as pathological traits, and large part of this variability is under the control of genetic loci. Thanks to a better understanding of the extent and nature of human genetic variability and the subsequent availability of an increasing number of genetic markers, genetic mapping of several such quantitative trait loci, or QTLs, has been accomplished in the past 20 years or so using linkage and association analysis in family-based and population-based studies. Rather than alternative, such methods are complementary as each has optimal power of detecting genetic variants underlying variability of quantitative traits under different scenarios defined by the QTL allele frequencies and magnitude of genetic effects. We describe how to apply such analyses to whole-genome or candidate-gene genetic marker data to correlate genetic variability to quantitative trait variability for the purpose of gene mapping and identification.

Key words: Quantitative trait locus, Linkage analysis, Association analysis

1. Introduction

Many traits of medical interest are quantitative rather than binary (affected vs. unaffected). A classic example is obesity, where someone is defined as obese when his or her body mass index (BMI), measured as (weight in kg)/(height in m)^2, exceeds the value of 30. In other cases, quantitative traits are used to measure risk factors for medical conditions, such as blood pressure in cardiovascular disease or bone mineral density in osteoporosis. For many such traits, a large part of the variability among individuals is attributable to underlying genetic variation (1). Evidence suggests that, for the purpose of gene mapping and identification, greater power is achieved by treating a quantitative trait as a continuous variable rather than classifying individuals into discrete categories identified by often arbitrary cutoffs (2). The identification of genes

Scott A. Rifkin (ed.), *Quantitative Trait Loci (QTL): Methods and Protocols*, Methods in Molecular Biology, vol. 871,
DOI 10.1007/978-1-61779-785-9_15, © Springer Science+Business Media New York 2012

controlling such quantitative traits is relevant not only to the trait itself, but also potentially to the correlated disease, as the same genes underlying normal variation may have genetic risk alleles directly involved in susceptibility to the disease. Furthermore, understanding the mechanisms underlying the quantitative trait distribution and variability may also clarify the disease risk mechanism and its causes, and possibly identify new treatments and therapies.

Gene identification for quantitative traits in humans traditionally follows the same positional cloning or candidate-gene approaches utilized in the study of disease (binary) phenotypes (3). Typically pedigrees are collected where the trait can be measured in order to perform a linkage analysis to identify candidate loci, in this case quantitative trait loci (QTLs). Given the limited resolution of linkage analysis, it is often necessary to follow this with fine mapping through an association study of markers located in the critical regions, possibly using family-based association tests in the same pedigrees utilized in the linkage study. Variants of candidate genes can also be studied directly for association to a quantitative trait in unrelated individuals using the measured genotype approach: comparing means of the trait in groups of subjects defined by the genotypes at the markers of interest. With the advent of the high-density SNP genotyping arrays, unbiased genome-wide association studies (GWAS) in large cohorts of unrelated individuals have become the standard approach to identify common variants responsible for variation of complex genetic traits, including quantitative traits. As more and more of these traits are studied with this approach, it is becoming evident that the common variants that can be directly identified by the standard GWAS only explain a small fraction of their so-called narrow-sense heritability (the proportion of their variance that can be attributed to additive genetic factors) (4). The expectation is that deep sequencing of candidate chromosomal regions identified by linkage or GWAS will provide a more exhaustive representation of the genetic variation underlying variation of quantitative traits. Until the more extensive whole-exome or whole-genome sequencing approaches become widely available, targeted deep sequencing following gene mapping by linkage or association analysis will still be a valuable approach for identifying genetic variation underlying variation of quantitative traits.

Linkage and association analyses are complementary approaches that can help identify genetic variants with different characteristics with respect to their allelic frequencies and effects on trait variability. In fact, it has been shown both by theoretical studies as well as applications of these methods that linkage has most power to detect rare variants of large effect on trait variation, whereas association is more valuable in the identification of more common variants with small effects (5). Since both types of variants are likely to contribute to the genetic architecture of all human traits, there is value in applying both types of analyses when the appropriate genetic data are available.

In this chapter, we will describe the steps that may be involved in the statistical analysis of studies aimed at identifying genetic variants responsible for variability of a disease-related quantitative trait. Specifically, the work we will describe includes a linkage and linkage disequilibrium study and a GWAS. Although not all similar studies will necessarily involve all the same steps, and some may involve different ones, the studies outlined below are fairly typical examples of how to carry out a gene mapping study for a human disease-related quantitative trait.

2. Data and Methods

2.1. Linkage Analysis and Fine Mapping by Family-Based Linkage Disequilibrium Analysis

2.1.1. Experimental Data

Data Format and Input Files for Statistical Analysis

In the following section, we will explain how one can perform a quantitative trait (QT) linkage analysis using the software Merlin (6) and test for linkage disequilibrium (LD) between markers in a candidate region and a QT using the software QTDT (7), in addition to other support software. Both Merlin (http://www.sph.umich.edu/csg/abecasis/Merlin/) and QTDT (http://www.sph.umich.edu/csg/abecasis/QTDT) are available for free download and run under several operating systems. We will assume they are run in a DOS Command Prompt window on a PC, but the commands are identical under all operating systems. All the commands that we will illustrate are run by simply typing them at the prompt, provided that the input files reside in the same directory that is opened at the prompt and the program executables have been properly installed so that they can be accessed from that same directory. There are many more commands for both Merlin and QTDT than the ones described here, and the reader is encouraged to consult the software web pages for more detailed description and updates.

Data for linkage analysis usually come in the form of phenotype (s) on the trait(s) under study and genotypes for multiple markers in related individuals from one or more families. In some cases, a single extended pedigree may be large enough to provide sufficient statistical power to find linkage (see Note 1); in most cases, however, a dataset will include multiple families independent from each other. The structure and size of each family will vary, but at the least will be comprised of one sibpair with or without parents. Also note that there is some limit in the size of families (number of family members) that Merlin can analyze and this is defined by the bit size of the pedigree, or twice the number of individuals with ancestors in the pedigree minus the number of pedigree founders. The default bit size for Merlin is 24, and larger pedigree will be skipped unless this can be increased.

Most analysis software used in linkage and association analysis, including Merlin and QTDT, expect phenotype information and genotype data for each individual in each family to be included in a file with a specific format, usually referred to as the *ped* file. The ped file is a text file that contains one row of data for each individual in the dataset (see Note 2). The first five columns of the ped file have a fixed format and must include the following items, one after the other and separated by at least one space, for each individual in each pedigree:

```
Pedigree ID (must be different for each pedigree)
Individual ID (must be different for each person in the
same pedigree)
Father ID (0 if person is a founder, i.e. his/her par-
ents are not included in pedigree)
Mother ID (0 if person is a founder, i.e. his/her par-
ents are not included in pedigree)
Sex (1 = male, 2 = female)
```

The next columns contain phenotype data (traits and covariates) and marker genotype data for that individual, and do not need to be in any specific order. Phenotypes for quantitative traits and covariates are entered as their numeric values. The default missing value codes for Merlin and QTDT are –99.999 or *x*. Marker genotypes are generally coded as 1 1, 1 2, 2 2, for homozygous for first allele, heterozygous, and homozygous for second allele in the case of biallelic SNPs, respectively, and 0 0 if missing.

Additional input data necessary for analysis using Merlin and QTDT are in the form of a so-called *dat* file. The dat file contains a list of all the traits, markers, and covariates included in the ped file, in the same order in which they are in the ped file. Quantitative traits are preceded by T, covariates by C, and genetic markers such as SNPs or microsatellites are preceded by M. In addition to the ped and dat file, Merlin (but not QTDT) also needs a so-called *map* file to be able to perform a multipoint linkage analysis using the correct marker map information. The map file contains as many rows as there are markers to be included in the analysis (these are not necessarily all the markers in the ped and dat files), and each row contains the chromosome number, the marker name, and its genetic map position. For very dense SNP maps, where a genetic map position is often not available, a useful albeit rough approximation to the genetic map position in cM is given by the markers' physical map position in base pairs divided by one million. Marker map positions that can be used in linkage analysis are usually provided by the same companies that develop the marker set or array for genotyping (see Note 3). Finally, if the sample size is not large enough to allow reliable allele frequency estimation from the genotyping data, a file specifying the expected marker allele frequencies in the general population should be provided when using Merlin (see Note 4). For most markers, these could be retrieved in public databases such as HapMap (http://hapmap.ncbi.nlm.nih.gov/).

In a genome-wide linkage scan, genotype data on all available individuals are usually grouped by chromosome, so you will have 23 sets of ped, dat, map, and possibly allele frequency files, one for each chromosome. Examples of input files similar to those we are referring to in this section are available with the Merlin and QTDT documentation. Some of the output presented in the following sections was obtained using example files included in the Merlin and QTDT documentation web pages.

Data Quality Control

A fundamental step before carrying out a mapping study is to identify and filter out markers and subjects with insufficient data quality, as they can increase the false positive and false negative rates. Basic statistical tools are used to assess data quality, and the procedures are roughly similar for both linkage and association data. A first simple measure is given by the genotyping call rate by SNP and sample, for the identification of problematic markers and of samples with poor DNA quality, respectively. Typical thresholds are genotyping call rates greater than 95 or 99%. Public databases, such as HapMap for SNPs data, can also be used to check that the observed genotype frequencies are not significantly different from what is expected in a general population sample. Besides accounting for the presence of genotyping errors, filtering on the minor allele frequency (MAF) is recommended for association studies, as the sample size might not be large enough to detect the effect of rare alleles. In linkage analysis, markers with small MAF (<0.10) tend to provide very little information, and if data reduction is necessary (see Note 3), these usually can be safely removed from the dataset.

Deviation from Hardy–Weinberg equilibrium (HWE) gives a further indication of possible genotyping errors. When using family data, the HWE test should be performed using a selected subsample of unrelated individuals (for instance, using the pedigree founders). Finally, family-based designs allow testing for Mendelian inconsistencies. In addition to the identification of putative genotyping errors, interpretation of Mendelian errors helps in the identification of nonpaternities, sample mix-ups, unreported adoption, or twinning. The software Pedstats (8) (http://www.sph.umich.edu/csg/abecasis/PedStats/index.html) (see below for additional details on how to run Pedstats) can be used to identify Mendelian errors, detect departure from HWE test (`--HardyWeinberg option`), remove subjects according to a user-defined threshold on the number of missing genotypes (`--minGenos option`), and evaluate allele frequencies. Maximum likelihood allele frequency estimates can also be obtained with Merlin (`-fm parameter`). More subtle Mendelian inheritance errors can also be detected using the option `--error` in Merlin that compares the recombination frequencies observed in the pedigree with that expected from the genetic map distances.

2.1.2. Statistical Analysis

Trait Distribution

Many methods of linkage analysis for quantitative traits, including the variance component approach discussed here, assume a normal distribution of the trait under study (9). As a first step, it is useful to check this assumption by examining the trait distribution in the available subjects and evaluating whether a transformation of the raw phenotype data may be more appropriate (10). This can be done using any statistical analysis software. Pedstats is a computer software package that has been designed specifically to check the content of input files used in linkage and LD analysis as it takes as input the same ped and dat files that are used by Merlin and QTDT. In addition to some useful format and Mendelian inheritance error checking as described above, Pedstats also calculates statistics on any trait and covariate included in a ped file and its corresponding dat file. In the following examples, we will call these two files pedfile.ped and datfile.dat, respectively, but keep in mind that these names (as well as all other file names we will use, unless otherwise stated) are arbitrary and they can be anything you like. To run Pedstats and produce summary trait statistics, one would enter the following command at the prompt:

```
pedstats -p pedfile.ped -d datfile.dat --pdf
```

The first two parameters (`-p` and `-d`) specify the names of the input files. The `--pdf` option instructs Pedstats to calculate summary statistics from the input files and write them to the output file pedstats.pdf. This file contains a graphic summary of family structure (distribution of pedigrees by number of family members, number of generations, number of founders, and nonfounders); all traits and covariates distribution overall, by sex, and by founder status, in addition to sib-sib plots (Fig. 1); and distribution of marker allele frequencies for all markers (overall, by sex, and by founder status, in addition to proportions of homozygotes and heterozygotes). In the example of Fig. 1, the trait values seem fairly normally distributed, and we may therefore feel data can be analyzed without having to apply any transformation. However, often a more thorough statistical analysis requiring estimates of kurtosis and skewness and a goodness-of-fit test may be necessary to reach any definite conclusion about the trait's distribution and its approximation to the normal distribution.

Estimation of Heritability

The proportion of variance of a QT that can be explained by additive genetic factors is called its narrow-sense heritability. In contrast, its broad-sense heritability includes all possible genetic effects, e.g., dominant variance and polygenic interactions, in addition to the additive variance. The narrow-sense heritability (henceforth referred to simply as heritability) can be estimated from family

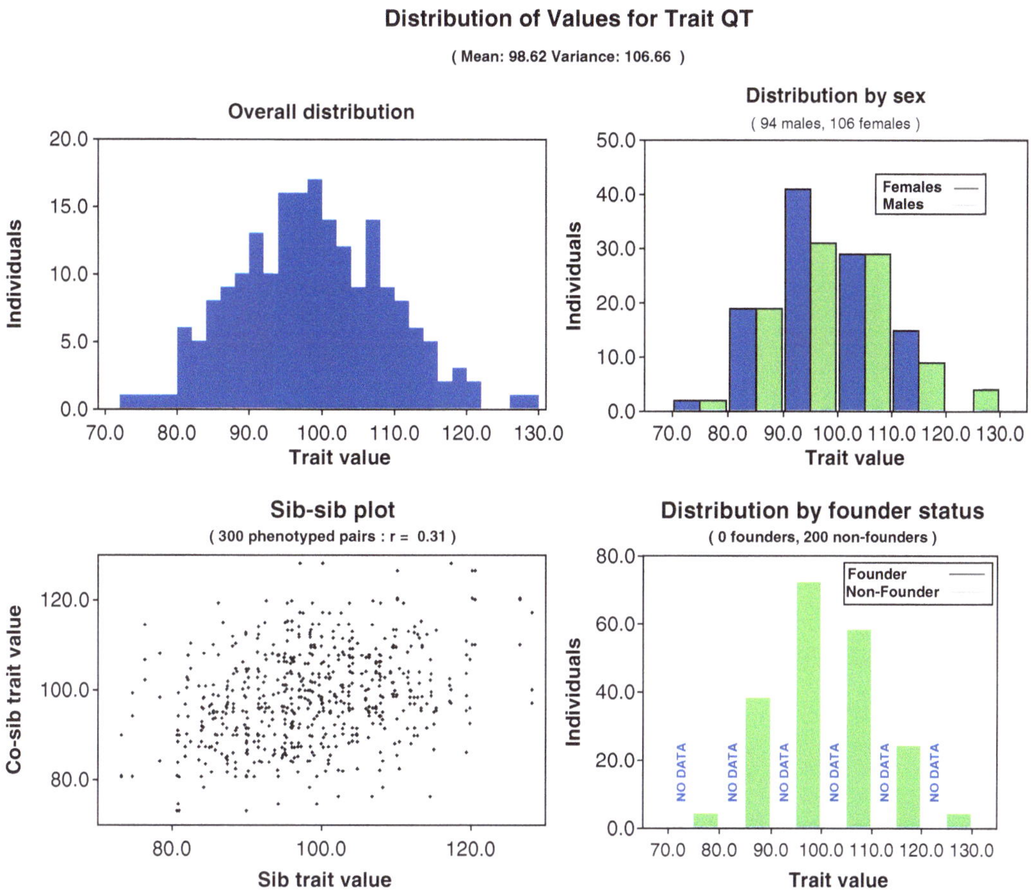

Fig. 1. Pedstats graphical output for quantitative trait summary statistics (pedstats.pdf file obtained with --pdf option).

data within the variance component framework implemented in the software QTDT. It is often useful to obtain an estimate of the heritability as it affects power to detect a QTL by both linkage and LD analysis. To estimate a trait's heritability using QTDT, one needs a ped file with information on pedigree structure and phenotype (trait) data, and a dat file listing the content of the ped file in the format described above. Then one can run QTDT by typing the command:

```
qtdt -p pedfile.ped -d datfile.dat -a- -we -veg
```

As in the previous example with Pedstats, the first two parameters (`-p` and `-d`) specify the names of the input files. The third (`-a-`) tells QTDT that we are not going to run an association test for the time being (association testing is the default in QTDT). The fourth (`-w`) specifies the variance model under the null hypothesis, which in this particular case (`-we`) includes only environmental effects (e). The alternative model is specified with -v, which in this case (`-veg`) includes both environmental (e) and genetic (g) effects. Comparing the two models will thus estimate the significance of genetic effects on variability of the trait, or its heritability.

The screen output of QTDT after issuing this command will look similar to Fig. 2. The bottom part includes the test of significance of genetic effects on the trait QT variability. The test is based on comparing the data likelihood under the null model of environmental effects only and the full (or alternative) model of environmental and genetic effects. The output reports the negative natural logarithm of the likelihood (-LnLk) under the two models (750.25 and 738.86 in this case), and the respective numbers of degrees of freedom (df), which depend on the sample size. The chi-square test at the bottom (with 1 df since there is only one additional parameter in the full model compared to the null one) is twice the difference in -LnLk between the two models. In the example of Fig. 2, there is a highly significant genetic effect on the QT trait variability, with a *p*-value of 2×10^{-6}.

The actual estimate of the heritability can be calculated from the content of the QDTD output file regress.tbl (Fig. 3). For each model (null hypothesis and full hypothesis), regress.tbl will give an estimate of the variance explained by the components included in the model. Under the full model, the two variances are the environmental variance (Ve, or 40.328 in Fig. 3) and the genetic variance (Vg, or 65.803 in Fig. 3). The ratio of Vg to the total variance is an estimate of the trait heritability (65.803/(40.328 + 65.803) = 0.62, or 62% in the example from Fig. 3).

Measuring Effect of Covariates on the QT Distribution

The distribution of many quantitative traits may be affected by variation in other variables, usually referred to as covariates. Typical examples of such covariates are age and sex, which are known to affect variability of almost all quantitative traits in humans. Both QTDT and Merlin allow for inclusion of covariates in the analysis so that their effect on variability of the QT can be properly accounted for. It is also possible, prior to a linkage or association analysis, to evaluate the effect of a covariate on the QT distribution in a dataset using a similar procedure to the one that we have utilized to estimate the QT heritability, even though QTDT does not implement such a test directly. In practice, one needs to estimate the likelihood of the data twice—one with and one without the covariate included in the model—and evaluate whether a model with the covariate fits the observations significantly better than a model without the covariate.

As sex is a variable that is usually present in the data (it is one of the pieces of information that should be included in the ped file), let's start by testing its effect on the QT distribution. For QTDT to

```
QTDT - Quantitative TDT 2.6.1
(c) 1998-2007 Goncalo Abecasis (goncalo@umich.edu)

This program implements tests described by
Abecasis et al, Am J Hum Genet 66:279-292 (2000)
Abecasis et al, Eur J Hum Genet 8:545-551 (2000)
and others

The following parameters are in effect:
           QTDT Data File :         datfile.dat (-dname)
       QTDT Pedigree File :         pedfile.ped (-pname)
     QTDT IBD Status File :            qtdt.ibd (-iname)
       Missing Value Code :             -99.999 (-xname)
               Covariates :                NONE (-c{p|s|u|-})
        Association Model :                NONE (-a[a|d|f|m|o|p|r|t|w|-])
     Full Model Variances :          NON SHARED (-v{e|c|g|n|t|a|d|-})
                          &           POLYGENIC
     Null Model Variances :          NON SHARED (-w{e|c|g|n|t|a|d|-})
  Parent of Origin Effects :                NONE (-o[f|t|m|p|-])
 Monte-Carlo Permutations :                   0 (-m9999)
              Random Seed :              123456 (-r9999)
        Numeric Minimizer :     NELDER AND MEAD (-n[f|n|p])
     Transmission Scoring :       FULL PEDIGREE (-t[n|p])

Additional Options
 --dominance, --snp, --multi-allelic, --deviates, --references,
 --exclude-founder-phenotypes, --p-values, --no-regress-tbl

Online documentation http://www.sph.umich.edu/csg/abecasis/QTDT
Comments, bugs: goncalo@umich.edu

The following models will be evaluated...
  NULL MODEL
     Means = Mu
 Variances = Ve

  FULL MODEL
     Means = Mu
 Variances = Ve + Vg

Testing trait:                               QT
==============================================

 Allele   df(0) -LnLk(0)   df(V) -LnLk(V)   ChiSq       p
    N/A     198   750.25     197   738.86   22.79  2e-006  (200 probands)

Run completed on Mon Sep 13 13:55:49 2010
1 tests carried out

The most significant result refers to:
    Trait: QT
    ChiSq: 22.793
  p-value: 2e-006

Overall Bonferroni significance level: 2e-006
```

Fig. 2. QTDT screen output for estimation of quantitative trait heritability.

```
Trait: QT
================================================================
Total Probands:    200
Family #1 Phenotypes - scores :  80.690  80.955  73.202  90.030

NULL HYPOTHESIS
---------------

Family #1 var-covar matrix terms [1]...[[Vg]]
Family #1 regression matrix...
       [linear] =
        [4 x 1]       Mu
            1.3   1.000
            1.4   1.000
            1.5   1.000
            1.6   1.000

Some useful information...
               df : 198
  log(likelihood) : 741.71
        variances : 130.303
            means :  98.626

FULL HYPOTHESIS
---------------

Family #1 var-covar matrix terms [2]...[[Ve]][[Vg]]
Family #1 regression matrix...
       [linear] =
        [4 x 1]       Mu
            1.3   1.000
            1.4   1.000
            1.5   1.000
            1.6   1.000

Some useful information...
               df : 197
  log(likelihood) : 738.86
        variances :  40.328  65.803
            means :  98.625
```

Fig. 3. QTDT output file regress.tbl for estimation of quantitative trait heritability.

work, we always need to specify a null model and a full model, so we would just run the same command we ran earlier:

```
qtdt -p pedfile.ped -d datfile.dat -a- -we -veg
```

to get an estimate of the likelihood of the data. We will need to use the likelihood including genetic effects, or LnLk(V) = 738.86 in Fig. 2, to correctly account for familial correlation and pedigree structures in the data. Let's now include sex as a covariate using the -c parameter followed by the letter s:

```
qtdt -p pedfile.ped -d datfile.dat -a- -cs -we -veg
```

```
QTDT - Quantitative TDT 2.6.1
(c) 1998-2007 Goncalo Abecasis (goncalo@umich.edu)

This program implements tests described by
Abecasis et al, Am J Hum Genet 66:279-292 (2000)
Abecasis et al, Eur J Hum Genet 8:545-551 (2000)
and others

The following parameters are in effect:
          QTDT Data File :         datfile.dat (-dname)
      QTDT Pedigree File :         pedfile.ped (-pname)
    QTDT IBD Status File :            qtdt.ibd (-iname)
      Missing Value Code :             -99.999 (-xname)
              Covariates :                 SEX (-c{p|s|u|-})
       Association Model :                NONE (-a[a|d|f|m|o|p|r|t|w|-])
    Full Model Variances :          NON SHARED (-v{e|c|g|n|t|a|d|-})
                         &           POLYGENIC
    Null Model Variances :          NON SHARED (-w{e|c|g|n|t|a|d|-})
 Parent of Origin Effects :               NONE (-o[f|t|m|p|-])
 Monte-Carlo Permutations :                  0 (-m9999)
             Random Seed :              123456 (-r9999)
       Numeric Minimizer :    NELDER AND MEAD (-n[f|n|p])
    Transmission Scoring :      FULL PEDIGREE (-t[n|p])

Additional Options
 --dominance, --snp, --multi-allelic, --deviates, --references,
 --exclude-founder-phenotypes, --p-values, --no-regress-tbl

Online documentation http://www.sph.umich.edu/csg/abecasis/QTDT
Comments, bugs: goncalo@umich.edu

The following models will be evaluated...
  NULL MODEL
     Means = Mu + sex
 Variances = Ve

  FULL MODEL
     Means = Mu + sex
 Variances = Ve + Vg

Testing trait:                         QT
=============================================

 Allele   df(0) -LnLk(0)   df(V) -LnLk(V)   ChiSq       p
    N/A     197   750.21     196   738.55   23.33  1e-006  (200 probands)


Run completed on Wed Sep 15 12:15:11 2010
1 tests carried out

The most significant result refers to:
    Trait: QT
    ChiSq: 23.327
  p-value: 1e-006

Overall Bonferroni significance level: 1e-006
```

Fig. 4. QTDT screen output for estimation of quantitative trait heritability with an additional covariate (sex).

If you compare the output in Figs. 2 and 4, you'll notice that sex is now included as a covariate in both the null and full model. This is also reflected in the number of df that are one less (196 vs. 197 for the full model) in Fig. 4 than Fig. 2. However, the likelihoods under the two models are basically identical (-LnLk(V) = 738.55 in Fig. 4

vs. 738.86 in Fig. 2), suggesting that sex has no significant effect on variability of this particular QT.

Let's suppose now we have new data on a covariate, i.e., age, included in the ped and dat files and we want to evaluate its effect on the QT variability. To estimate the likelihood without the covariate, you need to enter the command:

```
qtdt -p pedfile.ped -d datfile.dat -a- -c- -we -veg
```

where the parameter -c- exclude all covariates from the analysis. The output in this case will still be identical to the one in Fig. 2. To estimate the likelihood while accounting for the effect of the covariate, simply type the usual command:

```
qtdt -p pedfile.ped -d datfile.dat -a- -we -veg
```

which in this case will produce an output similar to the one in Fig. 5, with the covariate (AGE in our case) added to both the null and full model. You can now compare the likelihoods under the full for the model without and with the covariate and evaluate whether the second fits the observations significantly better than the first. Specifically, twice the difference between the -LnLk(V) of the model without the covariate and the -LnLk(V) of the model with the covariate has a chi-square distribution with 1 df (since there is only one less df in the model with the covariate compared to the model without it) and can be used to evaluate the difference in goodness-of-fit between the two models. In the example of Fig. 5, the -LnLk(V) of the model that includes AGE is 689.13 with 196 df, compared to 738.86 with 197 df for the model without AGE. The chi-square is thus 99.46 which, with 1 df, is highly significant ($p < 1 \times 10^{-17}$), suggesting a strong effect of the AGE covariate on variation of the QT (see Note 5).

Variance Component Linkage Analysis

In VC linkage analysis, the total trait phenotypic variance is partitioned into components attributable to the effects of the covariates (if available), the effect of the specific locus under scrutiny (the QTL), the residual additive genetic effects, and random environmental effects (which include measurements errors). A test for linkage is carried out by testing whether the QTL variance is significantly different from 0 by comparing the likelihood of this model with that of a restricted model in which the genetic variance at the same location is fixed at 0 (11).

To run VC linkage analysis, Merlin needs a ped, dat, and map file (usually one set for each chromosome in a genome-wide scan) in the format described above. An optional file containing marker allele frequencies can be specified with the option `-f` followed by the file name (see Note 4). Alternatively, allele frequencies can be estimated using maximum likelihood (`-fm`), by counting in founders (`-ff`) or in all individuals (`-fa`, the default), or assumed equal (`-fe`). Unless you have a large sample with

```
QTDT - Quantitative TDT 2.6.1
(c) 1998-2007 Goncalo Abecasis (goncalo@umich.edu)

This program implements tests described by
Abecasis et al, Am J Hum Genet 66:279-292 (2000)
Abecasis et al, Eur J Hum Genet 8:545-551 (2000)
and others

The following parameters are in effect:
          QTDT Data File :         datfile.dat (-dname)
      QTDT Pedigree File :         pedfile.ped (-pname)
    QTDT IBD Status File :           qtdt.ibd (-iname)
      Missing Value Code :            -99.999 (-xname)
              Covariates :      USER SPECIFIED (-c{p|s|u|-})
       Association Model :                NONE (-a[a|d|f|m|o|p|r|t|w|-])
    Full Model Variances :          NON SHARED (-v{e|c|g|n|t|a|d|-})
                         &           POLYGENIC
    Null Model Variances :          NON SHARED (-w{e|c|g|n|t|a|d|-})
 Parent of Origin Effects :               NONE (-o[f|t|m|p|-])
 Monte-Carlo Permutations :                  0 (-m9999)
             Random Seed :              123456 (-r9999)
       Numeric Minimizer :     NELDER AND MEAD (-n[f|n|p])
    Transmission Scoring :       FULL PEDIGREE (-t[n|p])

Additional Options
 --dominance, --snp, --multi-allelic, --deviates, --references,
 --exclude-founder-phenotypes, --p-values, --no-regress-tbl

Online documentation http://www.sph.umich.edu/csg/abecasis/QTDT
Comments, bugs: goncalo@umich.edu

The following models will be evaluated...
  NULL MODEL
     Means = Mu + AGE
 Variances = Ve

  FULL MODEL
     Means = Mu + AGE
 Variances = Ve + Vg

Testing trait:                              QT
=============================================

 Allele   df(0) -LnLk(0)   df(V) -LnLk(V)   ChiSq       p
    N/A     197   713.39     196   689.13   48.51   3e-012  (200 probands)


Run completed on Wed Sep 15 12:58:27 2010
1 tests carried out

The most significant result refers to:
    Trait: QT
    ChiSq: 48.506
  p-value: 3e-012

Overall Bonferroni significance level: 3e-012
```

Fig. 5. QTDT screen output for estimation of quantitative trait heritability with an additional covariate (age).

several typed founders, we recommend using the maximum likelihood procedure, which estimates allele frequencies using all available data, but accounts for the relationship among individuals belonging to the same family.

The command structure for Merlin is very similar to the one of QTDT, so the following command:

```
merlin -p pedfile.ped -d datfile.dat -m mapfile.map -
fm --vc --grid:1
```

will instruct Merlin to read the input files pedfile.ped, datfile.dat, and mapfile.map, estimate marker allele frequencies based on maximum likelihood, run VC linkage analysis (`--vc`), and calculate a lod-score every 1 cM along the marker map (`--grid:1`). In DOS, adding >outfile.out at the end will redirect the output from the screen to a file named outfile.out.

Other format options to consider are `--tabulate`, which generates tables summarizing key results in tab-delimited format, useful to examine results and create plots with programs like Excel; and `--pdf`, which sends output with lod-score plots to the file merlin.pdf (remember to rename this file if you are running multiple sets of input files or it will be overwritten every time you run Merlin again, or specify a different name using the option - -prefix). Options such as these should be typed on the same command line just after the file names, so the command:

```
merlin -p pedfile.ped -d datfile.dat -m mapfile.map -
fm --vc --grid:1 --tabulate --pdf>outfile.out
```

will create three output files: outfile.out (Fig. 6), merlin.pdf (Fig. 7), and merlin-vc-chr99.tbl (where in place of 99, there will be the chromosome number specified in the map file).

Following a summary of the parameters and options available and of those actually used, the bottom part of the outfile.out file in Fig. 6 contains the results of the VC linkage analysis. For each position along the marker map, Merlin reports an estimate of the trait's heritability (H2) explained by a linked locus at that position, the chi-square test of the hypothesis of linkage vs. no linkage at that position, and its corresponding lod-score and *p*-value. Since Merlin also reports an estimate of the trait's overall heritability (H2 = 86.86% in the example of Fig. 6), one can evaluate how much of the overall heritability is explained by a locus linked at any given position. In the example of Fig. 6 (see Note 6), the maximum lod-score is 4.29 at 30 cM, with a *p*-value < 0.00001 and a H2 of 68.49%. Given that the standard threshold for significance in linkage analysis is a lod-score >3, this would be considered significant evidence for a QTL in this position. The file merlin-vc-chr99.tbl will include the same information contained at the bottom of outfile.out in a tab-delimited format useful to import into spreadsheets like Excel to create other graphical output.

By default, VC linkage analysis expects that families are unselected for the trait under study, that is they represent a random sample from the population. However, a single proband

```
MERLIN 1.1.2 - (c) 2000-2007 Goncalo Abecasis

References for this version of Merlin:
   Abecasis et al (2002) Nat Gen 30:97-101        [original citation]
   Fingerlin et al (2004) AJHG 74:432-43          [case selection for association studies]
   Abecasis and Wigginton (2005) AJHG 77:754-67   [ld modeling, parametric analyses]
   Fingerlin et al (2006) Gen Epidemiol 30:384-96 [sex-specific maps]
   Chen and Abecasis (2007) AJHG 81:913-26        [qtl association analysis, qtl simulation]

The following parameters are in effect:
                    Data File :     datfile.dat (-dname)
                Pedigree File :     pedfile.ped (-pname)
           Missing Value Code :         -99.999 (-xname)
                     Map File :     mapfile.map (-mname)
           Allele Frequencies : ALL INDIVIDUALS (-f[a|e|f|m|file])
                  Random Seed :          123456 (-r9999)

Data Analysis Options
         General : --error, --information, --likelihood, --model [param.tbl]
      IBD States : --ibd, --kinship, --matrices, --extended, --select
     NPL Linkage : --npl, --pairs, --qtl, --deviates, --exp
      VC Linkage : --vc [ON], --useCovariates, --ascertainment,
                   --unlinked [0.00]
     Association : --infer, --assoc, --fastAssoc, --filter, --custom [cov.tbl]
     Haplotyping : --best, --sample, --all, --founders, --horizontal
   Recombination : --zero, --one, --two, --three, --singlepoint
       Positions : --steps, --maxStep, --minStep, --grid [10.00], --start, --stop
     LD Clusters : --clusters [], --distance, --rsq, --cfreq
          Limits : --bits [24], --megabytes, --minutes
     Performance : --trim, --noCoupleBits, --swap, --smallSwap
          Output : --quiet, --markerNames, --frequencies, --perFamily,
                   --pdf [ON], --tabulate [ON], --prefix [merlin]
      Simulation : --simulate, --reruns, --save, --trait []

Estimating allele frequencies... [using all genotypes]

Phenotype: QT [VC] (100 families, h2 = 86.86%)
==================================================================
            Position       H2    ChiSq     LOD  pvalue
               0.000   35.68%     3.50    0.76    0.03
              10.000   51.44%     8.83    1.92  0.0015
              20.000   57.37%    12.18    2.65  0.0002
              30.000   68.49%    19.74    4.29 0.00000
              40.000   66.09%    16.79    3.65 0.00002
              50.000   64.70%    11.97    2.60  0.0003
              60.000   58.28%     9.31    2.02  0.0011
              70.000   64.54%    11.40    2.48  0.0004
              80.000   52.02%     7.46    1.62   0.003
              90.000   32.03%     3.13    0.68    0.04
             100.000   19.44%     1.10    0.24    0.15
             110.000   10.50%     0.36    0.08     0.3
             120.000    5.77%     0.12    0.03     0.4
             130.000    0.00%     0.00    0.00     0.5
             140.000    0.00%     0.00    0.00     0.5
             150.000    0.00%     0.00    0.00     0.5
             160.000   13.84%     0.67    0.15     0.2
             170.000   16.53%     0.89    0.19     0.2
             180.000   11.50%     0.45    0.10     0.3
             190.000   20.34%     1.48    0.32    0.11
             200.000   21.12%     1.29    0.28    0.13

Variance component analysis tabulated to [merlin-vc-chr99.tbl]
Graphical output in file [merlin.pdf]
```

Fig. 6. Merlin screen output for variance component linkage analysis of a quantitative trait.

ascertainment correction is available in Merlin through the option `--ascertainment`. Additionally, the effect of covariates may be incorporated in the analysis by use of the `--useCovariates` option (those specified by the letter C in the dat file).

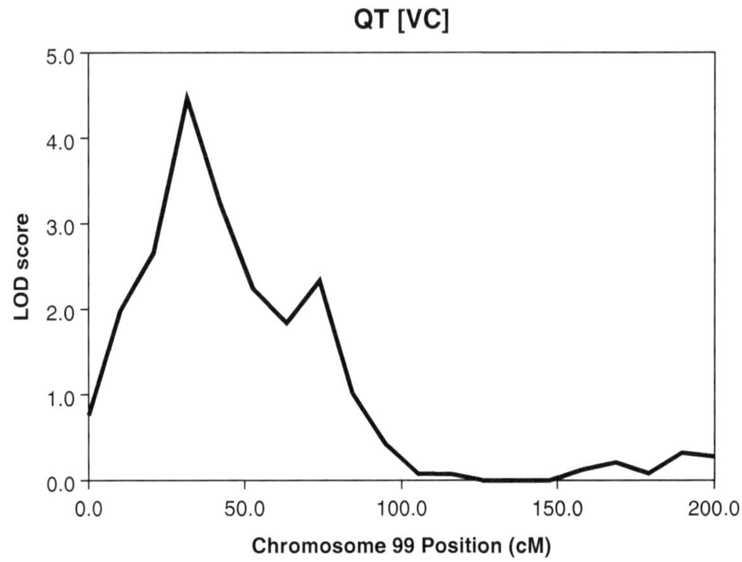

Fig. 7. Merlin graphical output (merlin.ped file) for results of variance component analysis of the QT trait and chromosome 99 marker data.

Critical Region and Fine Mapping by Linkage Disequilibrium Analysis

In classic linkage analysis, significant evidence for linkage to a given locus is achieved when the maximum lod-score is greater than 3. For the purpose of following up the results of a significant linkage study, it is useful to calculate the extent of the critical region—the genomic region that is most likely to contain the quantitative trait gene. One way to do this is by means of a support interval, which is analogous to the confidence interval that would be attached to a parameter's point estimate in classic statistical analysis. According to this method, the critical region is defined by all the points on the marker map that have a lod-score greater than the maximum lod-score minus 3, or those included in the 3-unit support interval (12). With high-density SNP data, which will have a spacing of less than 0.5 cM, the best way is to identify the SNPs corresponding to those points. For more sparse data, one could calculate the lod-score every 1 cM as illustrated above and then identify the critical region by its genetic map position.

In the data used for the analysis reported in Figs. 6 and 7, the 3-unit support interval would cover the genomic region from 6 to 81 cM along the genetic marker map. The large size of this interval clearly illustrates one of the limitations of linkage analysis: its resolution and therefore the precision of the estimate of the putative QTL location is usually poor. Therefore, as a follow-up to the linkage analysis and for the purpose of fine mapping the QTL location, it is often useful to carry out a linkage disequilibrium analysis of markers in the support interval, which may identify a smaller critical region or in some cases even point to a specific gene in the critical region. One way to do this is to use the same data used in the linkage analysis to test for association with the available markers located in the critical region; however, given that LD rarely extends over 100 Kb (which roughly corresponds to 0.1 cM), one will usually need higher density marker data than those needed for linkage analysis in order to carry out a meaningful test of LD.

Family-based tests of QT association can be performed with QTDT within the variance component framework. In order to properly account for the relationship among members of the same family, an additional input file must be created containing the observed identity-by-descent (IBD) sharing among all pairs of relatives in a given family. This can be done using a Merlin option:

```
merlin -p pedfile.ped -d datfile.dat -m mapfile.map --
ibd
```

which will create the file merlin.ibd. For consistency with the other file names, we will rename this file ibdfile.ibd. If you open this file, you will see that for each pair of individuals in each family and each marker, there are three numbers included between 0 and 1, and these represent the probabilities that those two individuals share 0, 1, or 2 alleles IBD at that particular marker. Once you have the merlin.ibd file, the command:

```
qtdt -p pedfile.ped -d datfile.dat -i ibdfile.ibd -
wega -snp
```

will perform the association test and produce an output similar to that in Fig. 8. The option `-snp` will identify the markers as biallelic (if this is the case, but markers with more than two alleles can also be analyzed by QTDT using the default commands) and perform a test of a single allele. Otherwise, the default in QTDT is to test all alleles for association, which in the case of SNPs will produce two identical results. As in previous cases, twice the difference in -LnLk between the null and the full model is a chi-square test with 1 df. In the example of Fig. 8, all three SNPs tested reach nominal significance ($p < 0.05$), and two also pass a Bonferroni correction for the number of SNPs tested (three tests, $p < 0.017$).

In genetic association studies, false positive rates increase if a sample contains subjects from more than one population that differ in the trait distribution and marker allele frequencies, a phenomenon referred to as population stratification or substructure (13). In the test we have applied (the so-called orthogonal test, the default in QTDT) association is modeled by the "within" families (W) component of the mean. The "between" families (B) component allows for different means in different families and thus for the possible presence of population stratification. This test is thus robust to population stratification and it is the preferred test whenever one suspects that this may be present. There are, however, other tests implemented in QTDT that do not account for population stratification, but may be more powerful than the orthogonal

```
QTDT - Quantitative TDT 2.6.1
(c) 1998-2007 Goncalo Abecasis (goncalo@umich.edu)

This program implements tests described by
Abecasis et al, Am J Hum Genet 66:279-292 (2000)
Abecasis et al, Eur J Hum Genet 8:545-551 (2000)
and others
The following parameters are in effect:
            QTDT Data File :              sibs.dat (-dname)
        QTDT Pedigree File :              sibs.ped (-pname)
      QTDT IBD Status File :              sibs.ibd (-iname)
        Missing Value Code :               -99.999 (-xname)
                Covariates :        USER SPECIFIED (-c{p|s|u|-})
         Association Model :           ORTHOGONAL (-a[a|d|f|m|o|p|r|t|w|-])
      Full Model Variances :         NOT MODELLED (-v{e|c|g|n|t|a|d|-})
      Null Model Variances :           NON SHARED (-w{e|c|g|n|t|a|d|-})
                           &            POLYGENIC
                           &             ADDITIVE
 Parent of Origin Effects :                  NONE (-o[f|t|m|p|-])
 Monte-Carlo Permutations :                     0 (-m9999)
              Random Seed :                123456 (-r9999)
        Numeric Minimizer :       NELDER AND MEAD (-n[f|n|p])
     Transmission Scoring :        FULL PEDIGREE (-t[n|p])
Additional Options
 --dominance, --snp [ON], --multi-allelic, --deviates, --references,
 --exclude-founder-phenotypes, --p-values, --no-regress-tbl
Online documentation http://www.sph.umich.edu/csg/abecasis/QTDT
Comments, bugs: goncalo@umich.edu

The following models will be evaluated...
  NULL MODEL
     Means = Mu + AGE + B
 Variances = Ve + Vg + Va
  FULL MODEL
     Means = Mu + AGE + B + W
 Variances = Ve + Vg + Va

  Likelihood ratio statistic from Abecasis et al (AJHG, 2000)

Testing trait:                                QT
=============================================
Testing marker:                             SNP1
---------------------------------------------
 Allele   df(0) -LnLk(0)   df(T) -LnLk(T)   ChiSq       p
      2     194   681.22     193   674.58   13.28  0.0003  ( 164/200 probands)
Testing marker:                             SNP2
---------------------------------------------
 Allele   df(0) -LnLk(0)   df(T) -LnLk(T)   ChiSq       p
      2     194   683.68     193   678.30   10.76  0.0010  ( 152/200 probands)
Testing marker:                             SNP3
---------------------------------------------
 Allele   df(0) -LnLk(0)   df(T) -LnLk(T)   ChiSq       p
      1     194   684.99     193   682.61    4.76  0.0291  ( 168/200 probands)

Run completed on Tue Sep 21 16:41:43 2010
3 tests carried out
The most significant result refers to:
    Trait: QT
   Marker: SNP1
   Allele: 2
    ChiSq: 13.285
  p-value: 0.0003

Overall Bonferroni significance level: 0.0008
```

Fig. 8. QTDT screen output for results of orthogonal test of association of a quantitative trait.

test to detect association. Before we apply one of them, it is better to test whether there is any evidence of stratification in the data, and this can be done with the command:

```
qtdt -p pedfile.ped -d datfile.dat -i ibdfile.ibd -ap -
wega -snp
```

This option tests whether there is any evidence for additional components contributing to the mean that can be attributed to a "within" family component. If this is not significant, and there is therefore no evidence for stratification in the data, then one could use the more powerful "total" test of association in place of the "orthogonal" test with the option:

```
qtdt -p pedfile.ped -d datfile.dat -i ibdfile.ibd -at -
wega -snp
```

This test is usually more significant than the orthogonal test in the presence of association, but keep in mind that it is not robust to population stratification and can therefore increase your false positive rate if stratification is in fact present in your data.

2.2. Genome-Wide Association Study of Quantitative Traits in Unrelated Individuals

2.2.1. Experimental Data

Data Format and Input Files for Statistical Analysis

In the last 5 years, GWAS using high-density panels containing several hundred thousand SNPs have become an invaluable tool to detect the effect of common genetic variants on complex traits and disorders (14). GWAS are typically performed in cohorts of unrelated individuals who are classified as cases and controls in the case of a binary trait or have phenotype information at one or more quantitative trait of interest. In the case of a quantitative trait, preliminary data analysis to evaluate the trait distribution, heritability, and the effect of covariates could be performed prior to a GWAS analysis as described above for a linkage study under Subheading 2.1.2 (Subheading "Trait Distribution," "Estimation of Heritability," and "Measuring Effect of Covariates on the QT Distribution"). However, the large amount of data generated for GWAS requires specialized software to perform an association analysis. PLINK (15) is a widely used software package to perform statistical analysis for case–control and population-based association studies and has been specifically designed to deal with large GWAS datasets. PLINK is available for a number of different operating system including MS-DOS, in which case it will be run on a PC in a Command Prompt window in the same way as Merlin or QTDT. The program reads data in a variety of formats, offers a number of options for data handling, can perform a large number of analyses, and is continuously updated. Therefore, we will discuss here some of the main options available to perform a GWAS study for a QT, while the reader is strongly recommended to consult the extensive documentation provided in the program web site (http://pngu.mgh.harvard.edu/~purcell/plink/) for additional information.

The basic input files expected by PLINK are a ped and a map files. The ped file follows the same standard format that has been specified in the linkage section above, with the additional constraint that a single phenotype can be provided in the sixth column of the ped file. Default missing value is −9. Additional phenotypes can be listed using alternative phenotype files with the following information in a single line for each individual:

```
Pedigree ID (FID) Individual ID (IID) Phenotype1 Phenotype2 ... PhenotypeN
```

Phenotypes names can be specified in the first line of the phenotype file:

```
FID IID NamePhenotype1 NamePhenotype2 ... NamePhenotypeN
```

Covariate files can be created following the same rules.

Genotypic data can be provided after the sixth column of the pedigree file or using the same format described for the additional phenotypes and covariates. The markers should be biallelic and can be coded with numbers or letters, except for 0 that is the default missing value.

The map file format is different from the one described for linkage analysis and contains four columns by default, each separated by at least one space:

```
Chromosome, SNP name, Genetic distance (in cM), Physical distance (in base pairs)
```

However, usually PLINK ignores the genetic distance and the information in that column could be replaced by any number.

For the next examples, let's suppose we have two files, qtgwas.ped and qtgwas.map, containing a single QT and GWAS data (see Note 7). By using the PLINK syntax, both files can be read by the program using the `--file qtgwas` option.

Quality Control

Quality control is of vital importance in GWAS given the large amount of data that are usually included in such studies, in terms of both number of samples and genetic markers (16). PLINK produces several quality control statistics, whose results can be used to filter the data in the successive analyses. Call rate can be evaluated using the command:

```
plink --file qtgwas --missing
```

which generates two files, plink.imiss (missingness by individuals) and plink.lmiss (missingness by locus). The additional option `--cluster-missing` generates two files clustering the subjects according to the pattern of missingness that might help identifying potential batch effects.

Allele frequencies are calculated using the command:

```
plink --file qtgwas --freq
```

A measure of the genotype quality can be obtained by checking the concordance of the observed genotype frequencies with publicly available data (i.e., HapMap).

The test for HWE:

```
plink --file qtgwas --hardy
```

generates the plink.hwe file containing the genotypes count, the expected and observed heterozygosity, and the HWE test results (the user can chose between exact and asymptotic test).

Departures from HWE can be determined by genotyping errors or population stratification. However, HWE test is not a precise tool for genotyping quality control, and departure from HWE might be also a signature of true associations. Although a typical threshold for HWE is a $p < 10^{-7}$, given the large number of tests generated with a GWA panel, the threshold might be defined by using the observed distribution of the statistics (see for example ref. (17)).

Sex check can be assessed calculating the observed homozygosity for X chromosome markers:

```
plink --file qtgwas --check-sex
```

If homozygosity estimates are greater than 80%, subjects are classified as male, whereas for estimates under 20%, subjects are classified as a female. These data will be stored in a file named plink.sexcheck. Adding the `--out filename` parameter will generate a new file (with the name specified by "filename") where sex codes are replaced by those estimated using the chromosome X data.

Availability of genome-wide data allows the identification of cryptic relatedness within the sample. This is useful as standard statistical tests of association assume that subjects are unrelated, and their results may not be valid in the presence of cryptic relatedness. The aim is to identify pairs of individuals who look more similar to each other than expected by chance. This check can be performed by estimating the amount of identity-by-descent (IBD) between all pairs of subject in the sample using the command:

```
plink --file qtgwas --genome
```

This will generate the plink.genome file containing for each pair of subjects the probability of their sharing 0, 1, or 2 alleles IBD, the proportion of alleles shared IBD, the identity-by-state (IBS) distance, and a few other statistics. The proportion of alleles shared IBD is evaluated as $P(\text{IBD} = 2) + 0.5{*}P(\text{IBD} = 1)$, and for instance, its expected value is 0.5 between sibs. An additional parameter can be added to reduce the file size by limiting the output to those pairs sharing a minimum proportion of alleles shared IBD by using the `--min number` parameter, for instance `--min 0.05`.

To detect population stratification, we can follow the opposite approach by identifying those pairs of individuals who look more different from each other than expected by chance. For this, we can use the matrix of IBS distances calculated using the `--genome` command. The IBS distance between any pair of individuals is calculated as (IBS2 + 0.5*IBS1)/(SNP pairs) where IBS2 and IBS1 are the number of loci at which the two individuals share two and one alleles identical by state, respectively. The matrix of IBS distances can be used to generate a multidimensional scaling (MDS) plot to allow a visual inspection of population substructure. MDS is a dimensionality reduction technique, similar to principal components analysis, in which points in a high-dimensional space are projected into a lower-dimensional space while approximately preserving the distance between points. MDS allows the detection of meaningful underlying dimensions that explain the observed genetic distance among individuals in the sample. The MDS analysis is performed using the following command:

```
plink --file qtgwas --read-genome plink.genome --
cluster --mds-plot 2
```

where plink.genome is the file that has been generated using the –genome command and 2 is the number of dimensions (or principal components) to be extracted. Distance of our sample from a population of known ancestry can be also assessed, for instance by including in the analysis samples from the HapMap panels. This will allow us to better classify our sample and identify subjects likely to belong to a different ancestry than that self-reported or expected. MDS results will be written in the plink.mds file and can be plotted, for example, using the package for statistical computing R (http://cran.r-project.org/) with the following R commands:

```
mds<-read.table ("plink.mds", header=T)
```

To plot the first two dimensions:

```
plot (mds$C1, mds$C2)
```

Each point in the graph represents an individual, and the two axes are a reduced representation of the IBS matrix in two dimension.

In a homogeneous sample, we expect all the points (subjects) to cluster together. Subjects falling far from the rest of the group, or clustering with reference samples of different ancestry than expected in case we included them in the analysis, should be removed as the presence of individuals with different ancestry in the sample could lead to spurious associations.

Subjects and markers failing the quality control might be removed from the files. The command:

```
plink --file qtgwas --exclude exclusionMRK.txt
```

will eliminate from the files all the markers listed in the exclusionMRK file, while:

```
plink --file qtgwas --remove exclusionSBJ.txt
```

will eliminate from the files all the subjects listed in the exclusionSBJ file.

Alternatively, the user could decide to dynamically filter markers and subjects according to the results of the quality control results. Therefore, adding at the command line the options `--mind value`, `--geno value`, `--maf value`, and/or `--hwe value` will respectively apply a filter, based on the thresholds specified in "value," on the missingness per individuals, missingness per marker, allele frequency, and HWE.

2.2.2. Statistical Analysis

The association test in PLINK is performed by running the command:

Tests of Association

```
plink --file qtgwas --assoc
```

In the case of a quantitative trait, this command will run a regression analysis of our phenotype of interest against the SNPs genotypes recoded according to an additive model. This means that 1/1, 1/2, and 2/2 genotypes will be recoded into a 0, 1, 2 variable that will be used as independent variable in the regression. The `--assoc` command will generate the output file plink.qassoc containing for each SNP the value of the regression coefficient, the r^2 of the regression, the Wald test statistics, and corresponding *p*-value.

In addition to the additive model, which is the most widely used since it partially captures also dominance effects, it is possible to specify other models, such as the `--dominant` and `--recessive` one. Clearly, testing different models will increase the number of tests that should be taken into account when correcting the observed *p*-values for multiple testing. More complex models can be specified which, for instance, consider interactions with covariates, test for genotype–environment interaction, or condition on the genotype of a particular SNP. This latter test allows for conditioning on a variant known to affect the phenotype (thus removing its effect) to facilitate the identification of additional variants.

P-value calculation is based on the standard asymptotic distribution and can be inaccurate if some of the asymptotic theory conditions are not satisfied, for instance, because of the trait distribution, hidden patterns of nonrandom missingness of markers and/or phenotypes, or small sample size. Empirical *p*-values, based on the empirical distribution of the test statistic under the null hypothesis (in this case absence of association), can be more reliable, although their generation can be computationally intensive. Permutations could be used to verify the top identified associations by assessing their empirical significance, adding the `--perm` or the `--mperm` options to the command line.

Permutations will shuffle the phenotypes among subjects at random and evaluate the association test after each shuffling (thus under the hypothesis of no-association) to assess how likely it is to obtain the observed *p*-value by chance. The first option uses an adaptive permutation scheme, which means that once the empirical *p*-value seems stable, the permutations for that SNP will be stopped. The adaptive permutation will quickly discard SNPs with *p*-values above the significance level. Alternatively, using the `--mperm` option, we can specify a fixed number of permutations that will be performed, for instance: `--mperm` 10,000. With this option, all permutations requested will be performed for each SNP regardless of the outcome.

Inclusion of one of the permutation options will generate an extra file: plink.assoc.perm or plink.assoc.mperm, depending on the chosen permutation scheme. The empirical *p*-values will be based on how many times a permuted dataset Wald statistics is equal or bigger than the one observed using the original data.

Results from the association tests can be plotted in different ways for different aims. A commonly used plot to visualize the results is the so-called Manhattan plot, which shows the distribution of the association statistics through the genome, expressed as $-\log_{10}(p\text{-value})$ to facilitate the identification of significant findings, ordered by physical position and using alternative colors to distinguish between different chromosomes (Fig. 9). This plot, as well as a deeper exploration of the results, can be obtained using Haploview (http://www.broadinstitute.org/haploview). Haploview is a Java program (and therefore works with the Java runtime

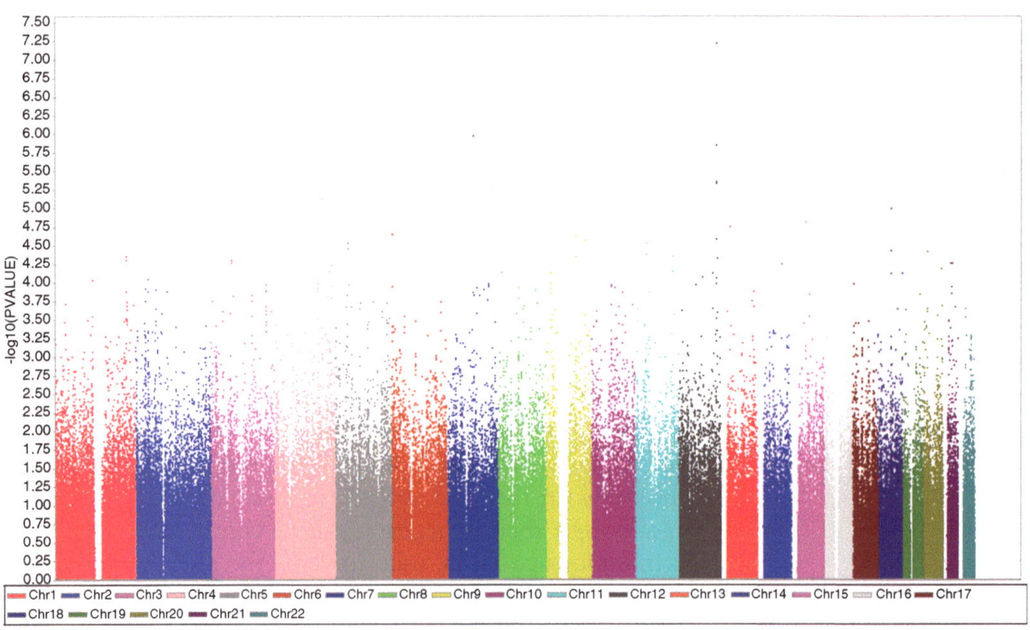

Fig. 9. Manhattan plot of GWAS results obtained from data generated by PLINK imported into Haploview.

environment that should be installed on the PC) that has been specifically designed for haplotype analysis and allows importing results from other programs including PLINK. Result files imported from PLINK (together with the map file to specify their physical position) can be filtered, plotted, and the associated regions can be explored though automatic download of data from the HapMap web site. The program web site includes extensive and clear documentation.

Another kind of plot is the qq-plot, mostly used to inspect the quality of the results. In a qq-plot, the observed statistics are plotted against the values expected under the hypothesis of no association (Fig. 10). The straight line represents the expected statistics under no association, while the dotted line reports what has been obtained from the analysis of our dataset. Association in a dataset should be identified as a few points on the top of the scale lying above the expectation line. If several points fall above the expected statistics line, for instance visualized as a line that suddenly diverges from the expectations as in Fig. 11, we can suspect our tests are globally inflated indicating some problems with the quality of the data.

The input data to obtain a qq-plot can be generated by PLINK by adding the `--adjust --qq-plot` parameters to the association

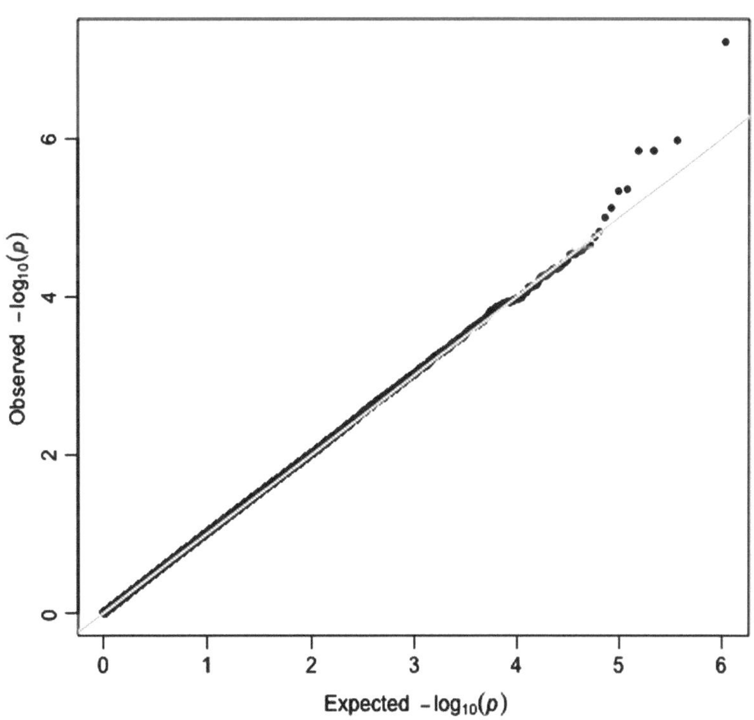

Fig. 10. QQ-plot of GWAS results obtained from data generated by PLINK imported into R.

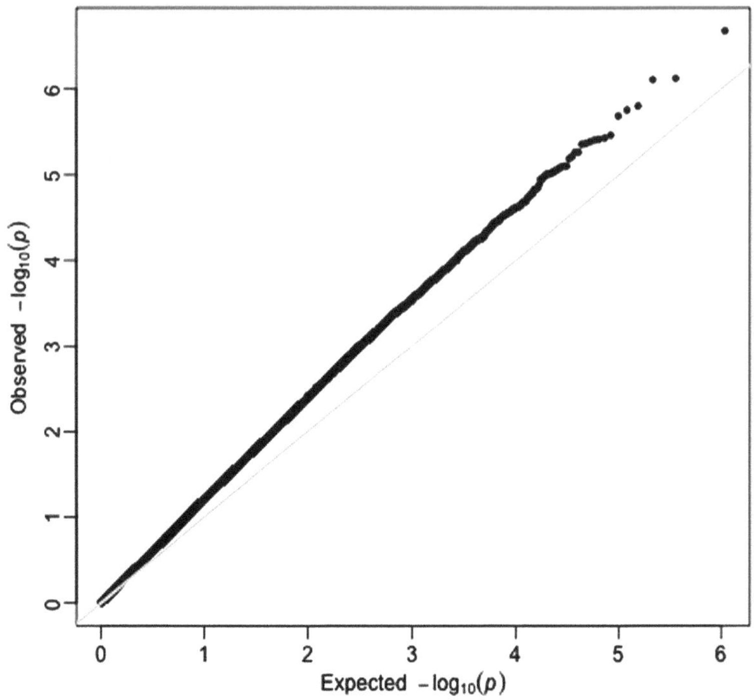

Fig. 11. QQ-plot of GWAS results obtained from data generated by PLINK imported into R showing a significant deviation of observed *p*-values from expectation.

command line. The plink.assoc.adjusted file can then be read in R to generate the qq-plot using the following commands:

```
data <- read.table(file = plink.assoc.adjusted, header = T)
plot(-log(data$QQ, 10), -log(data$UNADJ,10))
abline(a = 0, b = 1)
```

The last command will add the $y = x$ null line to the graph.

In case inflation of the test statistics is detected, we should go back to the quality control steps and try to find out what is causing it. A solution that could be adopted when the inflation is small and its cause cannot be identified and/or removed is to use the genomic control method and apply an overall (and sometimes conservative) correction to the whole set of tests (18). In the genomic control approach, a fixed value, usually the median observed chi squared statistic (which in the case of no systematic inflation is expected to be equal to 1), will be used to correct each test by dividing each test statistic by it. This procedure could be also automatically performed with PLINK adding the `--adjust --gc` options to the command line for association. If the inflation is determined by population stratification, or by any other identifiable factor that could be used to distinguish subgroups within the sample, these subgroups can be defined in a cluster file and the permutation tests conditioned to the cluster structure. A cluster file is defined by specifying for any subject an alphanumeric code, common for all subjects belonging to the same subgroup. The file columns contain the family ID, subject ID, and subgroup code, such as:

```
1 1 A
2 1 B
3 1 A
...
```

Adding the parameter `--within clusterName` will take into account in the association test the cluster structure contained in a file named clusterName.

Correcting Results for Multiple Testing

Increasing the number of tests also increases the probability that a highly significant statistic will appear among our results just by chance. This is obviously a problem in any GWAS where several hundred thousand SNPs are tested for association to the trait of interest. Several methods can be used to correct GWAS results for multiple testing, such as permutation testing, false discovery rate (FDR), Bayesian factor, and Bonferroni correction. When the association test is carried out with PLINK including the parameter `--adjust`, the output file plink.assoc.adjust will contain additional columns with Bonferroni, Holm, Sidak, and FDR corrections. All these corrections are rather conservative and assume that the tests are independent, which is not actually true given the LD structure of dependence among SNPs. The most conservative is the Bonferroni correction, which sets the threshold for significance to alpha/(number of tests). Therefore, if our desired overall significance level alpha is 0.05 and we perform 100,000 tests, after Bonferroni correction the threshold of significance level will be $0.05/100{,}000 = 5 \times 10^{-7}$. An additional option offered by PLINK is permutation testing, which is considered the gold standard for accurate multiple testing correction. Using the `--mperm` parameter, which allows specifying a fixed number of permutations, not only the nominal p-value can be calculated (thus the significance of each single test), but also the genome-wide significance level by taking into account the distribution of all maximum values obtained for all the tests in each permutation cycle. The output file plink.assoc.mperm will contain both values.

While permutation tests are computationally intensive, evaluating the genome-wide correction for multiple testing would require a reduced number of tests if compared with the assessment of the empirical p-value. If N permutations are performed, the smallest adjusted p-value is $1/(N + 1)$. Therefore, 1,000 permutations can potentially generate p-values as small as 0.001, while the genome-wide significance is declared beyond 0.05 or 0.01.

Markers reaching the desired level of significance will be further explored to identify the associated gene or chromosomal region. Resources such as BioMart (http://www.biomart.org) allow retrieving the closest gene to each SNP, the SNP position within the gene (e.g., intronic, exonic, etc.), and several other data that can be requested from the user through generation of dynamic queries. More detailed visual inspection of the region can be performed through Ensembl (http://www.ensembl.org/) or MapViewer (http://www.ncbi.nlm.nih.gov/projects/mapview/). A list of previously associated variants is contained in the Catalog of Published Genome-Wide Association Studies (http://www.genome.gov/26525384). More complex tools integrating data from the literature and public databases can help the often difficult process of mapping the identified association in the context of known genomic features, such as Grail (http://www.broadinstitute.org/mpg/grail/) or WGAViewer (http://people.genome.duke.edu/~dg48/WGAViewer/). An exhaustive list of tools and procedures to interpret the observed genotype–phenotype association are beyond the aims of this chapter, and the reader is referred to the vast literature on this topic (see ref. (19) and http://genepi_toolbox.i-med.ac.at/ for an interactive catalog of bioinformatics resources).

3. Conclusions

As stated at the beginning, the statistical analyses detailed here are just some of the options available for quantitative trait gene mapping, and the commands we illustrated are just a subset of those implemented within the software we have described. Several other useful and important tools should be considered by an investigator interested in genetic mapping, including SNP imputation, which can increase the density of genotyping "in silico" without the need for additional experiments (20); meta-analysis, to combine results from different studies, particularly important given the large sample sizes necessary to detect the small effects expected from common variants on complex traits (21); tests for interactions or epistasis among SNPs (22); pathway analysis, to look for enrichment of association signals in groups of related genes (21). While this chapter cannot be a substitute for papers describing the original methods and for software documentation, or the direct and specific advice of an expert, hopefully the material contained here should be enough to get the reader started on some of the main analyses and stimulate interest in learning more about these statistical approaches to quantitative trait gene mapping.

4. Notes

1. Power calculations help both the design and interpretation of linkage and association studies. The power of a study is the probability of detecting a true effect of a particular magnitude. Different factors influence the power of a QTL mapping study, mainly the sample size, the QTL effect size, the heritability of the trait under study, and the required level of statistical significance. An additional factor in indirect linkage or LD studies is the marker informativity determined by the marker allele frequency, the recombination fraction, and the LD between the marker and the underlying variant. The power of a study can be assessed either by asymptotic approaches or through simulations. Software packages have been developed to facilitate power calculations for quantitative traits, such as Genetic Power Calculator (23) for association with singletons and association and linkage with sibships of different sizes, or POLY (24) and PowQ (25) to assess the power of linkage studies in more general pedigrees.
2. In some cases, individuals need to be included in the ped file for whom data (genotype and phenotype) are not available, in order to correctly identify all relationships among available individuals. To give a simple example, if data are available on two sisters but not on their parents, it will still be necessary to include in the ped file a record (with all data missing) for their father and mother, because this will be the only way to identify the two individuals as being sisters (they are daughters of the same parents). If data were available for one parent only, a record will also need to be included for the other parent, even if that record will include all missing data.
3. Linkage analysis does not need the high-density marker data of common commercial genome-wide SNP panels to detect the recombination events happening in a few generations pedigree. Moreover, the presence of LD among markers has been shown to lead to overestimation of the identical-by-descent (IBD) sharing between pair of subjects, thus introducing some possible bias in the analysis and usually increasing the type 1 error rate (26). Although Merlin integrates an algorithm to cluster markers in LD and use the cluster as a super-marker for IBD estimation (e.g., the `--cluster`, `--rsq`, and `--distance` options), genome-wide SNP data are typically pruned to generate a reduced subset of markers in approximate linkage equilibrium (LE) with each other. The PLINK program described in the GWAS section of this paper provides two commands that can be used to extract SNPs in LE by using either a multiple SNPs (`--indep`) or a pairwise (`--indep-pairwise`) approach.

4. When using Merlin, if marker allele frequencies are available from an external source such as HapMap, an optional input file can be included that contains two lines for each marker. The first line starts with M followed by the name of the marker (as in the corresponding map and dat files); the second line starts with F followed by the allele frequencies for all alleles at that particular marker. For example, for a biallelic SNP named rs00001 with a MAF of 0.3, the frequency file will include the following two lines:

```
M rs00001
F 0.7 0.3
```

This implies that in the pedfile, the most common allele at this SNP is coded "1" and the least common one is coded "2." If this is not the case and alleles were coded as, for example, nucleotides, the following equivalent format may be used if, for the same SNP rs00001, T was the major and C was the minor allele:

```
M rs00001
A T 0.7
A C 0.3
```

In general, after the first line containing the marker name, one can have as many lines starting with A as there are alleles at that particular marker, followed by the allele name and its frequency. Examples of additional formats for the allele frequency file are included in the Merlin documentation.

5. If your files do include one or more covariates, QTDT will always include them in all the analyses unless you specify that they have to be excluded using the parameter `-c-`. However, if you include sex as a covariate using the `-cs` parameter, this will also exclude the other covariates from the analysis (that is only sex will be included even if you have other covariates in the ped and dat files); so to include in your analysis sex and all the covariates present in the input files, you should use the parameter `-csu` for sex (s) and user-specified (u) covariates.

6. In the interest of space, the `--grid` option used to produce the output of Fig. 6 was set to 10, but we do recommend that you set it to 1 or less, depending on the number and spacing of markers. In fact with high-density SNP data, it is often more informative to calculate the lod-scores at each marker position. Since this is the default in Merlin, the way to obtain this is simply not to include the `--grid` option.

7. Since flat text files containing GWA SNP data can be extremely large, PLINK can convert these data in a compact and faster accessible binary format. The basic command to convert from standard to binary format will be:

```
plink --file qtgwas --make-bed
```

which will read the ped and map file and create a binary bed file with genotype information, and two smaller bim and fam file containing information on markers and subjects, respectively.

References

1. Mackay TF (2001) The genetic architecture of quantitative traits. Annu Rev Genet 35:303–339
2. Blangero J (1995) Genetic analysis of a common oligogenic trait with quantitative correlates: summary of GAW9 results. Genet Epidemiol 12:689–706
3. Mackay TF, Stone EA, Ayroles JF (2009) The genetics of quantitative traits: challenges and prospects. Nat Rev Genet 10:565–577
4. Manolio TA, Collins FS, Cox NJ, Goldstein DB, Hindorff LA et al (2009) Finding the missing heritability of complex diseases. Nature 461:747–753
5. Botstein D, Risch N (2003) Discovering genotypes underlying human phenotypes: past successes for Mendelian disease, future approaches for complex disease. Nat Genet 33 (suppl):228–237
6. Abecasis GR, Cherny SS, Cookson WO, Cardon LR (2002) Merlin—rapid analysis of dense genetic maps using sparse gene flow trees. Nat Genet 30:97–101
7. Abecasis GR, Cardon LR, Cookson WO (2000) A general test of association for quantitative traits in nuclear families. Am J Hum Genet 66:279–292
8. Wigginton JE, Abecasis GR (2005) PEDSTATS: descriptive statistics, graphics and quality assessment for gene mapping data. Bioinformatics 21:3445–3447
9. Allison DB, Neale MC, Zannolli R, Schork NJ, Amos CI, Blangero J (1999) Testing the robustness of the likelihood-ratio test in a variance-component quantitative-trait loci-mapping procedure. Am J Hum Genet 65:531–544
10. Etzel CJ, Shete S, Beasley TM, Fernandez JR, Allison DB, Amos CI (2003) Effect of Box-Cox transformation on power of Haseman-Elston and maximum-likelihood variance components tests to detect quantitative trait loci. Hum Hered 55:108–116
11. Blangero J, Williams JT, Almasy L (2001) Variance component methods for detecting complex trait loci. Adv Genet 42:151–181
12. Terwilliger J, Ott J (1994) Handbook of human genetic linkage. The Johns Hopkins University Press, Baltimore
13. Tian C, Gregersen PK, Seldin MF (2008) Accounting for ancestry: population substructure and genome-wide association studies. Hum Mol Genet 17(R2):R143–R150
14. Manolio TA, Brooks LD, Collins FS (2008) A HapMap harvest of insights into the genetics of common disease. J Clin Invest 118:1590–1605
15. Purcell S, Neale B, Todd-Brown K et al (2007) PLINK: a tool set for whole-genome association and population-based linkage analyses. Am J Hum Genet 81:559–575
16. Balding DJ (2006) A tutorial on statistical methods for population association studies. Nat Rev Genet 7:781–791
17. Wellcome Trust Case Control Consortium (2007) Genome-wide association study of 14,000 cases of seven common diseases and 3,000 shared controls. Nature 447:661–678
18. Devlin B, Roeder K (1999) Genomic control for association studies. Biometrics 55:997–1004
19. Coassin S, Brandstätter A, Kronenberg F (2010) Lost in the space of bioinformatic tools: a constantly updated survival guide for genetic epidemiology. The GenEpi Toolbox. Atherosclerosis 209:321–335
20. Browning SR (2008) Missing data imputation and haplotype phase inference for genome-wide association studies. Hum Genet 124:439–450
21. Cantor RM, Lange K, Sinsheimer JS (2010) Prioritizing GWAS results: a review of statistical methods and recommendations for their application. Am J Hum Genet 86:6–22
22. Cordell HJ (2009) Detecting gene-gene interactions that underlie human diseases. Nat Rev Genet 10:392–404
23. Purcell S, Cherny SS, Sham PC (2003) Genetic power calculator: design of linkage and association genetic mapping studies of complex traits. Bioinformatics 19:149–150
24. Chen WM, Abecasis GR (2006) Estimating the power of variance component linkage analysis in large pedigrees. Genet Epidemiol 30:471–484
25. Falchi M, Borlino C (2006) PowQ: a user-friendly package for the design of variance component multipoint linkage analysis studies. Bioinformatics 22:1404–1405
26. Huang Q, Shete S, Amos CI (2004) Ignoring linkage disequilibrium among tightly linked markers induces false-positive evidence of linkage for affected sib pair analysis. Am J Hum Genet 75:1106–1112

Chapter 16

Quantitative Trait Locus Analysis in Haplodiploid Hymenoptera

Jürgen Gadau, Christof Pietsch, and Leo W. Beukeboom

Abstract

This article describes QTL analyses for solitary (*Nasonia*, a parasitoid wasp) and social hymenopteran species (honeybee and bumblebee). These exemplar QTL analyses determined the genetic basis of morphological, behavioral, and colony level traits. Mapping populations were derived either from lab crosses between highly inbred strains (*Nasonia* spp.), lab crosses of individuals caught in the field (bumblebees), or offspring from artificially inseminated queens from a managed honeybee population. Using these examples, we demonstrate the importance of a clear understanding of the life history, breeding, and reproductive system of the organism used for a QTL analysis, e.g., haplo-diploidy or reproductive division of labor in social insects. We lead the reader step by step through the process of multiple QTL analyses and describe potential problems and roadblocks (e.g., data handling, statistical, and biological problems) that can obscure or severely impair the results of a QTL study and how to detect and deal with those problems.

In particular, we provide a way to empirically estimate the Beavis effect for a larger QTL mapping population and how to estimate a more accurate value of the explained phenotypic variance of each detected QTL using a resampling procedure.

Key words: MapQTL, Multipoint, *Nasonia vitripennis*, *Bombus terrestris*, *Apis mellifera*, Haplodiploid sex determination, Colony level traits, Epistasis, Beavis effect

1. Introduction

A quantitative trait locus (QTL) is a genomic region that harbors a locus (coding gene, cis- or trans-regulatory unit, etc.) that explains a significant proportion of the variance in a quantitative trait in a mapping population. QTL analysis is therefore a method to understand the genetic architecture of an observed phenotype and can, if done correctly, reveal the minimum number of loci (QTLs) involved, quantify the amount of explained phenotypic variance per locus, and determine whether multiple loci interact and the direction of the effect of each "allele." Once we know where QTLs are located in a genome, we can narrow down the region of interest

Scott A. Rifkin (ed.), *Quantitative Trait Loci (QTL): Methods and Protocols*, Methods in Molecular Biology, vol. 871, DOI 10.1007/978-1-61779-785-9_16, © Springer Science+Business Media New York 2012

using different methods (e.g., marker-assisted introgression, fine mapping using more markers and more individuals, etc.). However, very few studies have actually gone the whole nine yards, i.e., from phenotype to QTL to gene/s and finally to nucleotide substitution (1).

This article will walk the reader through QTL analyses done in parasitic wasps (*Nasonia* spp.) and two social insects (bumble bees = *Bombus terrestris*; and honeybees = *Apis mellifera*) (2–4). It will in the end touch on some specific techniques that were used in *Nasonia* spp. and the honeybee to go from a phenotype to a candidate gene.

The principles of a QTL analysis are the same no matter whether the focal species of a study is a plant or animal (Fig. 1). However, it is important to understand and modify individual components of a QTL analysis according to the underlying genetic and reproductive system of the organisms and take advantage of any feature of an organism that may interfere positive or negative with a positive outcome of a QTL analysis, e.g., haplo-diploidy in Hymenoptera

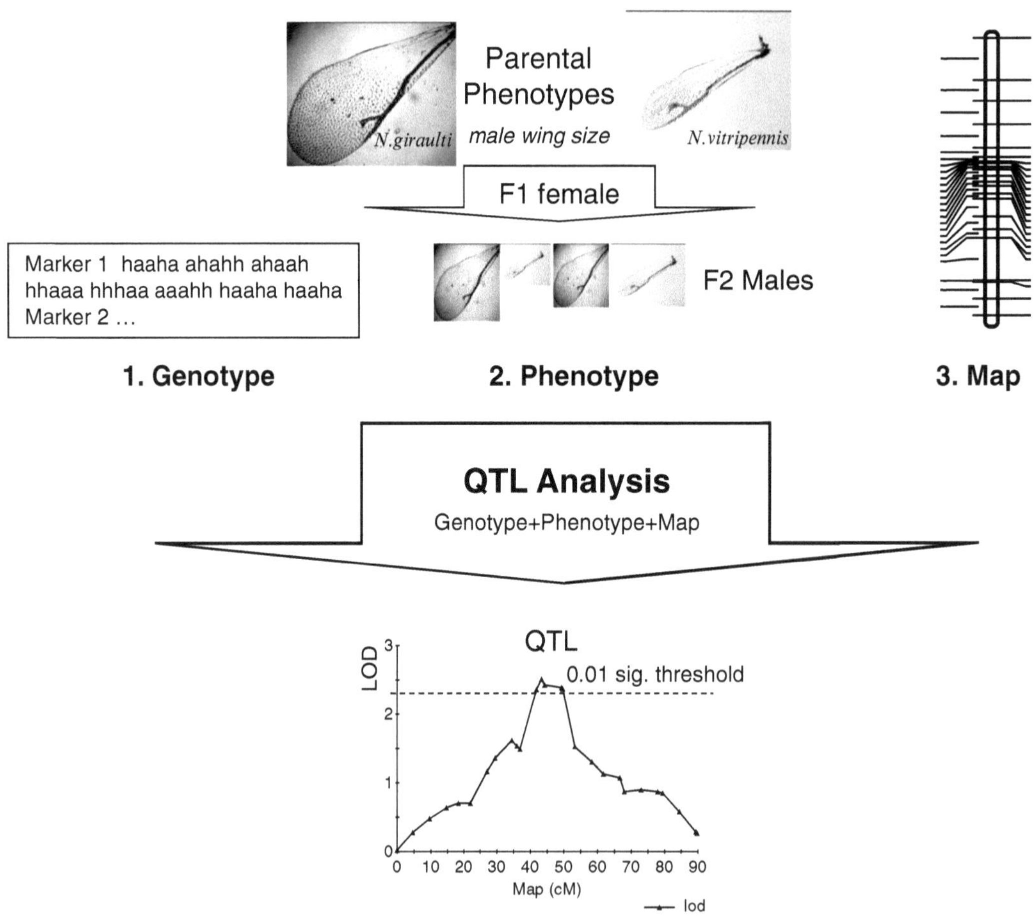

Fig. 1. Principle of a QTL mapping analysis. Three data sets (phenotype and genotype measured for each individual of the mapping population and the genomic order of the markers used for genotyping (linkage map) are combined to perform a QTL analysis.

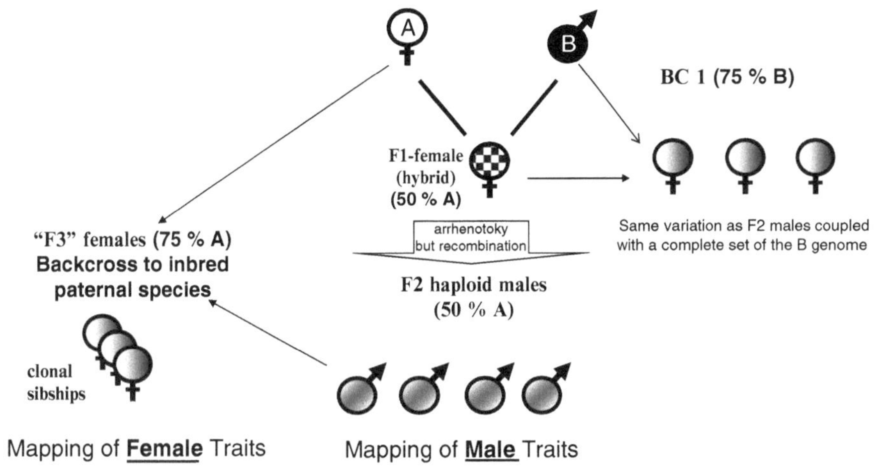

Fig. 2. Standard breeding schemes to quickly map genes for species differences in males and females of *Nasonia*. The standard strains ASYMC (*Nasonia vitripennis*), RV2 (*Nasonia giraulti*), and IV7 (*Nasonia longicornis*) have been inbred in the laboratory (sister/brother matings is the standard) for many years and are essentially homozygous at most loci (own unpublished data). Hence, F1 hybrid females have completely homogenous genome sets of both parental lines. All gametes produced by the F1 female are unique mixtures of the two parental genomes because of recombination during oogenesis. Note that male offspring of F1 females are identical to their mothers' gametes because they develop from unfertilized eggs and are haploid. A backcross of F1 females to any of the parental lines produces females whose genome is a complete set of her mate and a unique mixture of the genomes of the F1 females parents. To generate genetically almost identical F3 females, one has to backcross a F2 male with either line. Backcrosses of F2 haploid males produce clonal sibships, i.e. all females are identical and harbor one recombinant genome and one complete parental genome.

(see below). These features might in some instances make an organism an interesting model for certain questions. For example, haploid organisms are good for studying epistasis and genera with interspecific hybridization make it possible to study the genetic architecture of species differences or speciation (see below).

All examples used in this chapter are drawn from the insect order Hymenoptera which has some unusual life history and reproductive features. In particular, we rely heavily on our own work done in the parasitic wasp *Nasonia*, which produces viable and fertile F1 hybrid females and F2 hybrid males (Fig. 2). The single most important Hymenopteran feature to consider for a genetic analysis is the haplodiploid sex determination mechanism. All functional Hymenopteran males are haploid and have been produced parthenogenetically by arrhenotoky (5). Oocytes undergo a normal meiosis and, after the egg is ready to be laid, the mother can either fertilize it by allowing sperms to leave the spermatheca or not, i.e., hymenopteran females can actively determine their offsprings' primary sex ratio. Once unfertilized eggs are laid, they start to develop into haploid males; fertilized eggs will produce females. The consequences of haplo-diploidy for linkage mapping and QTL analysis are significant. First, there is no intralocus interaction in males (recessive, dominance, etc.) because males are haploid, i.e., the effect of an allele on a phenotype is fully expressed. This makes haploid males excellent study systems to test for epistasis (defined here as loci that do not interact additively) because there are only four possible genotypes for any two-locus interaction with two possible alleles at each locus. Second, maternal effects can be excluded if all males of a mapping population were derived from a single female. Third, most social hymenoptera like bees, wasps, and ants have a single queen who produces hundreds or thousands of male offspring, and virgin females of *Nasonia* can be repeatedly rehosted to generate hundreds of males, i.e., there is normally no shortage of individuals for a QTL analysis. Fourth, males have no fathers, and all offspring produced by a male inherit the same genetic material (see Note 1, Fig. 2)

2. Materials

Three data files are usually necessary to perform a QTL analysis (Fig. 1). First, we need a phenotype measure for all individuals (phenotype data), and second, a genotype for the same individual. The genotypes are then used to generate a linkage map, which is the third data set. A QTL analysis could technically be performed without a linkage map. However, more sophisticated mapping strategies (e.g., interval mapping) rely on linkage information. Once QTL are detected, it is possible to estimate the significance and explained variance of each QTL (Fig. 1).

2.1. Organisms

2.1.1. Nasonia spp.

Nasonia are parasitoid wasp that parasitizes fly pupae. All four described species of *Nasonia* are reproductively isolated from each other by cytoplasmic incompatibility based on the different *Wolbachia* endosymbiont strains each species harbors. However, they can produce viable and fertile hybrids once they are cured from their *Wolbachia* endosymbionts (6, 7). Highly inbred strains of all four species have been kept in the lab and are available on request from multiple labs (see http://www.rochester.edu/College/BIO/labs/WerrenLab/WerrenLab-NasoniaResearch.html).

2.1.2. Bombus terrestris

B. terrestris is a common European bumble bee which is classified as primitive eusocial because it forms annual instead of perennial colonies. Bumble bee queens that mated in the fall are the only individuals that overwinter, and they found their colonies anew in early spring. Initially colonies grow and do not produce virgin queens or males, i.e., they only produce worker offspring, until they switch to the production of reproductive brood (males and queens) in early to late summer. After the reproductive brood has left the colony for mating, the colony dissolves, and all worker eventually die. *B. terrestris* and several other bumble bees are cultured commercially for pollination in greenhouses and can be ordered online both in Europe and the US (e.g., http://www.koppertonline.com/). Note that *B. terrestris* cannot be imported into the US; instead of *B. terrestris,* the US breeders use *Bombus occidentalis* (Western US) or *Bombus impatiens* (Eastern US). The genome of *B. terrestris* is sequenced and an assembled and annotated genome should be come publicly available in 2012 (http://www.hgsc.bcm.tmc.edu/project-species-x-organisms.hgsc).

B. terrestris can be bred in the laboratory by combining males and virgin females in a small box (e.g., 10 × 10 × 10 cm). Since they have a single locus sex determination system and mate only once (5), inbreeding will instantaneously lead to the production of 50% of diploid males (5), which will reduce the productivity of a colony and complicate QTL mapping. Diploid males are genetic females (diploid and derived from a fertilized egg) that have developed into a phenotypic male because the individual inherited two similar alleles at the sex determination locus. Hence, laboratory populations need to be replenished regularly with field collected/queens.

2.1.3. *Apis mellifera*

The honeybee *A. mellifera* is a highly eusocial bee that proliferates by colony fission, i.e., the old queen and roughly half of the worker force leave the nest before the new queen has hatched. Once the new queen hatches, she kills all other newly emerging queens and leaves for mating flights. After she has mated with up to 40 males, she starts laying worker eggs to replenish the work force of her colony due to the exodus of the old queen. Honeybees have been cultivated or harvested by humans since prehistoric times, and bee hives or bees are available from commercial bee keepers. Honeybees have been introduced to the New World and are now cosmopolitan. Feral bee populations exist wherever commercial bee keeping is practiced in their native range in Southeast Asia and Africa. Artificial insemination of honeybee queens is a regularly used and widespread technique which allows for controlled breeding (8).

2.2. Phenotype

It is very important to measure the phenotype reliably, and ideally, at least two investigators should determine/measure the phenotype independently. For example, all morphological measures of wing size differences described below were based on pictures taken from wings spread on microscopic slides under a dissecting scope using the same magnification (40×) and measured using a computer program (e.g., Image-Pro Express, Media Cybernetics, Inc). The measurements were taken twice independently which allowed us to estimate the error due to measurement.

Behavioral phenotypes (e.g., male courtship behavior in *Nasonia* spp.) should be videotaped if possible, which allows repeated measures of the phenotype and the detection of subtle behavioral variations. For behavioral observations, it is very important to keep the environment as constant as possible and do all observations within a limited time frame, e.g., for the male courtship behavior we restricted our observations to the late mornings or early afternoons in a room with constant light and temperature within 2–3 months.

2.3. Generating a Linkage Map

Molecular markers used for linkage mapping range from AFLP (Amplified Fragment Length Polymorhpism), RAPD (Randomly Amplified Polymorphic DNA), microsatellites, to SNP (Single Nucleotide Polymorphism) (9–11). The first two marker types are the most unreliable but will generate many markers without any previous genomic information. These marker types will probably no longer play a significant role in genome mapping or QTL analysis due to the arrival of novel cheap next-generation sequencing and genotyping techniques. Microsatellites are codominant and reliable markers, but it is currently difficult and expensive to genotype many microsatellite loci simultaneously. Simultaneous genotyping is possible using SNP markers. Microarray or PCR-based techniques that can genotype thousands of SNP markers are well established. The disadvantage of SNP markers is their relative low number of alleles (maximum of four alleles) compared to microsatellites, which are typically characterized by many alleles and a high heterozygosity rate. This is especially important in intraspecific crosses or crosses between individuals that have a reduced genetic variability due to inbreeding. Hence, microsatellites may remain important markers for fine mapping or in highly inbred systems.

Marker systems based on new-generation sequencing techniques like RAD-Mapping (Restriction site Associated DNA sequencing) will probably be the markers of the future (12). RAD-Mapping does not need any previous genomic information and produces a large number of codominant markers (sequences) for a large number of individuals simultaneously. RAD markers are short DNA sequences that are the result of a restriction digestion and targeted amplification of short restriction fragments for multiple individuals simultaneously using an individual specific sequence tag to differentiate between the alleles of multiplexed DNA samples (for more details see (9)).

We will briefly discuss the program MultiPoint, which is a commercially available linkage mapping program. MultiPoint is able to handle a large number of markers (http://www.multiqtl.com/) simultaneously. For a complete list of mapping programs, see the webpage (http://linkage.rockefeller.edu/soft/). Independent of which mapping program one uses, the first thing to determine is what type of cross is used because this will be the first question asked by any program.

Mapping using haploid males is analogous to a backcross; two alleles (two genotypes in the case of a backcross; a homozygote and a heterozygote genotype) are segregating in a mapping population and the expectation is a 50:50 ratio of both alleles. Usually, it is necessary to determine the phase of a marker in each cross, i.e., whether it has been inherited from the grandfather or grandmother. This is normally done by genotyping the parents and grandparents simultaneously. All three species discussed here can be bred in the laboratory and hence all mapping can be done with the phase known. For species that cannot be bred in the laboratory, phase-unknown mapping techniques have been developed especially for Hymenoptera or haploid-mapping populations (13).

Once a genetic linkage map has been produced based on the individuals of a mapping population, the QTL analysis can be performed.

2.4. QTL Analysis Using MapQTL® 4.0 (Wageningen)

Three data sets (genotype, phenotype, and map) are necessary to perform a QTL analysis with MapQTL (14). It is extremely important to always keep the genotype and phenotype data correctly lined up. QTL analyses based on randomized data sets, i.e., where the genotypes are randomized relative to the phenotypes, are used to generate significance thresholds via permutation tests (14).

The technical and practical basis of a QTL analysis (interval, mqm, etc.) are described elsewhere (Chapter 6). Here we concentrate on some roadblocks and surprising results we have experienced during our studies and how we dealt with them.

The most frustrating result, after all formatting problems have been solved and the first QTL analysis has been run, is that no significant QTL is detected. This happened to us repeatedly and it almost always turned out to be an error in one of the three data files that happened during the reformatting process (adding a cell, column, or row effectively randomizes the data set). Hence, we usually save all intermediate formatting steps and make detailed notes on how the data were transformed.

In those cases where we did not get a significant QTL for a phenotype with high heritability, we could solve the problem by adding additional markers and/or individuals (Figs. 2 and 3). These phenotypes were probably "classic" quantitative traits, i.e., the genetic basis of this trait consists of many loci each with a small phenotypic effect, interacting additively. Hence, to detect those, we needed to increase both the coverage of our genome (= more markers to land some close to the genes causally involved) and detection power (= more individuals to be able to get a significant QTL for a QTL explaining a small proportion of the observed phenotypic variance).

Once a significant QTL is found, we need to estimate its significance and the true percentage of explained variance of the observed phenotypic variance in the mapping population.

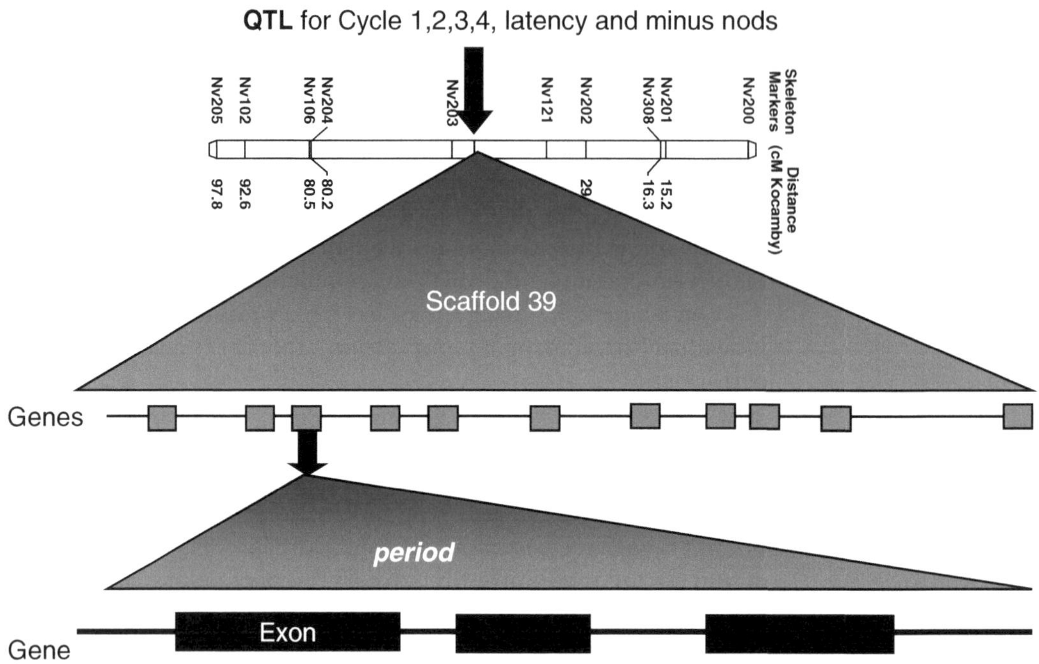

Fig. 3. From a candidate region to a candidate gene—example given is the region around a QTL for cycle time and other frequency-dependent phenotypes and the colocalization of the gene *Period* known to be involved in courtship behavior modulation of *Drosophila*.

2.5. Significance and Confirmation of Previously Described QTL

The best way to determine significance thresholds is a permutation test. MapQTL runs by default 1,000 permutations on a randomized data set for each measured phenotype (see Note 2), i.e., it performs 1,000 independent, interval QTL analyses. The result (output in MapQTL 4.0) is a cumulative list of LOD (logarithm of odds) scores for 1,000 QTL analyses per phenotype and linkage group, i.e., the program runs 1,000 interval mapping QTL analysis, and for each run, it reports the highest LOD score per linkage group and the highest genome-wide LOD score found. In a randomized data set, there should be no real signal and all LOD scores reflect statistical artifacts. The distribution of these 1,000 permutations allows us to determine 95 or 99% confidence intervals for each trait (=LOD score at 95% of the cumulative distribution). Usually, the 99% LOD score thresholds for a given cross should be comparable between different phenotypes. In some cases in *Nasonia*, we encountered extremely high 99% confidence thresholds, for our QTL analysis e.g., genome-wide 99% LOD thresholds of 5.4 rather than the usual 2.6–2.9. In all of these cases, it turned out that this was due to a small number of extreme outliers in the phenotype data (one was a simple typo, the other was an extreme transgressive phenotype, i.e., a phenotype that was 5 standard deviations outside of both parental phenotypes). Once we eliminated these outliers from our data, the 99% confidence thresholds returned to "normal" values, i.e., values in the range we found for all other QTL in the same mapping population.

Significant QTL should ideally be confirmed in a second independent mapping population. The easiest way to do this is to phenotype more individuals at the same time and partition the population a priori into two independent populations. QTL with large effects can normally be confirmed with two mapping populations of 96 individuals each (see Note 3). For example, the wing size QTL on chromosome 4 in *Nasonia*, which explains about 40% of the phenotypic variance of wing size in F2 hybrid males of *Nasonia vitripennis* and *Nasonia giraulti*, was detected in every QTL analysis done so far. For QTLs with smaller effect, the two mapping populations can be combined to increase the detection probably.

Lander and Kruglyak (15) proposed a three level classification of suggestive, significant, and highly significant QTLs, based on their significance level. Significant and highly significant QTLs had genome-wide *p*-values of 0.05 and 0.01, respectively. A suggestive QTL is a region that shows an effect, but is not significant. The last level is quite ambiguous, but it is helpful if multiple QTL analyses are performed on the same trait. Some QTLs might cross the significance level in some populations but not in others and then it is helpful to check whether the LOD scores in those mapping populations without a significant QTL at this position show elevated LOD scores.

2.6. Candidate Genes and Fine Mapping

A growing number of species have an assembled and annotated genome. In species with this resource, it is possible to use a denser map (more markers) and more individuals (increase in recombinant individuals) to identify potential candidate genes by associating a QTL position in the genome and genes in this region ((16), Fig. 3). Once candidate genes have been identified, they can be confirmed by fine mapping (see below). This is usually a three-step process. The first step is the generation of a map with a much higher marker density within the confidence interval of a QTL, i.e., the confidence interval for the position of a QTL along a linkage group (see Note 4). To fine map a QTL position, the marker density should be below 1 cM. This is necessary to narrow down the region to a reasonable size with approximately 50–100 genes that could be responsible for the observed QTL effect. The second step is to identify individuals who have a recombination within this region. The third step is to map all genetic markers on the physical genome sequence and align the genotypes of all individuals with a recombination in the region of interest. A comparison of the phenotypes and genotypes of those recombinant individuals will further narrow down the region of interest and ideally result in a small number of candidate genes. Candidate genes are usually chosen because the function they have in another organism suggests that they may also affect the currently analyzed trait. For example, a QTL for *cycle time* in *Nasonia*, a male courtship behavior trait, has been located in an area of the genome that contains a circadian rythm gene *period*. Period has already been shown to play an important role in courtship behavior of *Drosophila melanogaster* males. Hence, it is a strong candidate gene (Fig. 3). However, to ultimately confirm candidate genes, they have to be either knocked out or down depending on the technology available for the organism.

3. Methods

3.1. QTL Mapping of Species Differences in Nasonia spp.

Morphology—Male Wing Size (standard QTL mapping—epistasis)

Male wing size differs significantly between three of the four described *Nasonia* species. A QTL analysis on F2 hybrids between the two species, *N. vitripennis* and *N. giraulti*, that have the largest difference in male wing size resulted in multiple highly significant QTLs (Fig. 1 breeding scheme; Figs. 2 and 3 in (2)). This approach was chosen to maximize the phenotypic difference between the parents of our mapping population. Although we were able to use an interspecific cross between species that showed a large phenotypic difference (nature did the selection for us), it is always a good idea to maximize the phenotypic differences between the parents of a mapping population either through selective breeding or selection of extreme phenotypes as parents for the mapping population. In general, the larger the phenotypic difference between the two parental lines/parents, the higher the chance to detect QTL.

The QTL analysis of male wing size was based on a linkage map comprising 91 RAPD markers (2, 9). The map was produced using MapMaker 2.0 (http://linkage.rockefeller.edu/soft/). Fine mapping using SNP markers and other techniques confirmed both the marker order and QTL position (17) for two of the identified QTL (on Chromosome 1 and 4 in (9)). The genetic locus involved in the major QTL on chromosome 4 leading to a 45% male wing size increase has been determined to be a noncoding region between two genes (*prospero* and *dsx*) (18). The concrete mechanism of how these sequence differences in this noncoding regions achieve their phenotypic effect is still unknown.

Gadau et al. (2) measured four phenotypes (wing length, wing width, head width, and seta density) in a F2 hybrid male population (*N. vitripennis x N. giraulti*) and performed QTL analysis on all four traits and one composite phenotype, normalized wing multiple ((wing length x wing width)/head width). They detected 15 QTL by interval mapping and mqm mapping and epistatic interactions for all traits except wing width. Epistasis was detected using the program Epistat (19) (http://527270.sites.myregisteredsite.com/epistat.htm). This program essentially screens for pairwise epistatic interactions (= loci that have a nonadditive effect on the phenotype). Usually the two interacting loci have no or just a small significant effect on their own, but show a significant or larger effect when analyzed together. For example, the two loci 407-1.01 (chromosome II) and 323-098 (chromosome IV) interact epistatically and more specifically conditionally, i.e., all individuals of the mapping population that are fixed for a giraulti allele at locus 407-1.01 show a similar phenotype no matter whether they have a vitripennis or giraulti allele (27.36 vs. 26.50) at the interacting locus (see Table 4 in (2)). However, individuals who have a vitripennis allele at locus 407-1.01 differ significantly between individuals having a giraulti or vitripennis allele at the interacting locus 323-0.98. Hence, the phenotypic effect of the alleles at locus 2 (323-0.98) is conditional on the allelic composition at locus 1 (407-1.01). Haplodiploid individuals are ideal to study epistasis because two-way interactions have only four possible genotypes in haploid individuals. Hence, for any given population size, haploid individuals give us much more statistical power to detect epistasis than diploid individuals (see Note 5).

3.2. Beavis Effect: An Empirical Estimate of the Optimal Number of Individuals Determining the True Effect of a QTL in Nasonia

Beavis (20, 21) first noted that QTL analyses usually overestimate the effect of a QTL because the same data set is used to locate a QTL and to estimate its effect (% explained variance). Since only those QTLs that cross a predetermined threshold are reported, the distribution from which significant QTLs are reported in the literature is truncated. In other words, QTLs that have such a small effect are not detectable in a small mapping population (approximately 100 individuals) are only reported if by chance they surpass the detection threshold due to a statistical sampling effect that overestimates their true effect. Hence the true phenotypic effect of a detected is usually overestimated (20). Those QTLs are often not confirmed by independent QTL analyses because in different mapping populations they may not make the significance threshold. Beavis (21) estimated that with 100 individuals the phenotypic effect of a QTL is often hugely overestimated, with 500 individuals estimation comes fairly close, and with 1,000 individuals his simulations approached a convergence of the true and estimated effect, i.e., percent explained phenotypic variance.

We performed an empirical test of the Beavis effect on a data set of 500 haploid F2 hybrid males in *Nasonia* for which we determined QTLs for male courtship behavior (22). For that purpose, we resampled 100 times: 100, 150, 200, 250, 300, and 350 males from the mapping population of approximately 500 individuals and performed interval QTL analyses on each sample, i.e., 100 interval mapping on 100 males, 100 interval mappings on 150 males, etc..

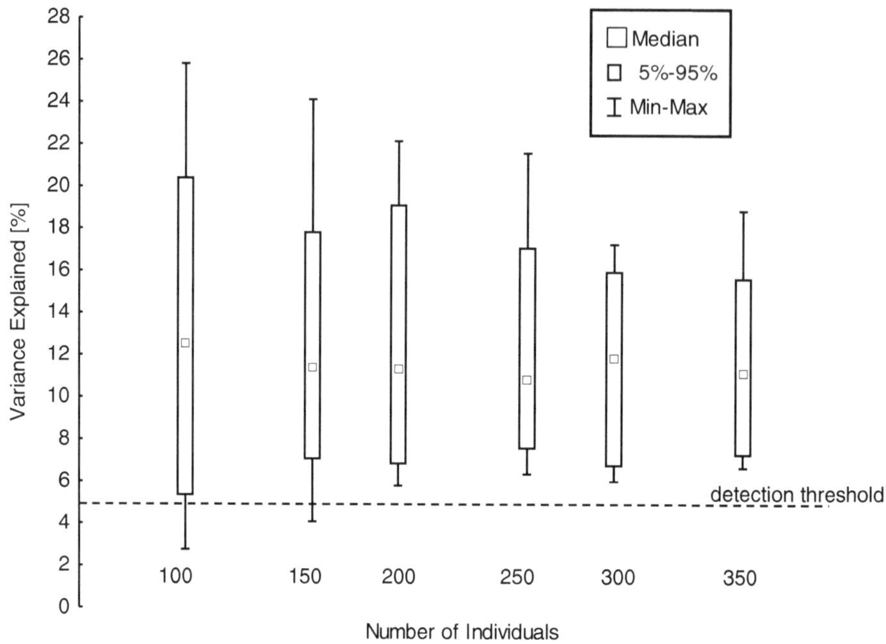

Fig. 4. Effect of increasing size of the mapping population on explained phenotypic variance (Beavis effect (20, 21)). The graph shows a summary of one of our empirical tests of the Beavis effect. From a pool of 500 genotyped and phenotyped individuals, we resampled 100 times 100, 150, 200, 250, 300, 350 individuals. For each sample size, we performed 100 QTL analyses based on the 100 randomly assembled individuals. Both the range and percentiles shrink as sample size increases, and as Beavis predicted, it is more likely to overestimate the effect of a QTL on the phenotype with smaller samples sizes because the lower end of the distribution will never be recorded as a significant QTL. Interestingly, in some cases with smaller numbers of individuals (100 and 150 individuals), we even failed to detect a QTL in a significant number of permutations (the LOD scores fell below the detection threshold = permutation based significance threshold).

Each time, we determined the percent explained variance. For our data set, the range of the explained variance declined for all traits when we went from 100 individuals to 350 individuals. The only exceptions were two traits that explained from the beginning (i.e., with 100 males) more than 20% of the observed phenotypic variance in our mapping populations. However, the change in phenotypic variance explained leveled off much more quickly than the 500 or even 1,000 individuals suggested by Beavis' simulations (21, 22). Hence, for *Nasonia* a mapping population of about 250–300 individuals should give us a rather accurate estimate of the true effect of a QTL.

One example of our analysis is shown in Fig. 4. The range of the variance explained and percentiles (5–95) both become smaller as we increase sample size. The median for all sample sizes hovers around 12%, i.e., one can get the correct value with small sample sizes. However, with 100 and 150 individuals, we did not detect a significant QTL in some subsamples and significantly overestimated the true effect by more than 100% in others. With 350 individuals, none of the subsamples fell below the detection limit and many fewer subsamples overestimated the explained variance, and when they did, it was not as dramatic.

3.3. QTL Mapping in Social Hymenoptera: *Bombus terrestris* and *Apis mellifera*

QTL analyses in social insects have to accommodate important differences in comparison to QTL analyses in solitary insects. First, usually only one or very few individuals reproduce (queens) and the males (in ants, bees, and wasps) are often absent because the queen mated once at the beginning of the colony founding years ago. Second, the phenotype for the QTL analysis may not be measured in individuals for which we have the genotype but on the colony level, e.g., division of labor. Third, most social insects cannot be bred in captivity. The advantages of social Hymenoptera are that a queen can produce thousands of offspring, and their haplodiploidy makes phase unknown mapping possible (13, 23).

3.3.1. QTL Analysis of a Complex Trait in a Social Insect 1: Disease Resistance (*Bombus terrestris*)

Wilfert et al. (4) performed a QTL analysis of a host parasite (*Crithidia bombi*) interaction in *B. terrestris*. They analyzed parasite infection intensity (measured as the number of *C. bombi* spores in the endgut of *B. terrestris* males) and the strength in the general immune response of the host (measured as encapsulation reaction to a novel antigen, i.e. a short nylon thread implanted for 24 h).

In order to use haploid males, the authors had to first prove that there are no differences in the immune responses of *B. terrestris* workers and males. Once they showed that there is no significant difference in the reaction of both castes, workers and males, to an infection with a standard dose of the parasite, a QTL analysis could be performed on haploid males. This made the QTL and epistasis analyses more powerful.

Multiple QTLs were detected that interacted mostly epistatically (4). The authors used three independent populations to locate QTLs for those two phenotypes, but they could not confirm a single one of their QTLs in another mapping population. This might be due to at least two factors. First, all detected QTLs had relatively small phenotypic effects (<5%, Tables 1 and 2 in (4)). Hence, detection probability is low and a QTL found in one mapping population may fall below the detection probability in another population (see Subheading 3.2). Second, the queens that produced the mapping populations were genetically very diverse, i.e., all queens were caught in the field and started colonies from which males were drawn in the laboratory. Since the parasite is constantly evolving to escape the host's defenses, it is plausible that there is significant genetic variation in the host population leading to the segregation of many loci and alleles in any given wild population. Hence, it may not be surprising that each queen might have a unique blend of QTLs to deal with a significant parasite. The next step in this study would be to follow particular matrilines or patrilines, i.e., breed some of the offspring of the original mapping population and redo the QTL analysis in another one or two generations. The next generation of males (grandsons) should share at least 50% of their grandmother's alleles. If there truly is allelic variation for host resistance, it should show up again.

3.3.2. QTL Analysis of a Complex Trait in a Social Insect 2: Honeybee (Apis mellifera) Foraging Behavior

Worker honeybees forage for pollen and nectar to provision their colony. Pollen and nectar (converted into honey) is stored in separate areas of the combs usually outside of the comb area used as brood cells. It has been repeatedly shown that workers specialize either on pollen or nectar foraging (24, 25) (see Note 6). Hunt et al. (3) mapped QTLs for pollen foraging, i.e., QTLs that explain why some workers predominantly forage for pollen after they became foragers.

To map this individual level trait, they first conducted a two-way selection for five generations for a colony level trait: *amount of stored pollen* (high line stores large amounts of pollen; low line stores small amounts of pollen). They then crossed a queen from their low pollen hoarding strain with a male from the high pollen hoarding strain to produce a F1 queen that had an equal amount of high and low pollen hoarding genes. The F2 haploid male offspring of this F1 queen were recombinants of low and high pollen hoarding genomes. These males were crossed individually with queens from the high pollen hoarding selection line. The resulting queens were equivalent to a BC1 (backcross one) being either homozygous or heterozygous for high/low pollen hoarding or high/high pollen hoarding alleles, respectively. These queens were allowed to build up a colony and the amount of pollen stored by each colony was determined once colonies matured. For the QTL analysis of pollen hoarding, the colony phenotype *amount of stored pollen* and the F2 haploid male (mates of the F1 queens) genotypes were used since the important genetic variation between those queens/colonies was derived from the queens' mates (F2 males). Note that all queens were derived from the highly inbred high pollen hoarding line and were supposedly homozygous with respect to alleles increasing pollen storage in a colony. Using this approach, the authors could identify two major QTLs which they named *pln 1* and *pln 2* that explained 59% of the observed variance in pollen storage between their test colonies. However, this might be an overestimation because their sample size was rather small ($n = 38$ colonies, see Subheading 3.2).

To confirm the effect of *pln1* and *pln2* on individual foraging behavior, Hunt et al. (3) determined the individual foraging behavior of workers (phenotypes measured were: *weights of pollen* and *nectar load* of a returning forager) that were offspring from another F1 queen (high x low line) mated with a single high pollen line male. The resulting allelic composition for this cross would again be workers that are high/high or high/low for *pln1* and *pln2*. Foragers of this cross were first phenotyped after their first foraging trips and than genotyped for markers for loci linked to the two

QTLs *pln1* and *pln2*. The results confirmed that being homozygote (high/high) or heterozygote (high/low) at markers linked to *pln1* or *pln2* had a significant effect on the individual behavior of honeybee foragers.

The selection lines are still available and kept alive by Robert E Page Jr (Arizona State University, School of Life Sciences) and have been subjected to many further analyses. For example, it turned out that *pln2* especially is highly pleiotropic and affects many behavioral traits (26).

4. Notes

1. Diploid males are due to matched matings in species with a single locus complementary sex determination (sl-CSD) system (4). However, they are usually due to artificial inbreeding in the laboratory and are otherwise rarly observed in natural populations. Diploid males are easy to detect in genetic studies using many molecular markers (standard for QTL analyses) since they show the same heterozygosity pattern as females with the exception of markers linked to the CSD locus.
2. More than 1,000 permutations never resulted in any significant difference in the 95 or 99% threshold in the few instances we tried it on our own data sets. However, one can test this on ones' own data set using one or two QTL.
3. Since all PCR machines have a 96-well plate format, it is more convenient to use 96 instead of 100 individuals.
4. Currently, there is no good way to determine a confidence interval for the position of a QTL along a linkage group/ chromosome. Most studies use a drop of 1-LOD score to estimate confidence intervals for the true QTL location.
5. A BC1 (backcross 1) mapping population has the same number of possible genotypes in a two-locus interaction, but there is always the possibility that the two alleles of one locus interact in the heterozygote individuals.
6. Many forager bees bring back some of both, i.e., pollen foragers often also carry some nectar and nectar foragers some pollen. However, usually it is very clear who prefers to collect what.

References

1. Korstanje R, Paigen B (2002) From QTL to gene: the harvest begins. Nat Genet 31: 235–236
2. Gadau J, Page RE Jr, Werren JH (2002) The genetic basis of the interspecific differences in wing size in *Nasonia* (Hymenoptera; Pteromalidae)—major QTL and epistasis. Genetics 161:673–684
3. Hunt GJ, Page RE Jr, Fondrk MK, Dullum CJ (1995) Major quantitative trait loci affecting

honey bee foraging behavior. Genetics 141: 1537–1545
4. Wilfert L, Gadau J, Schmid-Hempel P (2007) Natural variation in the genetic architecture of a host-parasite interaction in the bumblebee *Bombus terrestris*. Mol Ecol 16:1327–1339
5. Cook JM, Crozier RH (1995) Sex determination and population biology in the hymenoptera. Trends Ecol Evol 10:281–286
6. Breeuwer JAJ, Werren JH (1995) Hybrid breakdown between 2 haplodiploid species—the role of nuclear and cytoplasmic genes. Evolution 49:705–717
7. Breeuwer JAJ, Werren JH (1993) Cytoplasmic incompatibility and bacterial density in *Nasonia vitripennis*. Genetics 135:565–574
8. Laidlaw HH, Page RE (1998) Queen rearing and bee breeding. Wicwas Press, Cheshire
9. Gadau J, Page RE Jr, Werren JH (1999) Mapping of hybrid incompatibility loci in *Nasonia*. Genetics 153:1731–1741
10. Niehuis O, Gibson JD, Rosenberg MS, Pannebakker BA, Koevoets T, Judson AK, Desjardins CA, Kennedy K, Duggan D, Beukeboom LW, van de Zande L, Shuke DM, Werren JH, Gadau J (2009) Recombination and its impact on the genome of the haplodiploid parasitoid wasp *Nasonia*. PLoS One. doi:10.1371/journal.pone.0008597
11. Sirviö A, Pamilo P, Johnson RA, Page RE Jr, Gadau J (2010) Origin and evolution of the dependent lineages in the genetic caste determination system of *Pogonomyrmex* spp. Evolution. doi:10.1111/j.1558-5646.2010.01170.x
12. Baird NA, Etter PD, Atwood TS, Currey MC, Shiver AL, Lewis ZA, Selker EU, Cresko WA, Johnson EA (2008) Rapid SNP discovery and genetic mapping using sequenced RAD markers. PLoS One 3(10):e3376
13. Wilfert L, Gadau J, Schmid-Hempel P (2006) A core linkage map for the bumblebee *Bombus terrestris*. Genome 49:1215–1226
14. Van Ooijen JW, Boer MP, Jansen RC, Maliepaard C (2002) MapQTL® 4.0 Software for calculation of QTL positions on genetic maps. Plant Research International, Wageningen
15. Lander ES, Kruglyak L (1995) Genetic dissection of complex traits: guidelines for interpreting and reporting linkage results. Nat Genet 11:241–247
16. Gleason JM, Richie MG (2004) Do quantitative trait loci (QTL) for a courtship song difference between *Drosophila simulans* and *D. sechellia* coincide with candidate genes and intraspecific QTL? Genetics 166:1303–1311
17. Gadau J, Niehuis O, Peire A, Werren JH, Baudry E, Beukeboom LW (2008) Jewel wasp, *Nasonia* spp. In: Wayne H, Kole C (eds) Genome mapping and genomics in animals. Springer, Heidelberg
18. Loehlin DW, Oliveira DCSG, Edwards R, Giebel JD, Clark ME, Cattani MV, van de Zande L, Verhulst EC, Beukeboom LW, Munoz-Torres M, Werren JH (2010) Non-coding changes cause sex-specific wing size differences between closely related species of *Nasonia*. PLoS Genet 6(1):e1000821
19. Chase K, Adler FR, Lark KG (1997) Epistat: a computer program for identifying and testing interactions between pairs of quantitative trait loci. Theor Appl Genet 94:724–730
20. Beavis WD (1994) The power and deceit of QTL experiments: lessons from comparative QTL studies. In: Proceedings of the Forty-Ninth Annual Corn & Sorghum Industry Research Conference. American Seed Trade Association, Washington
21. Beavis WD (1998) QTL analyses: power, precision, and accuracy. In: Patterson AH (ed) Molecular dissection of complex traits. CRC Press, New York, pp 145–162
22. Gadau J, Pietsch CP, Beukeboom LW (submitted) Genetic architecture of courtship behavior in *Nasonia*
23. Gadau J, Gerloff CU, Krüger N, Chan H, Schmid-Hempel P, Wille A, Page RE Jr (2001) A linkage analysis of sex determination in *Bombus terrestris* (L.) (Hymenoptera: Apidea). J Hered 87:234–242
24. Calderon WR, Page RE Jr (1988) Genotypic variability in age polyethism and task specialization in the honey bee *Apis mellifera* (Hymenoptera: Apidae). Behav Ecol Sociobiol 22:17–25
25. Page RE Jr, Robinson GE (1991) The genetics of division of labour in honey bee colonies. Adv Insect Physiol 23:117–169
26. Hunt GJ, Amdam GV, Schlipalius D, Emore C, Sardesai N, Williams CE, Rueppell O, Guzman-Novoa E, Arechavaleta-Velasco M, Chandra S, Fondrk MK, Beye M, Page RE (2007) Behavioral genomics of honeybee foraging and nest defense. Naturwissenschaften 94: 247–267

Index

A

Advanced intercross 17, 32, 33, 35–38, 112
Affymetrix data analysis 47–48
Allele frequencies 34, 35, 38, 61, 64, 194, 196, 267, 268, 281, 284–286, 292–294, 297, 301, 307, 310
Animal QTLdb................................ 122, 130–133, 138, 142, 145, 166, 167
Apis mellifera 314, 317, 325–327
Association analysis 270

B

Backcross 3–15, 17, 81, 91–93, 97, 104, 105, 108, 109, 112, 114, 206, 207, 210, 231, 248, 250, 251, 315, 318, 326, 327
Bayesian methods................................20, 160, 255–256
Beavis effect 323–325
Bivalent 246, 247, 249–253, 258
BLAST 57, 69, 141
Bombus terrestris 314, 316–317, 325–327
Breeding design..37
Bulk segregant analysis 8–9, 41–53

C

Candidate genes 122, 139, 282, 321–322
Causation 176–178, 185–188
Change of reference 192, 198
Chromosome substitution strains 11–13
Co-expression network 274–275
Colony level traits 326
Composite interval mapping (CIM).................... 20–22, 27, 28, 75–118
Consensus map.. 150–152
Crossover 7, 10, 12–13, 15, 31, 248

D

Database design... 123–133, 138
Data modeling.. 125–133, 143
dbSNP.. 56–58
Development 4, 11, 34, 56, 58, 62, 104, 139, 146, 198, 205, 227–230, 234–237, 249–252, 258
Drift 34–36, 58, 63, 232
Dynamical system 237, 239

E

Empirical Bayes 20, 25, 27, 183, 184, 187
Epistasis/gene interaction 76
Expression QTL (eQTL)..................175–188, 265–277

F

False positives 84, 89, 105, 188, 267–269, 271
$F_{2:3}$ design 17, 20, 26
Fine mapping.....................................4, 6–7, 11, 17, 19, 23, 48, 51, 282–299, 314, 318, 321–322
Fixed effects... 25, 153–156, 161–163, 167
F_2 population 17–20, 23, 26, 36, 37, 83, 97, 113, 114, 193, 195, 206, 207, 231
Functional mapping 140, 227–241

G

Gene expression data 175, 237, 267, 270
Gene mapping 281–283, 308
Gene regulatory network...................................175–188
Genetic cross 44–46, 177, 178, 188
Genetic effect 5–7, 17, 22, 27, 146, 191–203, 228, 230, 234, 236, 241, 253, 286, 288, 290, 292
Genetic model 20, 22–23, 25, 27, 28, 192, 197, 199–202, 206–208, 210, 213, 249, 253
Genome sequencing 62, 236, 282
Genome-wide association study (GWAS)...... 56, 58, 63, 68–69, 282, 283, 299–308
Genome-wide threshold 84, 87, 88, 90, 93, 94, 97–98
Genomic map distances 65
Genomic mismatch scanning (GMS)...................41, 42, 45, 49–52
Genotypic values 193–199, 201, 202, 214

H

Haplodiploid sex determination 315
Hapmap 266, 267, 285, 301, 302, 305, 310

Scott A. Rifkin (ed.), *Quantitative Trait Loci (QTL): Methods and Protocols*, Methods in Molecular Biology, vol. 871, DOI 10.1007/978-1-61779-785-9, © Springer Science+Business Media New York 2012

Hardy–Weinberg equilibrium (HWE) 64, 70, 192, 196, 268, 269, 276, 285, 301, 303
Heritability 26, 67, 70, 195, 200, 203, 211, 219, 221, 223, 282, 286–291, 293, 294, 299, 309, 319
Heterochiasmy 10, 15

I

Identical-by-descent (IBD) 231, 232, 297, 301, 309
Immortalized F_2 (IF_2)population 19
Inbred line 4, 18, 107
Interspecific cross 14–15, 322
Interval mapping 17, 20–22, 27, 28, 75–118
Introgression 4–7, 9–11, 13, 15, 314

L

Likelihood 20–22, 24–25, 27, 83, 94, 113, 114, 118, 130, 135, 152, 179–182, 184, 187, 217, 231, 233, 254, 255, 258, 285, 288, 290–294
Linkage analysis 63, 231, 235, 246, 248–252, 256, 258, 282–300, 309
Linkage disequilibrium (LD) 31, 33, 56, 63–64, 229, 232, 271, 283–299
Linkage drag 4, 12
Linkage map 33, 35, 94, 95, 122, 129, 139, 140, 232, 235, 253, 314, 316, 318–319, 322
Literature review 153
LOD score 22, 130, 135, 151, 180, 182, 185, 296, 320, 321, 324, 327

M

Mapping population 4, 5, 7–11, 49, 229, 232, 235, 254, 313, 314, 316, 318–319, 321–325, 327
Mapping power 8, 9, 34, 38
Mapping resolution 9, 34–36, 38
MapQTL 319, 320
Marker
  density 24, 33, 36, 56, 63, 64, 66, 68, 122, 146, 209, 321
  selection 10, 68, 85, 86, 115
Markov chain Monte Carlo (MCMC) 164, 212, 214–216, 219, 222, 224, 255
Meiosis 177, 186, 206, 246–249, 258, 315
Merlin 283–286, 288, 292, 294–296, 299, 309–310
Meta-analysis 121–143, 145–169, 308
Microarrays 42, 44–49, 51, 52, 175, 176, 265–267, 274, 276, 318
Minor allele frequency (MAF) 60–62, 64, 69, 70, 268, 269, 276, 285, 303, 310
Mixture model 152, 153, 157–158, 164, 229, 253, 254
Model selection 98–101, 103–105, 115, 117–118, 146, 179–182, 185, 187, 201, 202, 208–209, 230, 235
Multiple alleles 194, 197, 200, 202, 249
Multiple interval mapping (MIM) 20, 27, 28, 75–118
Multiple-marker test 276
Multiple QTLs 325
Multiple testing 271–272, 275, 303, 307–308
Multiple traits 210, 213, 219–221, 223
MultiPoint 24, 212, 284, 318
Multivalent 246, 247, 249, 251, 253, 258
Multivariate model 207–209, 213
MySQL 122, 124, 131–133, 137, 143

N

Nasonia vitripennis 315, 321
National Center for Biotechnology Information (NCBI) 56, 276
Natural and orthogonal interactions (NOIA) model 191–203
Near isogenic lines (NILs) 3–15, 17, 20
Non-parametric models 169

P

Pedigrees 234, 282, 286, 309
Phenotype 5, 20, 26, 31, 33, 41, 46, 48, 51, 52, 55, 61, 70, 75, 112, 193, 194, 198, 206, 215, 236, 237, 247, 249, 257, 258, 268, 270, 271, 283, 284, 286, 299, 300, 303, 308, 309, 313–326
Pleiotropy 205–206, 208, 223–224
Ploidy 245, 247, 250, 251, 257–258
Polyploidy 245
Pooled mapping 41, 49
Protein–protein interactions 239–241

Q

QTL Cartographer 20, 22, 75–118
Quantitative trait locus (QTL) 121, 265, 313–327

R

R (statistical software package) 210–212
Random effects 153, 155–157, 161, 163, 164, 167

Recombinant inbred lines (RILs) 4, 17–19, 31–39, 81, 92, 93, 108, 112, 231, 232
Relational database....................122–126, 128–130, 143
Residual heterozygous line..19
Restriction site associated DNA sequencing (RAD-mapping) 318
R/qtlbim 20, 206, 209–210, 215, 219

S

Single-marker test 270, 276
Single nucleotide polymorphism (SNP)..........9, 26, 41, 47, 52, 55–70, 266–269, 271, 274, 282, 284, 285, 297, 299, 300, 302–304, 308–310, 318, 322
Statistical model 81–83, 91–92, 96, 97, 147, 153–159, 188, 192, 206, 228, 231, 236, 241, 245–259
Statistical power 115, 268, 276, 283, 323
Structural equation modeling 181–183
Subject list for QTL book 123
Systems biology..236–241

T

Trait distribution...................... 282, 286, 297, 299, 303

Y

Yeast genomic DNA preparation 42, 44, 46

MIX
Papier aus verantwortungsvollen Quellen
Paper from responsible sources
FSC® C105338

If you have any concerns about our products,
you can contact us on
ProductSafety@springernature.com

In case Publisher is established outside the EU,
the EU authorized representative is:
Springer Nature Customer Service Center GmbH
Europaplatz 3, 69115 Heidelberg, Germany

Printed by Libri Plureos GmbH
in Hamburg, Germany